Equipment for DIAGNOSTIC RADIOGRAPHY

E. Forster
Formerly Principal, NW Lancashire School of Radiography, Lancaster

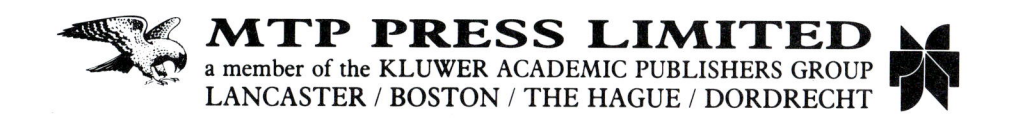

MTP PRESS LIMITED
a member of the KLUWER ACADEMIC PUBLISHERS GROUP
LANCASTER / BOSTON / THE HAGUE / DORDRECHT

Published in the UK and Europe by
MTP Press Limited
Falcon House
Lancaster, England

British Library Cataloguing in Publication Data

Forster, E.
  Equipment for diagnostic radiography.
  1. Radiography, Medical—Equipment and supplies
  I. Title
  616.07'57'028   RC78.5

  ISBN 0-85200-437-0 (Paperback)
  ISBN 0-85200-928-3 (Hardback)

Published in the USA by
MTP Press
A division of Kluwer Boston Inc
190 Old Derby Street
Hingham, MA 02043, USA

Library of Congress Cataloging in Publication Data

Forster, E. (Edward), 1923-
  Equipment for diagnostic radiography

  Includes index.
  1. Radiography, Medical—Instruments.
  2. Radiography, Medical—Equipment and supplies.
  I. Title. [DNLM: 1. Radiography—instrumentation.
  WN 150 F733e]
  RC78.5.F67 1985   616.07'57'028   85-14951

  ISBN 0-85200-437-0 (Paperback)
  ISBN 0-85200-928-3 (Hardback)

Copyright © 1985 MTP Press Limited

All rights reserved. No part of this publication
may be produced, stored in a retrieval
system, or transmitted in any form, or by any
means, electronic, mechanical, photocopying,
recording or otherwise, without prior permission
from the publishers.

Photosetting by Titus Wilson, Kendal

Printed by Butler & Tanner Limited, Frome and London

Contents

	Preface	vii
	Acknowledgements	viii
	List of contributors	ix
1	Mains electricity supply and distribution	1
2	Diagnostic X-ray circuits	11
3	Electronic devices	35
4	Exposure timers and specialized X-ray generators	44
5	Diagnostic X-ray tubes	56
6	Tube rating and tube supports	69
7	Control of scattered radiation, X-ray tables and bucky stands	85
8	Equipment for fluoroscopy and fluorography	101
9	Equipment for mobile, dental, accident and skull radiography	118
10	Tomography – theory and equipment	130
11	Organ (anatomically) programmed units, automatic film changers and other specialized X-ray equipment	140
12	Care, choice and installation of equipment	154
13	Computers and microprocessors	156
14	Protection and monitoring of patients and staff	162
15	Quality assurance of diagnostic X-ray equipment	168
16	Ultrasound	180
17	Nuclear medicine	189
18	Computerized tomography	199
19	Nuclear magnetic resonance imaging	210
20	Digital radiographic systems	217
	Appendix 1 Calculation of power	227
	Appendix 2 Measurement of angles	227
	Appendix 3 Symbols in common use on imaging equipment	228
	Appendix 4 Si units used in radiography	230
	Index	231

To Bessie – with a lifetimes' thanks

Preface

I hope this book, which covers the Equipment section of the DCR and HDCR syllabuses, will be of help not only to those students preparing for these examinations, but also for those taking the modular HDCR to be introduced sometime in the near future, and indeed to those returning to radiography after a break in service.

In addition to reading a wide range of technical literature, I would hope that students will relate this knowledge to the equipment they use in the Department. For example what type of equipment are they using? Who was the manufacturer? What sort of generator is it? What interlocks are present? What is the maximum loading of the tube? Is it a falling load generator?

Ask the Superintendent for permission to see the rating charts for your particular unit and study them carefully. With the help of the Superintendent find out which quality assurance tests are carried out on the equipment and ask for permission to participate in the procedures.

Remember, radiography is a practical subject – learning from books is of little value unless you apply it to the work you are doing – unless of course you are preparing for a change of job or promotion!

Finally, whether you are using this book to refresh your knowledge prior to returning to radiography after a break in service, or as part of your preparation for the DCR or HDCR, or indeed if you are using it in conjunction with a distanced learning course, may I wish you good luck and success in your endeavours.

Ted Forster

Acknowledgements

It gives me great pleasure to acknowledge the help given to me so generously by colleagues who have helped me throughout the 45 years of my radiographic and teaching career.

A special thank you must go to Dr F. Turner and Dr J. Meredith, two gentlemen who will be remembered with affection and gratitude, not only by myself but by the countless DCR and HDCR students who were fortunate enough to be taught by them.

To the training committee, who under the chairmanship of Dr J. Brown supported the work of the School from its inception – thank you.

To the Superintendents throughout the North-West, and in particular to the District Superintendents at Blackpool and Lancaster Mr S. Whitley and Mr B. F. Gale respectively, I extend thanks for the help and support given to me so willingly at all times.

To the X-ray firms especially Messrs Philips, Picker, Siemens, Siel and General Electric who have supplied photos or leaflets to illustrate the book I send my grateful thanks. My appreciation also goes to Mr B. F. Gale, Mrs B. Mingham and Mr D. B. Pilkington for the photos of equipment they so kindly sent me.

To the colleagues on the DCR/HDCR Boards of Examination, as well as the members of the Committee and working parties I was associated with, I send my thanks for their friendship and guidance.

My special thanks go to The College of Radiographers, in particular to the General Secretary Mr R. M. Jordan, the Members of Council and the various Presidents who have supported the work of the School for many years.

I would like to express my thanks to the individual contributors who wrote chapters 15 to 20, namely Richard Price (15), Val Challen (16), David Manning (17 and 19) and Nigel Spencer (18).

My grateful thanks also go to the excellent staff at the School of Radiography who often worked under adverse conditions helping to build up the School to its present eminence. My thoughts go particularly to David Jenkins, Diane Greenwood, John Raby, David Manning, Val Challen and to the present Principal Richard Price. A word also for the various school secretaries, in particular Mrs A. Rice for her invaluable work and pleasant demeanour which is so essential, as she is often the first contact visitors make with the School. As I was employed by the Lancashire Education Committee and combined my role as Principal of the School with that of Principal Lecturer at the College of Further Education I would like to express my appreciation for the support given to the School by the College Principal and the College Governors without whose help development of the School would have been difficult, if not impossible. Of course an immense debt of gratitude is also owed to the Hospital Authorities who recently provided the New School Building, making it one of the premier Schools in the country. Finally I would like to express my thanks to the staff of MTP, particularly Mr Lister for being such an immense help in the production of this book.

In conclusion I am acutely aware that I have missed out, by name, many of my good friends who have helped me with their guidance and friendship over the years. You know who you are – please accept these heartfelt thanks – from me to you.

List of contributors

V. CHALLEN, HDCR(R), Cert. Ed.
Senior Lecturer, NW Lancashire School of Radiography,
Lancaster, England

H. JARVIS, HDCR(R)
Superintendent Radiographer, Department of Neuroradiology
Manchester Royal Infirmary, Manchester, England

D. J. MANNING, MSc, Cert. Ed., TDCR, DNM
Senior Lecturer, NW Lancashire School of Radiography,
Lancaster, England

R. C. PRICE, MSc, TDCR, T.Cert
Principal, NW Lancashire School of Radiography,
Lancaster, England

N. M. SPENCER, HDCR(R)
Superintendent Radiographer, Department of Radiology,
Newcastle General Hospital, Newcastle-upon-Tyne, England

1
Mains electricity supply and distribution

GENERATION OF AN ALTERNATING CURRENT (AC) POWER SUPPLY	1
Principles of electromagnetic induction	2
Generation of a three-phase supply	3
DISTRIBUTION OF ELECTRICAL ENERGY	4
ELECTRICAL SUPPLY TO THE HOSPITAL	5
SUPPLY CABLE RESISTANCE COMPENSATION	5
MAINS SWITCH	5
FUNCTION OF THE FUSES	6
CIRCUIT BREAKERS	7
Thermal circuit breaker	7
Bimetal strip	7
Electromagnetic circuit breaker	8
Operation of the circuit breaker and 'on', 'off' switches in the X-ray circuit	8
ELECTRICAL INSULATION	9
EARTHING	9
HIGH TENSION CABLES	9
Shockproofing the high tension circuit	10

The range of diagnostic imaging equipment available today is very wide, extending as it does from the simple portable X-ray unit costing a few hundred pounds to highly complex computerized systems costing hundreds of thousands of pounds. Despite this variation in complexity and cost however, they all have one factor in common and that is their need for electrical energy. Without electrical energy in one form or another none of them can function. Some low powered X-ray units operate from batteries and are thus completely independent of the mains electrical supply, but apart from these all other imaging systems are dependent on the mains supply. With this in mind it would seem sensible and logical for us to start our studies by looking at the way in which electricity is generated at the power station and then distributed to users throughout the country.

GENERATION OF AN ALTERNATING CURRENT (A.C.) POWER SUPPLY

At the power station electricity is generated as a three-phase supply by utilizing the principle of electromagnetic induction. The reader will, no doubt, recall from studies in Physics that an e.m.f. (electromotive force) is induced into a conductor when there is relative motion between the conductor and a magnetic field. In the power station the necessary motive power may be supplied by burning coal or oil, or from heat produced by nuclear fission, or by water falling from a height; in each case the energy is used to drive a turbine which produces the necessary motion between conductor and magnetic field.

At the power station a direct current (d.c.) generator, called an exciter, feeds direct current through a coil, called a rotor, which rotates within a series of coils called a stator. The rotor is driven by a turbine and the resultant changes in the number of lines of magnetic force threading or linking with the stator cause an e.m.f. to be induced into its windings.

It is important to realize that electrical energy is not *created* at the power station. We know from the energy conservation principle that energy can be neither created nor destroyed although it can be changed from one form to another. Such an energy conversion takes place in the power station, the heat energy released by burning coal or oil being used to boil water and produce steam, which under pressure acts on the blades of a turbine causing it and the rotor to rotate. The magnetic field associated with the rotor sweeps past the stator windings inducing into them an e.m.f. As the consumers use more and more electric power the current drawn by the consumers increases, as does that which flows through the stator windings, and the magnetic field associated with the current flowing in the stator windings reacts with the magnetic field associated with the rotor so that the rotor tends to slow down. To maintain the speed of rotation of the turbine more energy is needed to turn it and this extra energy is provided by burning more coal or oil and therefore increasing the pressure of the steam which drives the turbine. In this way a balance is established between the energy used by the power station in the form of coal or oil and the energy provided by the power station in the form of electrical power. The electrical energy used by the consumer can never exceed the energy used by the power station and indeed will always be less as some energy is used in overcoming friction etc. in the turbine.

The output of a modern power station is very high. The nuclear power station at Heysham in England for instance has an output of 2 × 622 MW and is able to satisfy the needs of many thousands of industrial and domestic consumers. Before we consider how electrical energy is transmitted to these consumers however, let us look at the principles involved in generating an electric current and why we get an alternating supply.

Principles of electromagnetic induction

Imagine a single loop of wire rotating in a magnetic field (Figure 1.1). As the right hand side of the loop moves up

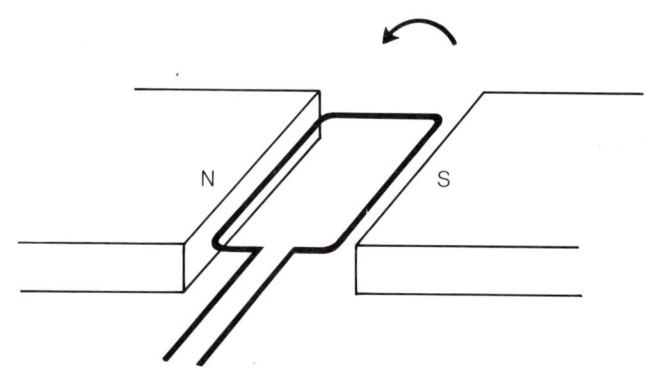

Figure 1.1 Conductor rotating in magnetic field

through the magnetic field the left hand side moves down. Whilst the loop is in the position shown, the loop is passing through the lines of magnetic force at right angles and the maximum number of lines of magnetic force are being 'cut' by the loop. Note that the induced e.m.f. is acting in *opposite* directions on each *side* of the loop but the effect in terms of electron current flow of the two opposing forces is additive as shown in Figure 1.2. Because of this only

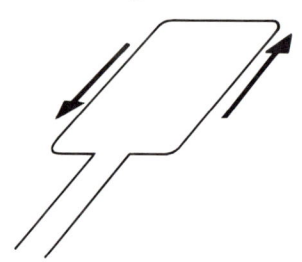

Figure 1.2 Direction of induced e.m.f.

one half of the loop need be drawn, the other half being indicated by means of a dotted line (Figure 1.3).

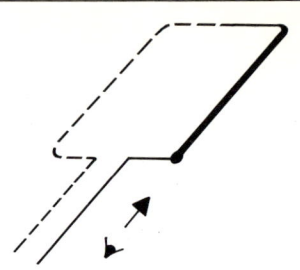

Figure 1.3 Because e.m.f.'s are additive only one half of coil need be shown

Consider Figure 1.4 and let us imagine that the coil moves down from position A to position B. The e.m.f.

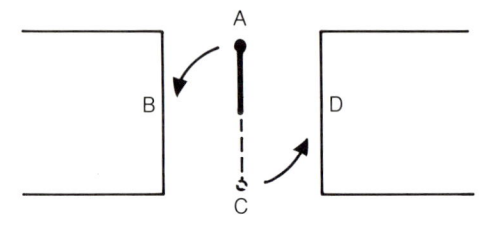

Figure 1.4 Coil rotating in magnetic field (only one half shown)

which is zero at A gradually increases to a maximum value at B and then reduces to zero value when it reaches C. As the coil moves up to position D the induced e.m.f. gradually increases and is at maximum value at D when it decreases until it reaches its original starting point at A. Note, however, that the coil is moving in the opposite direction from C to D, and that the direction of the induced e.m.f. is opposite to the e.m.f. induced between A and C. This is illustrated in Figure 1.5 and it will be noted that

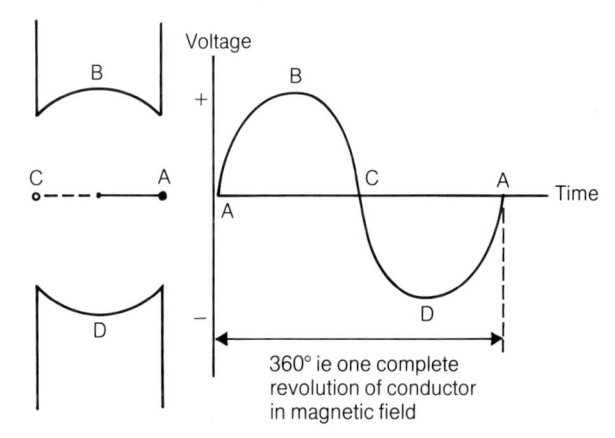

Figure 1.5 Voltage induced when coil makes one revolution in magnetic field

one revolution of the coil in the magnetic field induces an e.m.f. which rises from zero to maximum in one direction and then to maximum and zero in the opposite direction. The time taken for one pulse in one direction and one pulse in the opposite direction is the same time as the coil takes to make one complete revolution through the magnetic field.

So far we have considered the induction of a single phase voltage, i.e. one coil rotating in a fixed magnetic field. At the power station, however, electricity is generated as a three-phase supply. Let us therefore see how such a three-phase supply is produced.

Generation of a three-phase supply

In the case of the three-phase electrical generator three coils rotate simultaneously in a magnetic field. Each coil (consisting of two halves) is separated by an angle of 60° as shown in Figure 1.6 but as one half of each coil is producing an e.m.f. opposite in direction (but additive) to the other, we need, as before, show only one half of the coil (as a thick line) and the other half once again as a dotted line. Figure 1.6 illustrates the position of the three coils and of the voltages induced into each coil at different instants in time.

voltage) and its e.m.f. is reducing towards zero value (plotted as a positive value on the graph). Coil 3 is approaching the point where the voltage reaches its maximum value but is moving in the opposite direction to that of coil 2, and its e.m.f. is therefore plotted as a negative value on the graph.

Let us now consider this in terms of one complete revolution of coil 1. Starting from zero at point A the induced e.m.f. gradually increases until at point B (90° rotation of the coil) maximum voltage is being induced. The voltage now decreases as the coil approaches point C (180° rotation) at which point it is once again at zero value. The coil is now moving in the opposite direction and the e.m.f. once again increases as it approaches point D (270° rotation) but as the e.m.f. is now acting in the opposite direction it is plotted on the graph below the base line. The coil now approaches point A (360° rotation) and the voltage drops to zero as the coil completes one complete revolution. The same sequence of events occurs with coils 2 and 3, each coil having the same value of voltage induced into it as is induced into coil 1. It is apparent, however, that as each coil occupies a different position in the mag-

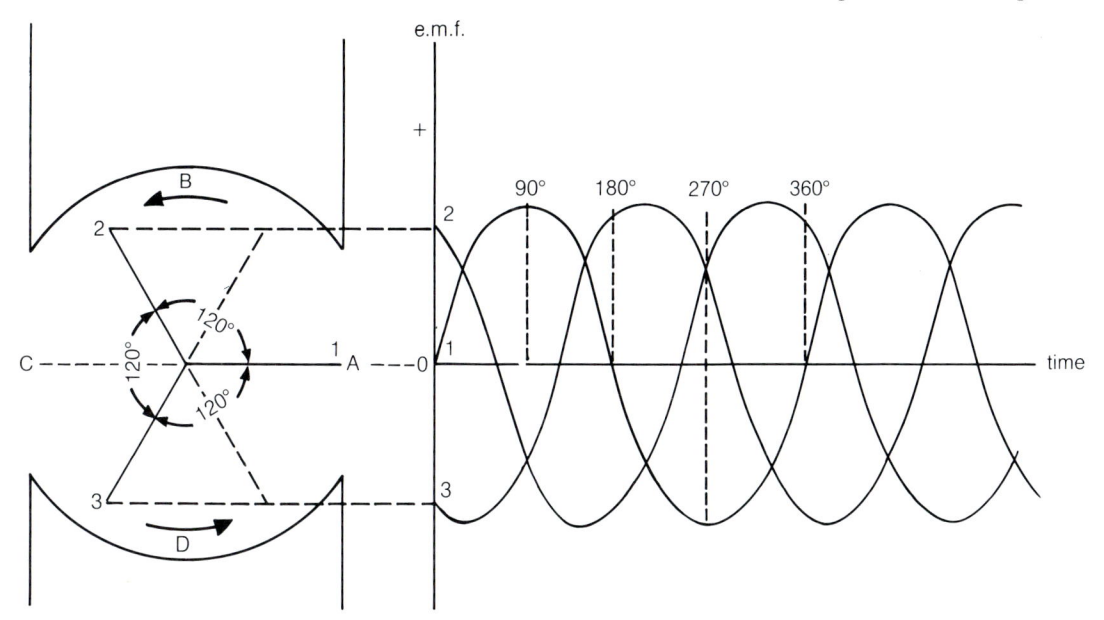

Figure 1.6 Generation of 3 phase voltage

The coils rotate at a frequency of 50 Hz (50 cycles per second) in the UK and in Europe, and 60 Hz in the USA.

Consider Figure 1.6 and imagine the coils have just reached their present position. Coil 1 is moving with the lines of magnetic force and consequently no e.m.f. is being induced (plotted at zero on the graph). Coil 2 has passed point B at which maximum voltage was induced (peak

netic field, maximum voltage cannot be induced in each coil *at the same instant in time*. The three induced e.m.f.'s are said to be 120° out of phase with respect to one another. This means that maximum voltage is attained by coil 1, one third of a cycle (120°) after maximum voltage has been reached by coil 2; and coil 2 reaches maximum voltage one third of a cycle after coil 3.

Phase Angle is the angle swept out by the coil to induce a given e.m.f.

DISTRIBUTION OF ELECTRICAL ENERGY

We have seen that at the power station a separate e.m.f. is induced into each coil and that each e.m.f. is 120° out of phase with respect to its neighbour. Each e.m.f. is stepped up at the power station to approximately 400 kV by the use of h.t. (high tension) transformers and transmitted to consumers throughout the country via overhead transmission lines. The conducting cable is usually aluminium (cheap and light) which surrounds a supporting steel cable. The h.t. supply is stepped down to lower working voltages by means of a step-down transformer before passing along underground cables to the consumer.

In the UK the consumer has the choice of a 240 V (phase voltage) or 415 V (line voltage). 240 V is normally supplied for domestic (low power) consumption. All three phases are used for certain equipment such as three-phase motors in industry or in the case of the X-ray Department, the three-phase (6-pulse) X-ray generator.

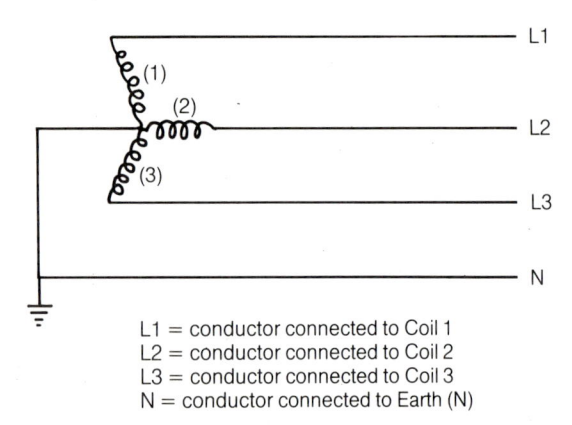

Figure 1.7 Mains supply lines from electrical generator

In Figure 1.7, the potential difference between L1 and neutral, L2 and neutral, and L3 and neutral is 240 V r.m.s. in each case, and is used for low power or domestic supply. When power consumption is high, however, as in the case of a major X-ray installation in the Department of Radiology, it is advantageous to use a higher voltage and thus obtain the necessary power with a lower current. This higher voltage of 415 V is obtained by connecting across any two live conductors, i.e. L1 and L2, L1 and L3, or L2 and L3 as shown in Figure 1.8.

The 240 V supply obtained from L1, L2 or L3 and neutral is called the *phase voltage*, whilst the 415 V obtained across two lines is called the *line voltage*. At first

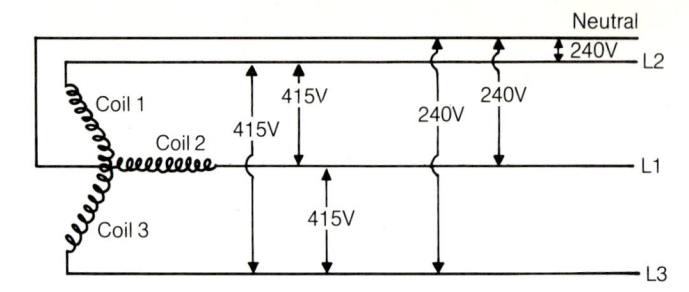

Figure 1.8 Two different voltages from a 3-phase supply

sight it would appear that the line voltage should be twice the phase voltage, i.e. 480 V rather than 415, but we must remember that the e.m.f.s induced into each coil are out of phase with one another. From Figure 1.9 it can be seen that when one e.m.f. (say from L1) is at peak value the other two (L2 and L3) are of equal value and opposite sign but are *less* than peak value.

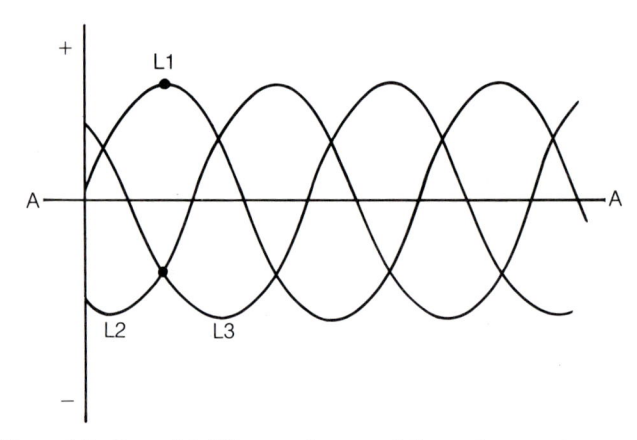

Figure 1.9 Potential difference between 3 lines when one is at peak value

The base line A–A is at zero value (neutral). L1 is at peak value positive to the base line whilst L2 and L3 are seen to be negative with respect to the base line and less than peak value. Now peak value is 1.414 × r.m.s. value. Therefore L1 has a peak positive value of 240 × 1.414 which is 339.36 V and the other two have a negative value of 175 × 1.414 which is 247.45 V. To find the potential difference we must subtract one from the other, 339.36 − −247.45, and as two minus values give a plus; the difference between 339.36 and −247.45 is 339.36 + 247.45 which is 586.81 V. However, as this is a peak value we must calculate the r.m.s. value and to do this we must divide the peak value by 1.414 (or multiply by 0.707) which gives us 414.87 or 415 to the nearest volt.

Note: Mathematically, assuming a true sine wave the r.m.s. value of L1 (240 V) is multiplied by $\sqrt{3}$, which is 1.73, to give the r.m.s. voltage across two live conductors i.e. 240 × 1.73 = 415.

MAINS ELECTRICITY SUPPLY AND DISTRIBUTION

ELECTRICAL SUPPLY TO THE HOSPITAL

The hospital is connected to the mains supply as shown in Figure 1.10.

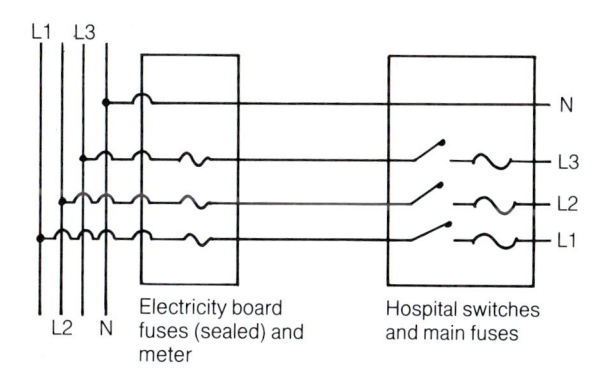

Figure 1.10 Electricity supply to hospital

The fuses A, B and C are Electricity Board fuses and are sealed by them to ensure that they are not interfered with. Next comes the meter, also belonging to the Electricity Board, which records the amount of energy consumed by the hospital. All the wiring from the meter onwards is the property and responsibility of the Hospital Authority. The Hospital Engineer determines which parts of the hospital will be supplied with a 240 V supply and which with 415 V or three-phase. In the X-ray Department, for example, we may use 240 V for lighting, electric fires, densitometers, etc. and for low-powered X-ray equipment such as dental or mobile units; 415 V for major 2-pulse units and all three phases for high-powered 6-pulse X-ray generators.

Note: The use of the line voltage (415 V) supply enables us to obtain the necessary power ($v \times i$) for an X-ray exposure with a lower current than would be possible using a 240 V supply. This means that the voltage drop along the supply cables, during an exposure, is much less which means that the reduction in voltage to the X-ray equipment during the exposure is less, and the kV across the X-ray tube is maintained closer to the selected value ($V_{drop} = I^2R$).

SUPPLY CABLE RESISTANCE COMPENSATION

Prior to installing new X-ray equipment it is important to ensure that the supply cable resistance does not exceed the maximum value quoted by the manufacturers. For example, the manufacturer of a particular unit may specify that the supply cable must not exceed 0.5 ohms at 415 V, or 0.35 ohms at 240 V. If this value is exceeded then the voltage drop along the cables will result in an unacceptable reduction in voltage to the equipment when an exposure is made. The manufacturer designs the X-ray equipment to operate satisfactorily with a supply cable resistance of the specified value and he then calibrates the equipment in the factory using the specified supply cable resistance, say 0.35 ohms at 240 V.

When the X-ray equipment is installed in the X-ray Department the supply cable resistance is measured and if it is found to be, say, 0.25 ohms, a resistance of 0.1 ohms is selected on the resistance compensator within the unit to bring the supply cable resistance up to the specified 0.35 ohms. The unit will now operate satisfactorily in precisely the same way it did when calibrated in the factory. As the X-ray unit is a fixture it is not necessary to alter the resistance compensator after installation.

MAINS SWITCH

The mains switch in the X-ray room provides a means of switching the current 'on' and 'off' by 'making' or 'breaking' each of the electrical conductors. The equipment is thus completely isolated from the mains supply when the switch is 'off'.

The switch gear is contained within an earthed metal box (Figure 1.11). The box has a hinged front, or door,

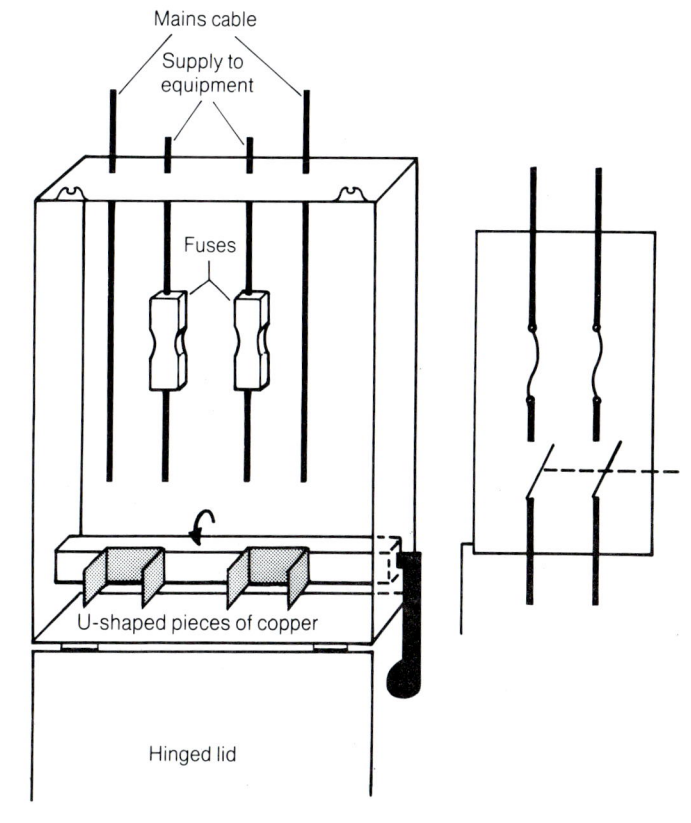

Figure 1.11 Diagrammatic and symbolic representation of mains switch

which can only be opened when the switch is in the 'off' position. The switch handle is attached to a bar of insulated material which rotates when the handle is moved up to the 'on' position, or down to the 'off' position. Fastened to the bar are two 'U' shaped pieces of copper (three if the supply is to a three-phase X-ray unit) which 'make' or 'break' the circuit according to their position. Also contained within the box are a number of fuses, the number being determined by the number of live conductors (i.e. three if there are three live phases, L1, L2 and L3, two if there are two live phases (line voltage) and one if there is one live conductor and neutral (phase voltage).

If possible, all electrical supplies to the equipment in an X-ray room, e.g. supply to the motor for tilting the table, supply to the television etc. as well as the electrical supply to the X-ray unit itself, should pass through one mains switch, so that the equipment can be switched off rapidly in case of accident.

FUNCTION OF THE FUSES

A fuse is the weakest part of a circuit and serves to protect the component parts of the circuit from damage due to overload. Electrical components are designed to carry a particular current or to withstand a particular voltage. Each electrical component is rated in terms of the maximum current it can safely carry and the maximum voltage it can withstand. If the current flowing through the component exceeds its rated value the component will probably suffer damage and may even be destroyed. Fuse wire is also rated in terms of the maximum current it can carry before it melts (e.g. 5 A, 10 A and 15 A fuse wire). The symbol for a fuse is shown in Figure 1.12. For example, if the current flowing through the X-ray circuit rises to such a value that it would constitute a hazard to a particular component (say a valve) then the fuse melts and breaks the electrical circuit. In this way the fuse protects the component parts of a circuit.

Figure 1.12 Circuit symbol for a fuse

Although the same current flows through all parts of a *series* circuit, the current in a *parallel* circuit splits, and the current flowing in one part of an electrical circuit may be quite different from that flowing in another. It is, therefore, necessary to protect different parts of the circuit with different gauges of fuse wire, e.g. 5 A, 15 A, 30 A, 100 A fuse wire, each gauge being appropriate to a particular fuse and capable of carrying a particular value of current. Figure 1.13 illustrates two different types of fuses and holders.

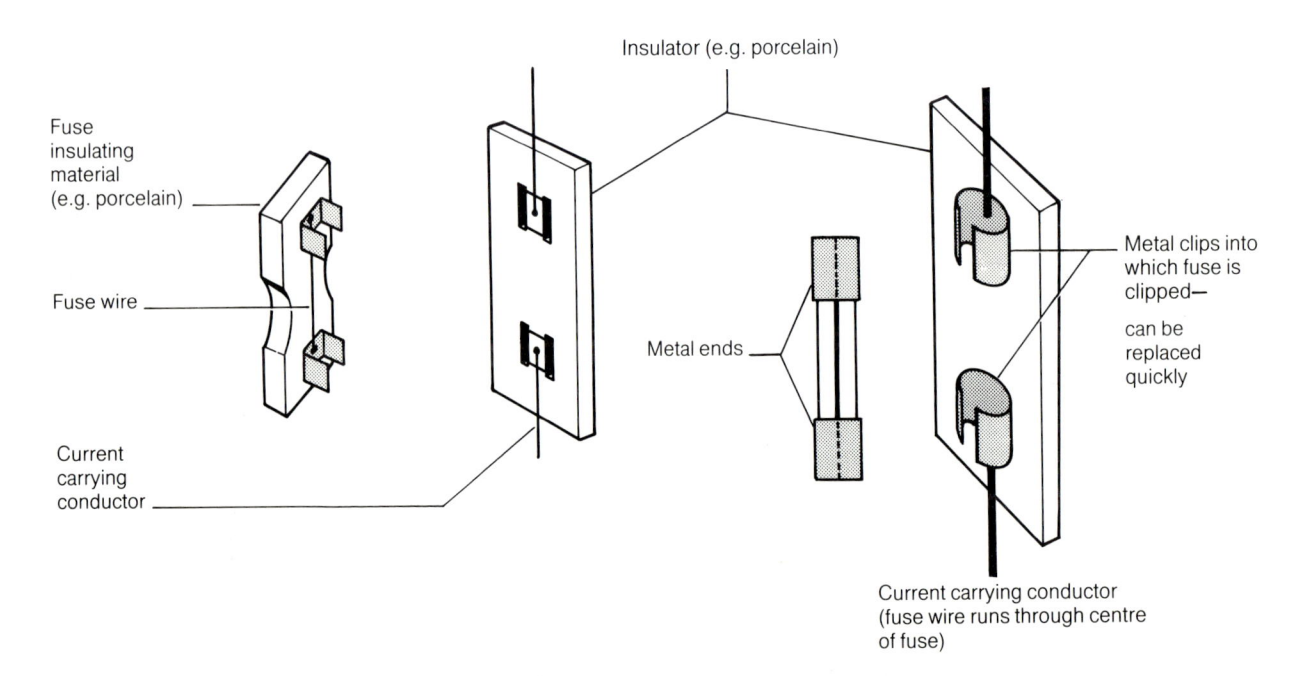

Figure 1.13 Different types of fuse and holder

MAINS ELECTRICITY SUPPLY AND DISTRIBUTION

As the fuse wire melts if the current through it rises above a certain critical value, it will be appreciated that it is necessary to attach the fuse to a non-inflammable base, or to situate the fuses in a fireproof box. Fuse wire wears thin with use and will eventually melt, even though the current through it is not excessive. Rewiring the fuse normally restores the circuit to normal functioning. If, however, the fuse wire melts again *after* replacement, it is essential that the equipment be inspected by a competent person and the cause of the fault located.

Never use a heavier gauge of fuse wire than that recommended, as this may cause damage to the circuit or its components.

CIRCUIT BREAKERS

Whilst fuses are used extensively in electrical circuits and provide adequate protection for the components in the circuit, they tend to be awkward to replace. Panels usually need to be removed from the unit to gain access to the fuse holder, the correct gauge of fuse wire must be available and a screwdriver must be to hand. Even if a spare fuse is kept with the equipment ready for immediate insertion, there is an inevitable delay before the X-ray unit is once more ready for use. This can be the cause of much frustration, particularly if the unit is being used in the operating theatre.

To overcome this difficulty, the manufacturer may use a circuit breaker rather than a fuse to protect the circuit and thus ensure that the current through the unit does not rise to an excessive value. The circuit breaker can be reset immediately by pressing a small button (usually coloured red) if the circuit breaker is of the thermal type, or by moving a switch handle in the case of the electromagnetic circuit breaker. (It should be noted that, although maximum current through the unit is limited by a circuit breaker, individual parts of the circuit will almost certainly be protected by fuses.) As already indicated, there are two types of circuit breakers, one thermal and the other electromagnetic.

Thermal circuit breaker

This type depends upon the effect of heat on a bimetal strip for its operation. Such a strip bends on heating and, in the thermal circuit breaker, bending of the strip causes a contact to open, which breaks the circuit. The bimetal strip is usually in series connection in the electrical circuit, its temperature being governed by the current flowing through it. As the current increases, the temperature of the bimetal strip rises, bending more the hotter it becomes. At a predetermined critical temperature the strip is bent to such an extent that it releases a mechanism which opens the circuit. Before considering the thermal circuit breaker further, however, let us find out a little more about the bimetal strip.

Bimetal strip

Whilst all metals expand on heating and contract on cooling, different metals experience different degrees of expansion for the same temperature rise. If very thin slices of two different metals, such as iron and brass, are welded together it is found that the compound strip bends on heating (Figure 1.14).

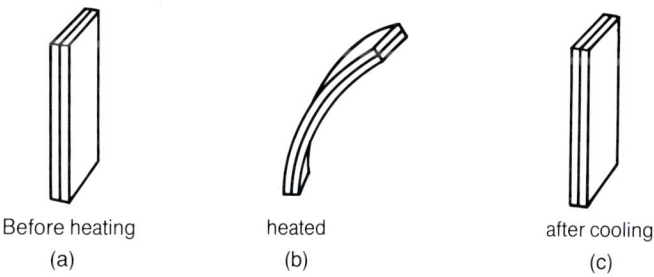

Figure 1.14 Bimetal strip when cold (a) and (c), and when heated (b)

Iron and brass have different coefficients of linear expansion*, brass expanding about 60% more than iron for the same temperature rise. As they are welded together and expand at different rates for the same temperature rise, the pressures cause the strip to bend, slowly at first, then more and more rapidly as the temperature rises. Conversely, as the strip cools the metals contract, once again at different rates, and the pressures within the strip cause it to gradually straighten until it returns to its original state.

A diagrammatic representation of a thermal circuit breaker is shown in Figure 1.15 which indicates the principle of operation of such a device.

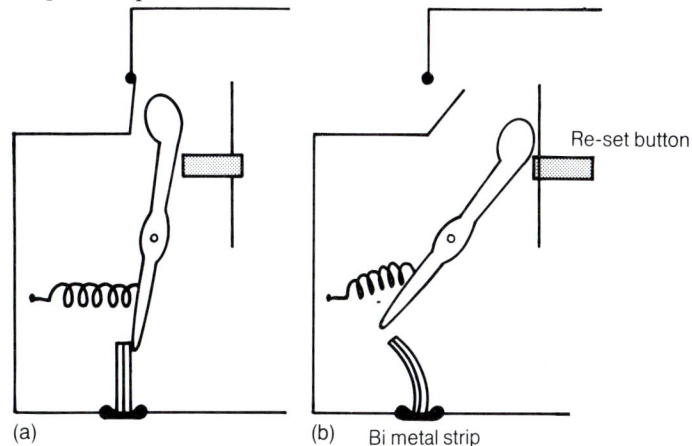

Figure 1.15 Thermal circuit breaker (a) set, and (b) overloaded

* *Coefficient of linear expansion* is the amount by which unit length (1 metre) of a particular substance increases when its temperature rises by 1 K (1 degree Kelvin).

It will be noted that current flowing through the circuit also passes through the bimetal strip. If the current rises to an excessive value, the strip bends and releases a spring-loaded arm, causing a contact to open, breaking the circuit. The same movement of the arm pushes a red button out. Current can now no longer flow through the circuit. When the bimetal strip has cooled and returned to its original shape, the circuit breaker can be reset by pressing the red button. This closes the contact and the bimetal strip, now in its original position, holds the spring-loaded arm in position keeping the contact closed. The circuit now functions normally. If the device breaks the circuit again, immediately after being reset, the equipment must be inspected by a competent person and the fault located.

The advantage of the thermal circuit breaker over a fuse lies in the ease with which it can be reset. It is, however, much slower in action than a fuse, as it takes longer for the metal strip to bend.

Electromagnetic circuit breaker

This device relies upon the magnetic effect of a current-carrying conductor for its operation. If the current flowing through a thick coil of wire, in series connection with the circuit, rises to an excessive value, the magnetic effect associated with the current causes a moveable metal core to be drawn into the coil (Figure 1.16). The metal then strikes a bar, which operates a trip mechanism, causing the circuit to be opened and current flow to be stopped. To prevent the current being switched off by transient rises in current, movement of the metal core into the coil may be impeded by pressure of oil in a small dashpot. In this way only a sustained rise in current will cause the trip mechanism to be operated and the current to be switched off. This type of circuit breaker is quickly made functional again by pressing a button. This resets the trip mechanism.

Operation of the circuit breaker and 'on','off' switches in the X-ray circuit

Pressing the 'on' switch (Figure 1.17) completes the circuit $N-S_1-$'on' switch$-$trip switch$-L_1$ (drawn in thin lines). Current flows through the coil, S_1, causing closure of contacts C_1, C_2 and C_3 which are ganged. The primary circuit (thick lines) is now complete and current flow to the autotransformer is established.

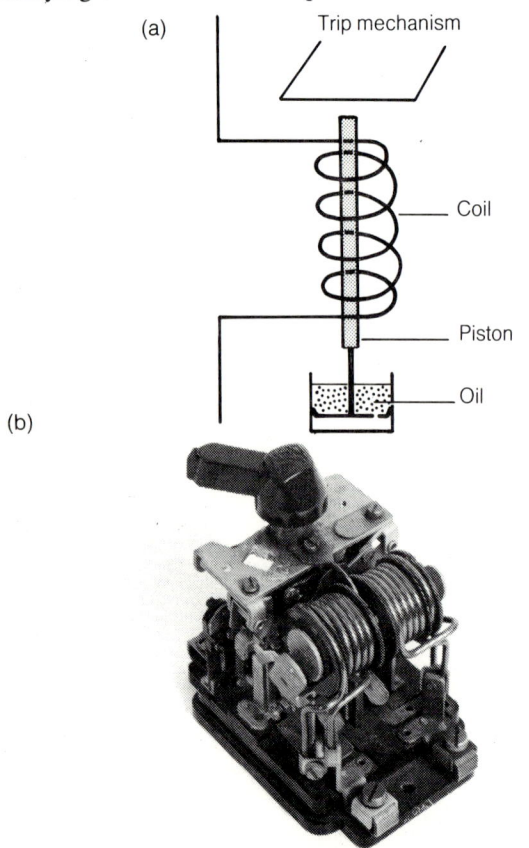

Figure 1.16 Electromagnetic circuit breaker, (a) diagram, (b) photograph

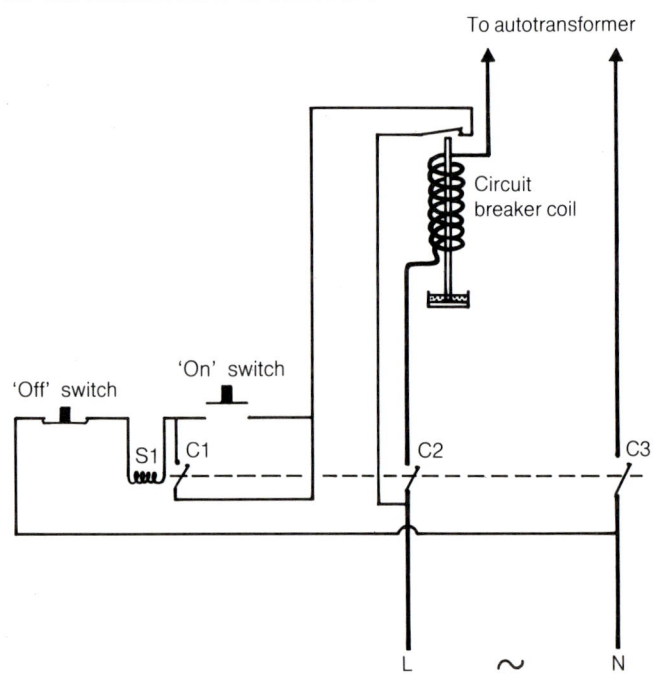

Figure 1.17 X-ray unit 'on' and 'off' switches and circuit breaker switch connected in circuit

Excessive current through the coil of the circuit breaker, which forms an integral part of the primary circuit, causes a moveable core to be drawn into the coil. Movement of the core operates the trip switch, which opens the circuit

MAINS ELECTRICITY SUPPLY AND DISTRIBUTION

$N-S_1-C_1-$trip switch$-L_1$ stopping current flow through S_1. Switches C_1, C_2 and C_3 are then opened and current flow through the primary circuit is terminated.

Circuit $N-S_1-C_1-L_1$ may also be opened by pressing the 'off' switch. Interruption of current flow through S_1 causes switches C_1, C_2 and C_3 to be opened, terminating current flow in the primary circuit. See also Figure 2.14 to see how this fits into the complete circuit.

ELECTRICAL INSULATION

To protect the user against the effects of electric shock, current-carrying conductors must be insulated, the amount of insulation being determined by the potential difference between the current carrying conductor to earth, or to other conductors at different potential.

Electrical conductors are usually made of copper. The greater the current to be carried by the conductor the thicker it must be (to minimize voltage drop) and the greater the potential difference between such a conductor and earth the thicker (or more effective) must be the insulating material surrounding the conductor if the user is to be adequately protected.

Most of the cables rated to carry current at 240 or 415 V are similar to the one shown in Figure 1.18. They are identified as live, neutral or earth conductors by the colour of the plastic sleeve which surrounds the conductor.

Live is coloured brown.
Neutral is coloured blue.
Earth is coloured green with yellow stripes.

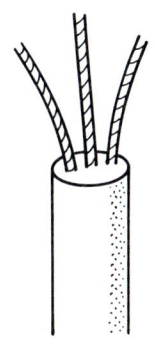

Figure 1.18 Low tension (mains voltage) electrical cable

Each cable (conductor and insulation) is rated in terms of the maximum current it can safely carry and the maximum voltage its insulation can withstand to earth.
Note: By convention low voltage = up to 1000 V (l.v.); high voltage (h.v.) = over 1000 V.

EARTHING

All metal parts of electrical equipment, *with the exception of the conductors themselves*, must be connected to earth (Figure 1.19). This ensures that breakdown in the insulation around the conductors does not present a serious hazard to the user. If the metal parts of a piece of equipment are accidentally connected to the electrical supply, due to breakdown of insulation, loose connections, etc., a current will flow between the metal and earth. If the metal is connected to earth via a good conductor the electron current will flow directly to earth. This current is usually large and 'blows' a fuse or trips out a circuit breaker, breaking the circuit and protecting anyone who may have been in contact with any metal part of the equipment, e.g. patient on the table, radiographer, etc.

If the metal parts of electrical equipment (excepting the circuit itself) are *not* connected to earth via a good conductor, a person touching the metal will act as a conductor and, as the human body is not a good electrical conductor, current flow to or from the earth through the body may not be sufficiently high to 'blow' a fuse or operate a circuit breaker. In these circumstances current continues to flow through the body, possibly with disastrous results.

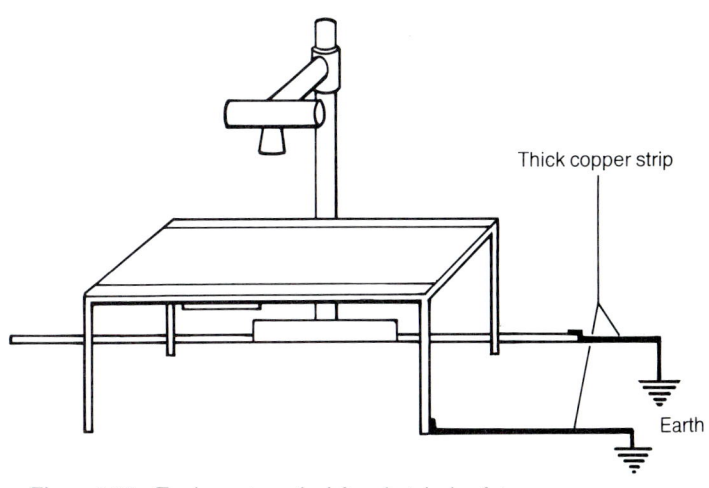

Figure 1.19 Equipment earthed for electrical safety

So far we have discussed shockproofing in terms of equipment operating at voltages of 240 V or 415 V. The cables carrying current to the X-ray tube, however, may be at potentials of up to 75 kV with respect to earth and therefore need special provision to make them shockproof.

HIGH TENSION CABLES

The high tension conductors are surrounded by thick rubber insulation which is then enclosed by a metallic braid.

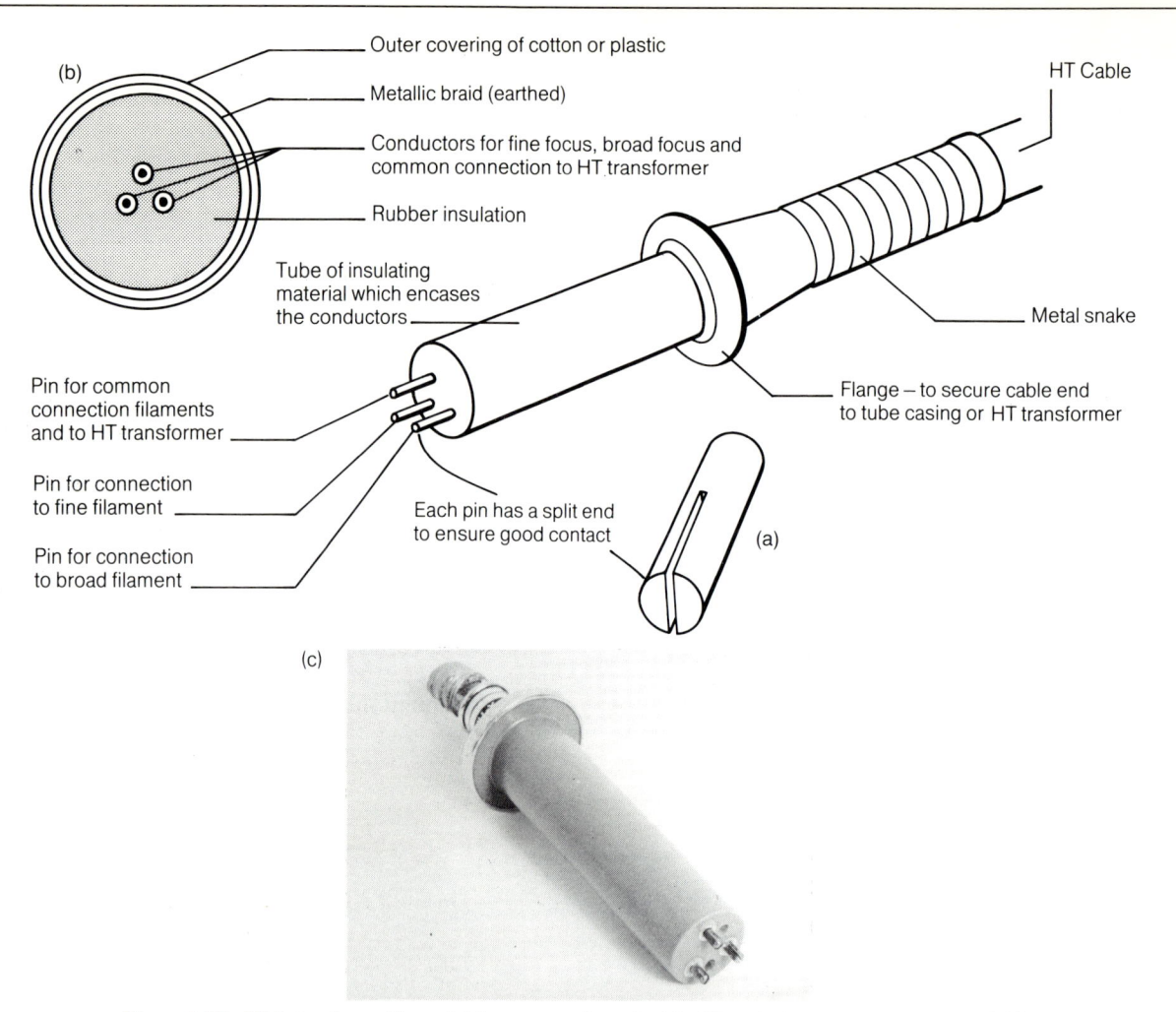

Figure 1.20 High tension cable end (a), cross section of cable (b) and photograph of cable end (c)

Figure 1.20. The metallic braid is continuous with the X-ray tube casing at one end and with the high tension transformer tank at the other, as shown in Figure 1.21.

Where the cable bends at an acute angle, e.g. when it leaves the h.t. transformer or enters the X-ray tube, it is enclosed within a metal snake. This prevents the cable from bending too severely and thus prevents damage to the conductors or the insulation.

Shockproofing the high tension circuit

From Figure 1.21 it will be noted that the complete high tension circuit is surrounded by insulating rubber or insulating oil and further enclosed within an earthed metal sheath or casing. In the event of breakdown of the insulation, the high tension current will discharge through the low resistance path to earth rather than through the high resistance path offered by the patient's or radiographer's body, thus protecting patients and staff.

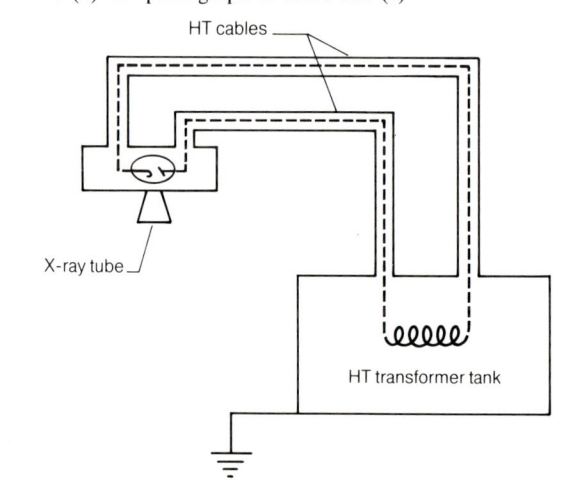

Figure 1.21 Ensuring safety against h.t. current by earthing X-ray tube casing, h.t. transformer tank and metal braid around h.t. cable insulation

2
Diagnostic X-ray circuits

THE X-RAY CIRCUIT	11
THE PRIMARY CIRCUIT	11
The autotransformer	12
The mains voltage compensator	12
Automatic mains voltage compensation	13
kV control	14
THE HIGH TENSION TRANSFORMER	14
TRANSFORMER REGULATION	16
TRANSFORMER RATING	16
Compensation for voltage drop in the supply cable	17
DIAGNOSTIC HIGH TENSION CIRCUITS	18
Inverse voltage reducer (primary circuit) used in self-rectified X-ray circuits only	21
Full-wave rectification two-pulse (single-phase using four rectifiers)	22
Single phase constant potential circuit using secondary switching	22
Preparing for an exposure	22
Making the exposure	22
Functioning of the secondary circuit	23
kV control – using high tension triodes	24
Three-phase circuit six-pulse (six rectifiers)	24
Functioning of the circuit	24
Advantages of the three-phase over single-phase circuits	25
Radiographic advantages of three-phase X-ray generators compared to those operating on single-phase	25
12-pulse (12 rectifier) circuit	25
POSITION OF METERS IN THE CIRCUIT	26
Reading meters	26
X-RAY TUBE FILAMENT HEATING CIRCUIT	27
kV COMPENSATOR	28
kV compensation when there is no prereading kV meter	31
THE mA CONTROL	31
TRIMMER RESISTANCE	32
FILAMENT STEP-DOWN TRANSFORMER	32
EXPOSURE SWITCHING (PRIMARY CIRCUIT)	33
The mechanical (electromagnetic) contactor switch	33

THE X-RAY CIRCUIT

We will consider the circuit of a simple X-ray generator from two aspects:

(1) *The primary circuit* which is at low tension, i.e. 240 or 415 V

(2) *The secondary circuit* which is at high tension, i.e. up to 75 kV peak with respect to earth.

The primary circuit includes the mains switch, fuses, circuit breaker, autotransformer, mains voltage compensator, kV control, primary contactor switch, pre-reading kV meter, primary winding of the high tension transformer, timer circuit, filament heating circuit and various compensating circuits. (See Figure 2.14)

The secondary circuit consists of the secondary winding of the high tension transformer, high tension rectifiers, the X-ray tube and the secondary winding of the filament heating transformer.

THE PRIMARY CIRCUIT

As we have already described the mains switch, and circuit breaker, etc. let us now move on to some other parts of the primary circuit starting with the autotransformer.

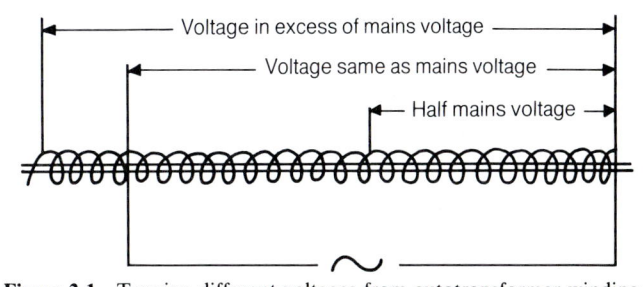

Figure 2.1 Tapping different voltages from autotransformer winding

The ratio of the voltage applied (Figure 2.1) to the autotransformer winding, to the voltage tapped from it, is equal to the ratio of the number of turns to which the mains voltage is applied, to the number of tapped turns.

$$\frac{\text{Applied voltage}}{\text{Tapped voltage}} = \frac{\text{No of turns to which mains voltage is applied}}{\text{No. of tapped turns}}$$

The autotransformer

This consists of a single winding of thick copper wire, wound on a closed iron core. Alternating current, which is rising, falling and changing in direction 100 times per second, flows through the winding. The magnetic field associated with the alternating current, which is also expanding, contracting and changing its polarity 100 times per second, is concentrated by the iron core. As the magnetic field expands it passes through the core and through the copper windings, inducing a voltage into each turn of the winding and also into the iron core itself. Voltages induced into the iron core cause eddy currents to flow in the core. These are reduced by laminating (slicing) the iron core, each slice being electrically insulated from the next. As the magnetic field collapses it once again induces a voltage into each turn of the autotransformer winding (and the core) but this time in the opposite direction.

Any desired voltage, from zero up to rather more than the input voltage, can be obtained by simply tapping off a particular number of turns.

Example (See Figure 2.2)

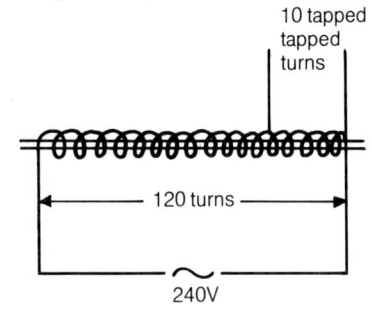

Figure 2.2

Applied voltage = 240 V
No. of turns to which voltage is applied = 120
Tapped turns = 10
Tapped voltage = x

$$\frac{240}{x} = \frac{120}{10}$$
$$120x = 240 \times 10$$
$$x = \frac{240 \times 10}{120}$$
$$x = 20 \text{ V}$$

In this example it can be appreciated that a voltage of 20 V is always obtained when ten turns of the autotransformer winding are tapped off *providing* the mains voltage remains constant at 240 V (r.m.s.). If, however, the mains voltage varies, as it does, over both long and short periods of time, then the tapped voltage also varies and we no longer get 20 V as anticipated but a voltage which is more or less than this, dependent on how much the mains voltage varies.

Let us calculate mathematically the effect on the tapped voltage of a change in the mains voltage from 240 V to, say, 210 V. Using the previous example,

Applied voltage now = 210 V
No. of turns to which the mains voltage is applied, still = 120
No. of tapped turns = 10
The tapped voltage now = x

$$\frac{210}{x} = \frac{120}{10}$$
$$120x = 210 \times 10$$
$$x = \frac{210 \times 10}{120}$$
$$x = 17.5 \text{ V}$$

A drop in mains voltage from 240 V to 210 V therefore results in a tapped voltage across ten turns of 17.5 V compared to 20 V obtained at 240 V even though the number of tapped turns remains the same in each case.

Now any desired kV may be obtained from the secondary winding of the *high tension transformer* by applying the appropriate voltage to the primary. If, for example, a high tension transformer with a turns ratio of 300:1 has 200 V applied to its primary winding, the output from the secondary will be $200 \times 300 = 60$ kV (assuming 100% efficiency). Providing therefore 200 V (no more, no less) is applied to the primary of such a transformer, the output will always be 60 kV. Similarly, of course, any other kV may be obtained by applying the appropriate voltage to the primary winding and *providing* the applied voltage remains *constant* we will always get the anticipated kV from the transformer secondary. Unfortunately, however, the primary voltage, which is obtained by tapping off a selected number of turns from the autotransformer varies with variation in the mains supply voltage. It is, therefore, essential, if the X-ray unit is to function reliably, to compensate for the effects of mains voltage variation.

The mains voltage compensator

The mains voltage compensator fulfils this function by ensuring that the voltage induced into each turn of the autotransformer winding remains constant, despite variations in mains voltage. This is achieved by varying the number of turns to which the mains voltage is applied (Figure 2.3).

DIAGNOSTIC X-RAY CIRCUITS

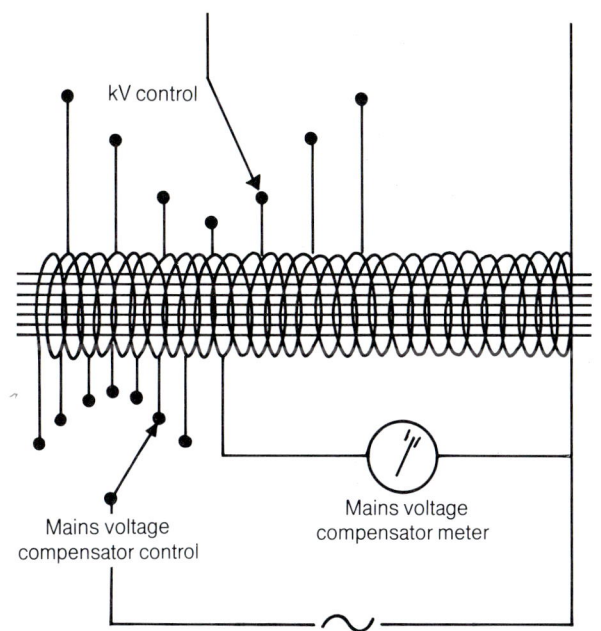

Figure 2.3 Autotransformer, mains voltage compensator and kV control

Considering the same examples as before
Applied voltage = 240 V
No. of turns to which voltage is applied = 120
Tapped turns = 10
Tapped voltage = 20 V
If, however, the applied voltage drops to 210 V
No. of turns to which voltage is applied remains 120
Tapped turns remain 10
Then tapped voltage now = 17.5 V
To restore the tapped voltage to 20 V (2 V per turn) we must vary the number of turns to which the mains voltage is applied.
By calculation
The applied voltage = 210 V
Tapped turns = 10
Tapped voltage = 20 V
No. of turns to which voltage must now be applied = x

As $\dfrac{\text{Applied voltage}}{\text{Tapped voltage}} = \dfrac{\text{No. of turns to which mains voltage is applied}}{\text{No. of tapped turns}}$

$$\frac{210}{20} = \frac{x}{10}$$
$$20x = 210 \times 10$$
$$x = \frac{210 \times 10}{20}$$
$$= 105$$

If, therefore, the reduced voltage of 210 V is applied to 105 turns (instead of 120 as previously), 2 V will be induced into each turn and 10 tapped turns will give us 20 V.

These calculations need not be made in practice, of course, as a voltmeter called a mains voltage compensator meter (Figure 2.4) is connected across a *fixed* number of turns of the autotransformer winding.

Consider our previous example. We required 2 V to be induced into each turn of the winding. A voltmeter connected across, say, 75 turns would indicate 150 V if the mains voltage was at its correct value of 240 V. (*Note*, the mains voltage compensator meter does *not* indicate the value of the mains voltage itself but the voltage induced across a specific number of turns.) If the mains voltage drops then the voltage induced into each turn of the autotransformer winding is less, the voltage across a given number of turns is reduced, and the mains voltage compensator meter indicates a voltage which is less than 150 V. Indeed, if the mains voltage drops to 210 V, 1.75 V is induced in each turn and the meter indicates a voltage of $1.75 \times 75 = 131$ V. The induced voltage is restored to its original value, 2 V per turn or 150 V across 75 turns, by applying the reduced mains voltage (210 V) to 105 turns of the autotransformer winding, instead of 120. It is not necessary to make any calculations, of course, as we know the correct voltage is being induced into each turn of the winding when the mains voltage compensator meter indicates 150 V. It is not even necessary for the meter to be calibrated in volts and may indeed by marked with only two red lines (Figure 2.4). When the pointer is between these lines we know that the correct voltage is being induced into each turn of the autotransformer winding and that when we tap off a certain number of turns we always get the correct voltage.

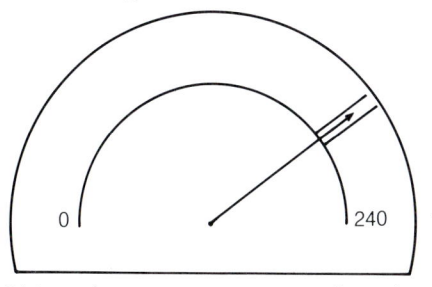

Figure 2.4 Mains voltage compensator meter (sometimes called line voltage compensator meter)

Automatic mains voltage compensation

Some modern X-ray units have no manually operated mains voltage compensator control. It should not be assumed, however, that because there is no manual control for the radiographer to operate that no compensation takes place. Indeed, a moment's thought will make it obvious that despite the lack of such a control, changes in mains voltage must be compensated for. In fact, the compensation is automatic in so far as changes in mains voltage cause a pivoted bar to operate a ratchet which in turn moves a contact so that more (or less) turns of the autotransformer are connected to the mains supply. The operation of the ratchet, which makes a clicking noise when in operation, can usually be heard as it functions, between exposures, to maintain a steady voltage (r.m.s.) from the autotransformer to the primary winding of the high tension transformer. When the unit is put into 'prep' before an exposure is made the compensator circuit is automatically switched off then switched back on again when the exposure is terminated. This is because the compensator cannot operate fast enough during an exposure and in any case the high primary current which flows during the exposure would damage the contacts on 'make' and 'break'.

kV control

Any kV, up to a specified maximum, may be obtained from the secondary winding of the high tension transformer by applying the appropriate voltage to the primary winding. The kV control is used to select the appropriate voltage from the autotransformer. This may be done by moving a rotary control which selects the appropriate number of turns from the autotransformer for application to the primary winding of the high tension transformer. This voltage may be indicated on a meter which measures the *primary* voltage but which may be calibrated in terms of the secondary voltage which will be induced during the exposure. Alternatively, a pointer may indicate the proposed kV on a scale or on more modern units a digital readout may be used.

For radiography a range of kV values from about 35 to a maximum of 100–150 kV is obtainable on most major units in steps of about 2 kV. Some other units provide fine and coarse control, the fine control allowing steps of 1 kV and the coarse control steps of 10 kV.

For fluoroscopy stepless or continuous control of kV is provided by using a variac transformer.

THE HIGH TENSION TRANSFORMER

The high tension transformer is a step-up transformer. It consists of a primary winding and a secondary winding, carefully insulated from one another and wound on a shell type metal core (Figure 2.5). The function of the high tension transformer is to provide the high voltages (up to 150 kVp in some units) needed for the production of X-rays in the X-rays tube.

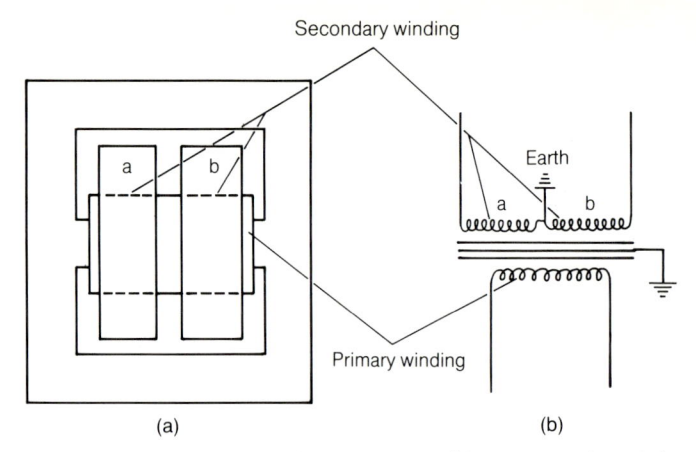

Figure 2.5 Diagrammatic (a) and symbolic (b) representation of the high tension transformer

The magnetic field associated with the current flowing in the primary winding is concentrated in the metal core. The shape of the core ensures a continuous path for the magnetic flux with maximum concentration within the core and minimum leakage to the air (Figures 2.6, 2.7)

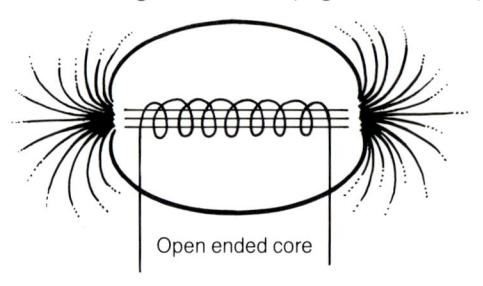

Figure 2.6 Magnetic flux leaking away in air

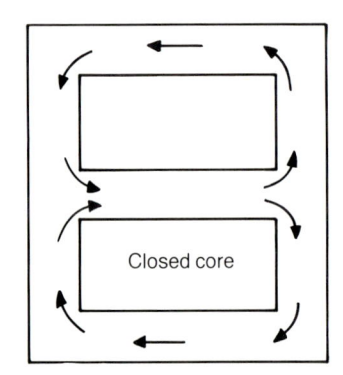

Figure 2.7 Continuous path for flux

The core is made of a metal alloy such as stalloy, an alloy of steel and silicon, and is built up in laminations or slices, each slice being electrically insulated from the next (Figure 2.8).

DIAGNOSTIC X-RAY CIRCUITS

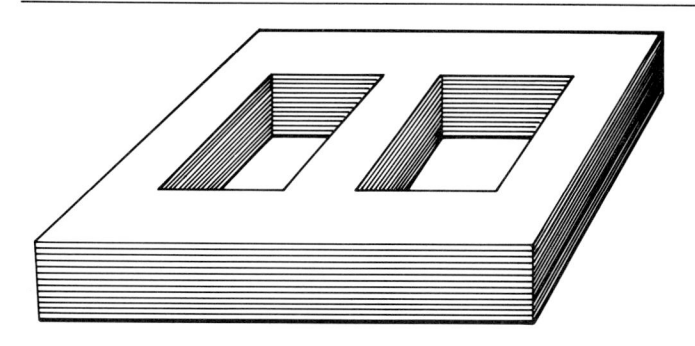

Figure 2.8 Laminated core of stalloy, each slice is electrically insulated from the next

Stalloy has a high magnetic permeability with low hysteresis loss, e.g. it magnetizes and demagnetizes easily. It also has a comparatively high inherent electrical resistance, which, coupled with the fact that the core is laminated, helps to reduce the value of eddy currents induced within the core. If the electrical resistance to these currents is small, as would be the case if the core was of solid iron, the induced currents would assume large proportions and cause the core to become red hot (Figure 2.9).

The primary and secondary windings are carefully insulated from each other and the entire transformer is placed in a metal tank which is filled with oil. The purpose of the oil is to provide electrical insulation and to convect heat from the transformer.

The primary winding is made up of a few hundred turns of thick copper wire. The wire is thick as it has to carry the high primary current which can momentarily rise to a value as high as 300 A at the beginning of the X-ray exposure. The copper wire, coated with a tough insulating medium such as shellac or enamel is wound onto a cylinder of insulating material, into which the core is later inserted (Figure 2.10).

The secondary winding, consisting of thousands of turns of thin copper wire, also coated with enamel, shellac or other insulating material is wound onto an insulating cylinder and fitted over the primary winding. Each layer of windings is insulated from the preceding layer by a sheet of insulating material, such as paper impregnated with wax or oil. The layers of windings are stepped, the narrowest step being nearest the surface. This prevents an outer turn slipping and coming into close proximity to an inner turn. It should be noted that whilst there is a difference of potential of only a few volts between adjacent turns there is a potential difference of thousands of volts between different layers of the windings, up to 75 kVp difference between the outer and inner layers of the secondary windings, and up to 150 kVp between the two sets of windings, one end being up to 75 kVp negative with respect to earth and the other up to 75 kVp positive to earth.

Between the primary and secondary windings there is a

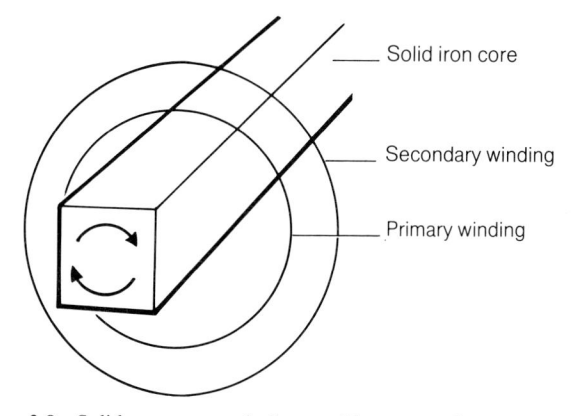

Figure 2.9 Solid core arrows indicate eddy current flow

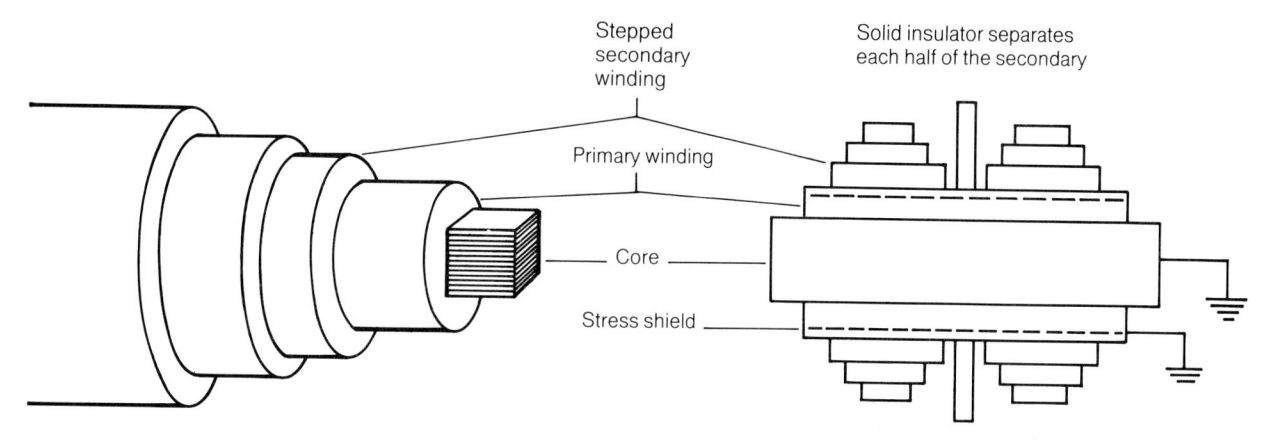

Figure 2.10 High tension transformer

stress shield, which is a thin sheet of copper, wrapped around the primary winding but carefully insulated from both it and the secondary winding. The stress shield is earthed and it forms a protective barrier between the secondary and primary windings preventing high tension current discharging to the primary circuit in the event of breakdown of the electrical insulation between the windings.

The secondary winding is in two parts being earthed at the centre point, the mA meter is in series connection with the secondary winding at the earthed midpoint making it possible to place the mA and mAs meter on the control unit. Connections to these meters are the *only* ones brought out from the secondary circuit to the control unit. All other meters and controls, including the pre-reading kV meter, are of course connected into the low tension primary circuit. It should be borne in mind that although the mA and mAs meters are connected into the secondary circuit, there is only a small voltage across either during an exposure.

The great advantage of a two-part secondary winding is that each of the high tension cables connecting the output of the transformer to the X-ray tube needs to be insulated to withstand only half the total kVp developed across the secondary winding. For example, if there is a difference of potential across the secondary winding of 100 kVp, one winding will be 50 kVp positive to the earthed centre point and the other will be 50 kVp negative to the earthed centre point. Because of this the electrical insulation around the high tension conductor need withstand only 50 kVp to earth whilst the voltage across the X-ray tube is 100 kVp.

TRANSFORMER REGULATION

Copper losses in the high tension transformer vary in direct proportion to the resistance of the windings and to the square of the current flowing through them. Such losses result in the production of heat in the windings and also in a reduction in the kilovoltage available across the high tension transformer secondary winding – and therefore across the X-ray tube. A proportion of the *anticipated* secondary voltage is lost in this way whenever an X-ray exposure is made, the proportion increasing as the mA is increased.

If the secondary winding is not connected to a circuit it is said to be in open circuit or 'no load' condition. In these circumstances no current flows in the secondary winding, there are no copper losses, no voltage drop, and in consequence the voltage available at the secondary winding is at its maximum value.

If, however, the secondary winding is connected to a complete circuit, i.e. to the X-ray tube, current flows, copper losses ensue, and there is a reduction in the voltage available across the X-ray tube. When maximum safe current is flowing in the secondary circuit (max. mA) the circuit is said to be operating under 'full load' condition, copper losses are at a maximum and voltage drop is also at maximum value. The difference between peak secondary voltage under 'no load' condition and peak secondary voltage under 'full load' condition is called the inherent voltage regulation and represents maximum voltage drop due to copper losses.

Transformer regulation is of importance in radiography because the voltage applied to the X-ray tube determines the intensity and the penetrating power of the resultant X-ray beam and, as we have seen, the voltage available across the X-ray tube *decreases* as the current *increases*.

Example

For a particular examination, factors of 100 kVp and 10 mA are selected. The tube current is small and therefore the reduction in transformer voltage (during the exposure) is also small and the voltage across the X-ray tube is 100 kVp less a *small* reduction due to transformer regulation.

If, however, 100 kVp and 400 mA are selected for a particular exposure, the tube current is larger and therefore voltage drop on load (during the exposure) is increased and the voltage available across the X-ray tube is 100 kVp less a *large* voltage reduction. The kVp across the X-ray tube will be much less than anticipated and unless compensated for the radiograph will probably be of no diagnostic value.

With most modern X-ray units, transformer regulation is compensated for by increasing the primary voltage to the high tension transformer when a higher value of mA is selected. This ensures that the kVp across the X-ray tube remains constant even though the tube current is changed.

Regulation may be expressed as a percentage using the following formula:

$$\text{Percentage regulation} = \frac{V_s \text{ (no load condition)} - V_s \text{ (full load condition)}}{V_s \text{ (no load condition)}} \times 100$$

(where V_s = secondary voltage).

TRANSFORMER RATING

The rating of a transformer is a statement of the maximum safe output of its secondary winding. If this rating is exceeded the transformer may overheat, causing breakdown in insulation, or burn out the winding.

DIAGNOSTIC X-RAY CIRCUITS

Transformers used for industrial purposes are usually operated continuously at a constant power output. The rating of such a transformer can therefore be expressed as a simple statement of the maximum safe output of its secondary winding in kVA (kilovolt–amperes).

The high tension transformer used in an X-ray circuit differs from its industrial counterpart in that it is used under a wide range of conditions. For example, a small current at high voltage flows continuously during fluoroscopy whilst a large current at high voltage flows for only a very short period of time during diagnostic exposures. It is, therefore, necessary to have a transformer rating which is more explicit than a simple statement of maximum output as a kVA value.

The rating of a high tension transformer in a diagnostic X-ray unit should include the following information:

(1) The maximum voltage (kVp) the transformer can safely deliver under 'no load' condition.

(2) The maximum current which may flow for a period of up to 1 second followed by a stated cooling time. This is called momentary or intermittent loading and applies to diagnostic exposures.

(3) The maximum current which may safely flow continuously. This is called continuous loading and applies to fluoroscopy or therapy use.

(4) The inherent voltage regulation when maximum current flows during intermittent loading. Such regulation should not exceed 15% of the maximum kVp under 'no load' conditions.

(5) The inherent voltage regulation at maximum continuous rating. This should not exceed 5% of maximum kVp under 'no load' conditions.

(6) The percentage permissible overload.

(7) Further information of a technical nature relating to insulation, maximum permitted temperature rise under certain conditions, etc.

Compensation for voltage drop in the supply cable

We have seen that the primary circuit of an X-ray generator is completely isolated from the secondary circuit, i.e. there is no direct electrical connection between primary and secondary circuits (Figure 2.11). Energy is *transferred* from the primary circuit to the secondary circuit of the high tension transformer by means of the changing magnetic field.

It is, therefore, readily apparent that all energy used in the secondary circuit, i.e. to produce X-rays etc., *must* be provided by the primary circuit and equally, of course, if there is a reduction in the power provided by the primary circuit the energy or power used in the secondary will also be reduced. Note that in an ideal circuit without losses secondary power *equals* primary power, it is *not* additive to it.

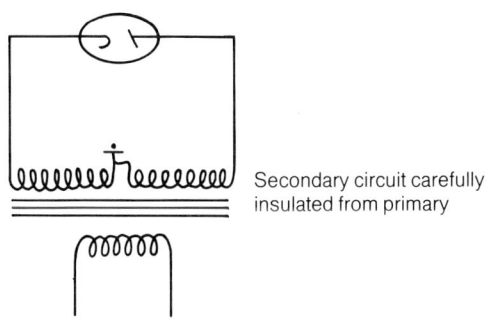

Figure 2.11 Secondary circuit carefully insulated from primary

If, for any reason, the power in the primary is less than anticipated, the power in the secondary will also be reduced. Such a reduction in secondary power will obviously create difficulties for the radiographer, i.e. less kV than anticipated with consequent results so far as film blackening is concerned. Some way must be provided to ensure that primary power is increased as secondary power is increased.

Now we know that kV is increased by increasing primary voltage, i.e. tapping off more turns from the autotransformer, and that changes in mains voltage are compensated for by varying the number of turns on the autotransformer to which the mains voltage is applied. We have also seen, however, that the supply cable to the X-ray unit has significant resistance and that the energy lost (as heat) in the cables varies proportionally to their resistance and to the square of the current flowing through them. Now, if the power used in the secondary is supplied by the primary it follows that as the secondary power is increased, by increasing kV and/or mA, the current in the primary must also increase; and that this will result in an increased loss of power (as heat) in the supply cables.

Say that an exposure is to be made using 50 mA at 100 kV, and that the secondary power $(v \times i) = 100\,\text{kV} \times 50\,\text{mA}$, i.e. 5000 W. From the previous discussion we know that if 5000 W of energy is to be used in the secondary it must be provided by the primary circuit.

Now the primary voltage is, say, 240 V and as power = $v \times i$ we can see that

$$i = \frac{\text{power}}{\text{voltage}}$$

or, i (primary circuit) $= \dfrac{5000}{240}$ Amperes

Therefore, primary current is about 21 A.

If, however, we alter the exposure factors to, say, 300 mA and 100 kV we now need a secondary power of $300 \times 100 = 30\,000$ W and as we have seen, the 30 000 W must be provided by the primary circuit.
Once again therefore,

$$i = \frac{\text{power}}{\text{voltage}}$$

$$i = \frac{30\,000}{240}$$

$$= 125 \text{ A}$$

The primary current is now six times the previous value. We saw on p. 17 that the supply cable resistance must not exceed the value specified by the manufacturer of that particular X-ray unit. Let us say that the resistance of the supply cable is acceptable to the manufacturer at $0.35\,\Omega$ (Figure 2.12).

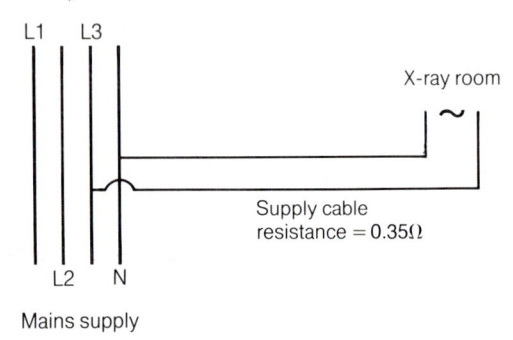

Figure 2.12 Supply cable resistance

Now the voltage drop along the cables $= i \times R$. Therefore, when exposure factors of 50 mA and 100 kV are used necessitating a primary current of 21 A the voltage drop along the supply cables $= 21 \times 0.35$ or 7.35 V, so the voltage to the equipment is $240 - 7.35 = 233$ V (approx.) and the primary power, instead of being 5000 W, is 4893 W, a reduction in power of about 2%. The power in the secondary is therefore 2% less than anticipated.

If we now consider the second case where the factors are increased to 300 mA at 100 kV necessitating a primary current of 125 A to provide power of 30 000 W, the voltage drop along the supply cables $= 125 \times 0.35 = 44$ V (approx.). The primary voltage is now reduced from 240 to 196 V and the primary power to 24 500 W. This is a reduction by 18% of the power to the secondary circuit (as opposed to 2% in the previous case).

Such variations in secondary power would be disastrous so far as the radiographer is concerned and some means must obviously be provided to restore the power to its original value.

The additional power needed to compensate for the power lost in the supply cable during the exposure is achieved by connecting a compensatory transformer into the circuit as shown in Figure 2.13.

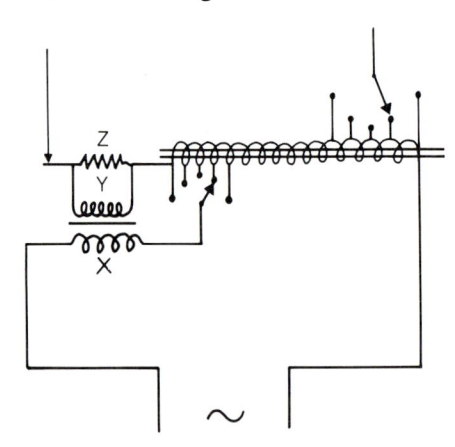

Figure 2.13 Supply cable resistance compensator circuit

The value of the e.m.f. induced into winding Y is determined by the current flowing in winding X. As the secondary power requirement is increased (by increasing kV and/or mA) the primary current also increases. The greater the primary current the greater is the power lost, as heat, in the supply cable, *but* the greater is the e.m.f. induced into Y. The voltage induced into Y causes a current to flow through resistor Z and the greater the current flow through resistor Z the greater the voltage developed across the resistor. As Z is in series with the autotransformer winding it follows that an increase in primary current causes an increase in the output voltage from the autotransformer. The values of the resistor Z and the ratio of the compensating transformer windings X and Y are such that the power lost in the cables is *automatically* compensated for, thus sustaining the correct power in the primary and therefore in the secondary.

It should be noted that had the equipment been connected to the 415 V supply rather than 240 V the primary current would have been smaller and in consequence the voltage drop in the supply cable would also have been reduced. It is for this reason that manufacturers quote a higher acceptable supply cable resistance for the 415 V supply compared to that quoted for 240 V.

The block diagram in Figure 2.14 shows how each of the components studied up to now fit into the primary part of an X-ray circuit.

DIAGNOSTIC HIGH TENSION CIRCUITS

Before we move on to study other aspects of the primary circuit, such as the pre-reading kV meter, timer, filament heating circuit, etc., let us look at the secondary circuit

DIAGNOSTIC X-RAY CIRCUITS

Thermionic vacuum triode valves and capacitors are present in some special circuits, e.g. constant potential generators.

The self-rectified (one-pulse) circuit is very simple and may be represented as shown in Figure 2.15.

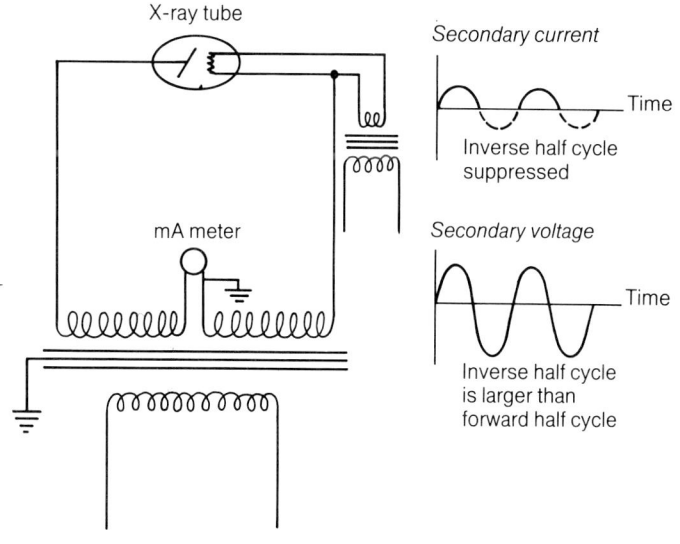

Figure 2.15 Voltage and current waveforms of a self-rectified X-ray circuit

This circuit is usually used with a stationary anode X-ray tube which acts as a rectifier as well as a producer of X-rays. Let us see how such a tube is constructed.

The stationary anode X-ray tube shown in Figure 2.16 is used in some (but not all) mobile units, most dental units and all portable equipment. Unlike the rotating anode tube which is described later it has no sophisticated associated circuitry and its great simplicity particularly suits it to low powered simple circuits. It consists essentially of a glass insert, containing a cathode and anode, and an oil-filled casing into which the insert is fitted.

The insert is an evacuated glass envelope made of specially toughened glass. It encloses the filament, made of tungsten wire, the focusing cup made of molybdenum or steel and the copper anode into which the tungsten target is embedded.

The tube casing, made of steel, contains the insert and is filled with oil. It provides a means of introduction for the high tension cables and provides a plane of reference for the positioning of the tube during radiography. It also provides attachment for cones, light beam diaphragm, etc.

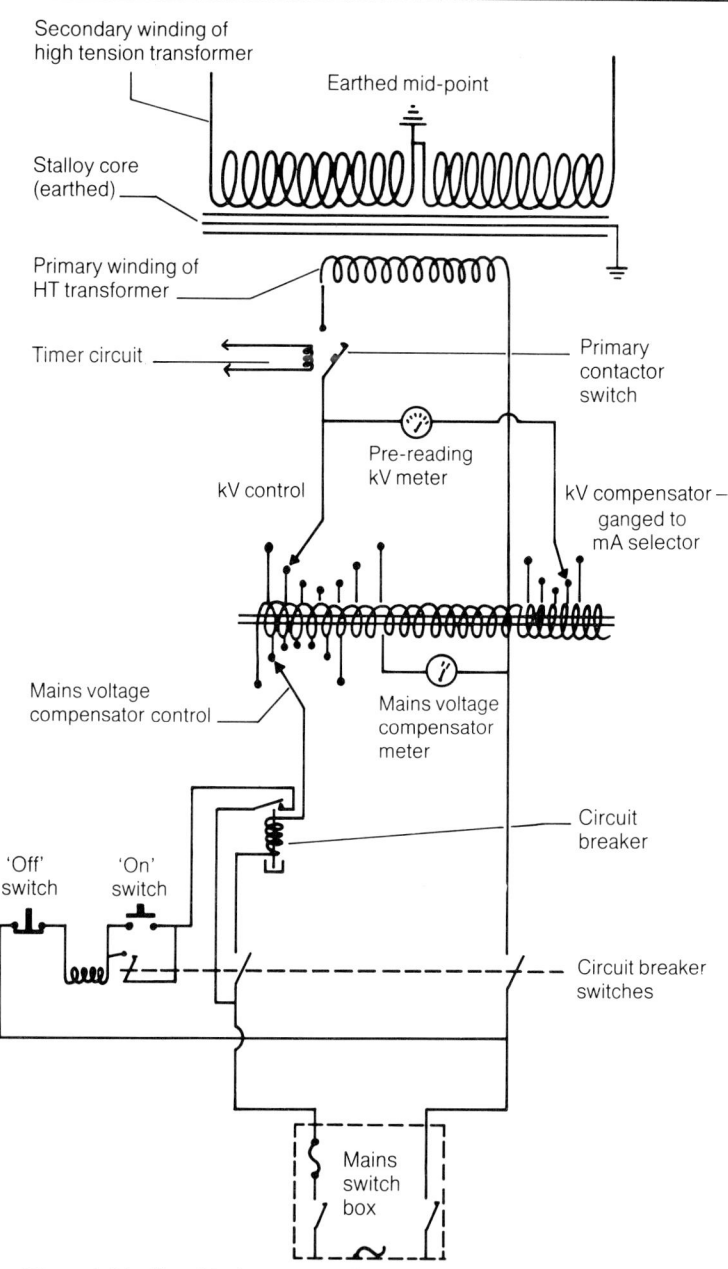

Figure 2.14 Simplified representation of the primary circuit of a basic X-ray unit

which consists of the secondary winding of the high tension transformer, some form of rectification, e.g. thermionic diode rectifying valves, solid state rectifiers, or indeed the X-ray tube itself, which may act as a rectifier as well as a producer of X-rays. The secondaries of the step-down transformers which supply the heating current to the filaments of the valves and the X-ray tube also form part of the secondary circuit, as do the mA and mAs meters.

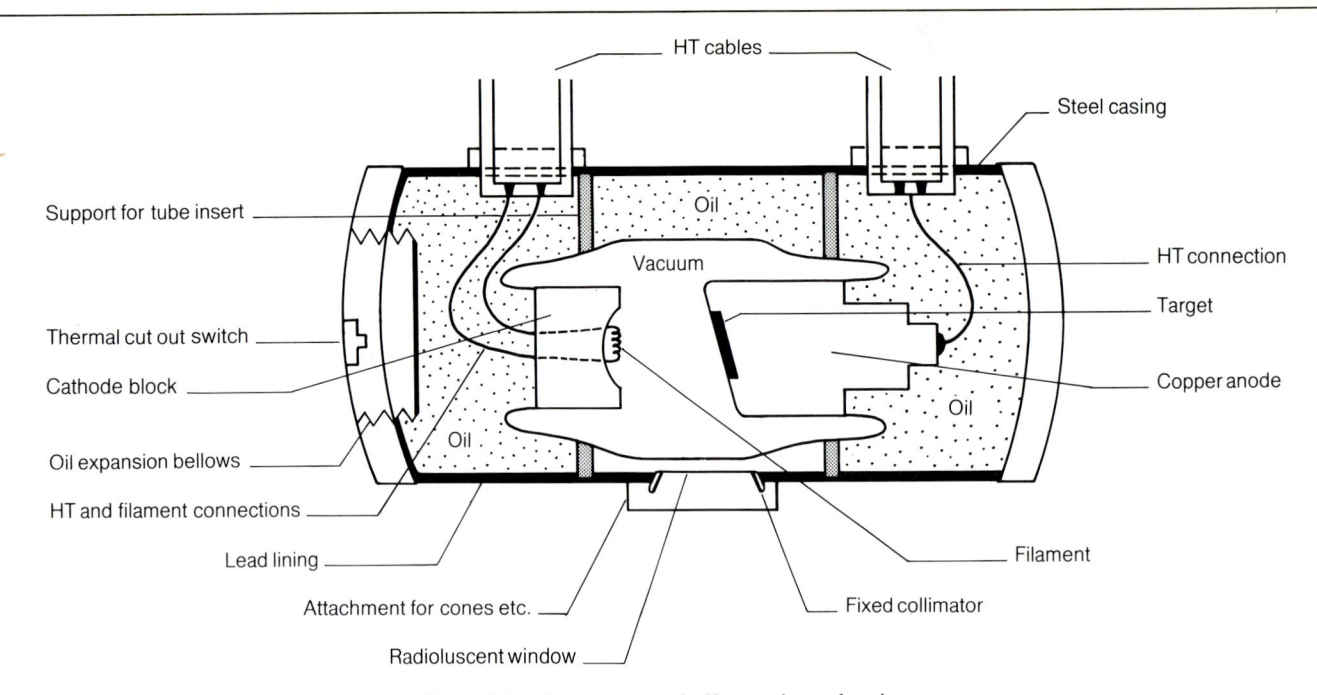

Figure 2.16 Stationary anode X-ray tube and casing

All radiation emitted by the target, *excepting* that which passes through the radiolucent window, is heavily attenuated by the lead with which the tube casing is lined.

In use, the oil within the casing becomes heated and expands. A bellows within the casing creates extra space as the oil expands and reduces the available space as the oil cools. It is necessary to avoid air bubbles being drawn into the oil as this may result in electrical spark-over during an exposure and possible puncture of the glass envelope.

When the bellows are fully contracted, due to pressure of the expanded oil, it is obvious that maximum space has been created and that any further increase in the temperature of the oil would damage the insert, due to implosion or to leakage of oil, either through the oil seal or the radiolucent window. Leakage of this nature could lead to the introduction of air bubbles as the oil cools and contracts. To eliminate this possibility the bellows, on maximum contraction, operate a cut-out switch which prevents further exposures being made until such time as the oil has cooled sufficiently for the bellows to re-expand. The function of the oil is to provide electrical insulation and to transfer heat from the anode to the casing.

A fan may be fitted to the outside of the tube casing to assist in the transfer of heat from the casing to the outside air. The tube casing is earthed making it shockproof.

The X-ray tube described uses high tension cables to carry current to and from the high tension transformer.

To obviate the need for such cables many mobile and all portable units have an oil-filled casing which incorporates not only the insert but the high tension transformer and indeed the entire secondary circuit (Figure 2.17). This arrangement provides a simple uncomplicated piece of equipment easily manoeuvrable and ideal for bedside radiography. In this unit the X-ray tube functions as a rectifier

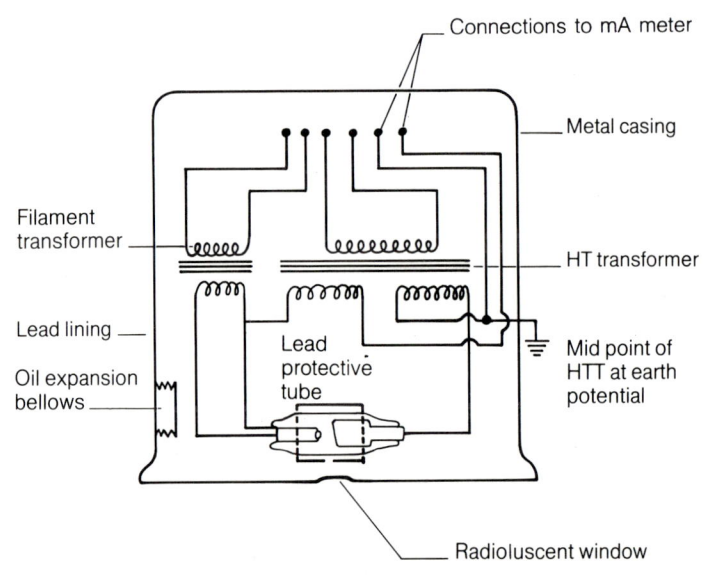

Figure 2.17 Single tank unit tube head

as well as a producer of X-rays. The rating of such a tube is low as the maximum 'safe' temperature of the anode is not that at which it would be adversely affected as a producer of X-rays, but the temperature at which it would emit electrons by the process of thermionic emission (1600 °C) and therefore cease to act as a rectifier.

So far we have considered only the self-rectified X-ray circuit in which the X-ray tube acts as a rectifier as well as a producer of X-rays. Such equipment has certain advantages over full-wave rectified equipment, e.g. simplicity, compactness, manoevrability, cheapness, etc. It also has some disadvantages. The major disadvantage is related to the use of the X-ray tube as a rectifier as well as a producer of X-rays. To function as a rectifier the temperature of the target must not exceed about 1600 °C, at which temperature it would emit electrons by the process of thermionic emission allowing a flow of electrons from target to filament during the inverse half cycle. Bombardment of the filament by these high speed electrons would rapidly raise the temperature of the filament and lead to its destruction.

It should be appreciated that if the temperature of the target is not to exceed 1600 °C the electrical energy, which is responsible for the temperature rise, must be limited. (Over 99% of electrical energy is converted into heat at the target of the tube, less than 1% being converted into X-rays.)

Heat produced at the target of the X-ray tube, measured in radiographic heat units may be calculated using the following formula:

Total heat units = kVp × mA (average) × time (seconds)

However, the *rate* at which electrical energy is converted into heat, i.e. heat units per second, at the target of the tube is the product of kVp and mA.

Heat units per second = kVp × mA (see footnote)

As the temperature of the target is determined by the product of exposure time and rate at which electrical energy is converted into heat at the target of the tube (other factors include the material from which it is made, rate of heat transfer, area on which heat is concentrated, etc.) it follows that kVp and mA (heat units per second) must be restricted if the temperature of the target is not to rise above the critical value of 1600 °C, at which temperature thermionic emission would occur.

It should be noted that a given diagnostic exposure, e.g. total energy expended, can be achieved by *either*, a high rate of heat production (kVp × mA) for a short time, *or*, a low rate of heat production (kVp × mA) for a long time.

Thus, when using a self-rectified X-ray unit the same

These radiographic heat units should not be confused with watts or joules per second. To convert heat units to watts see appendix.

radiographic contrast and density, e.g. kVp × mA s can be achieved as with a full-wave rectified major X-ray unit but the exposure *time* will be much longer and the mA much lower when using the self-rectified unit. This, of course, means that there will be increased danger of motional blur unless the part under investigation can be completely immobilized.

Other disadvantages include a reduction in tube rating (discussed later) due to high peak value of current compared with average value, and, when high tension cables are used, the increased insulation needed to overcome the problem of high inverse voltage. The latter difficulty is alleviated by using an inverse voltage reducer (Figure 2.18).

Inverse voltage reducer (primary circuit) – used in self-rectified X-ray circuits only

The inverse secondary voltage may be reduced to roughly the same value as the forward voltage by means of an inverse voltage reducer. This consists of a gas-filled diode valve (or solid state device) and a resistance, connected in series with the primary circuit as shown in Figure 2.18. During the forward half cycle when 'A' is negative and 'B' is positive, electron current flows freely through the valve (current flow rises rapidly to a high value due to ionization of the gas in the valve).

During the inverse half cycle when 'A' is negative and 'B' positive electrons are unable to flow through the valve and must perforce pass through resistance R, thus causing a reduction in inverse voltage.

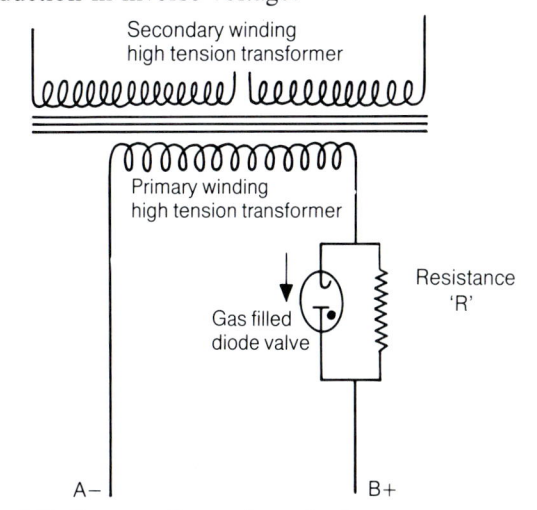

Figure 2.18 Inverse voltage reducer circuit

Absence of the resistor would lead to complete suppression of current flow in the inverse half cycle. This, however, would lead to difficulties, as the high tension transformer core would become permanently magnetized in one direction. The presence of the resistor ensures an inverse current flow which is equal to the forward current flow and therefore demagnetization of the transformer core.

This system is used in some self-rectified equipment, particularly if the high inverse voltage is likely to create problems, e.g. if the equipment is using high tension cables, or if the tube shield needs to be kept as small as possible.

If the secondary circuit is full-wave rectified, i.e. both half cycles of current are used, there is no need to use an inverse voltage suppressor.

Full-wave rectification two-pulse (single-phase using four rectifiers)

If the X-ray tube is relieved of its function as a rectifier, by rectifying the current before it reaches the X-ray tube, the temperature of the tungsten target may be safely increased beyond 1600 °C. In theory is should be possible to raise the temperature of the target to 3400 °C, at which temperature it would melt but in practice the maximum temperature is usually set at a lower value so that thermal stresses will not cause undue crazing of the tungsten surface. Vaporization of the tungsten is also reduced.

Current through the X-ray tube is made unidirectional in the following way. By the appropriate use of rectifiers in the secondary circuit the inverse half cycle of current is made to flow through the X-ray tube in the same direction as the forward half cycle. That is to say, the target of the X-ray tube is always positive and the filament always negative. The circuit is arranged as in Figure 2.19. *Note*: the high tension transformer is frequently drawn in block form as in the circuit on the right.

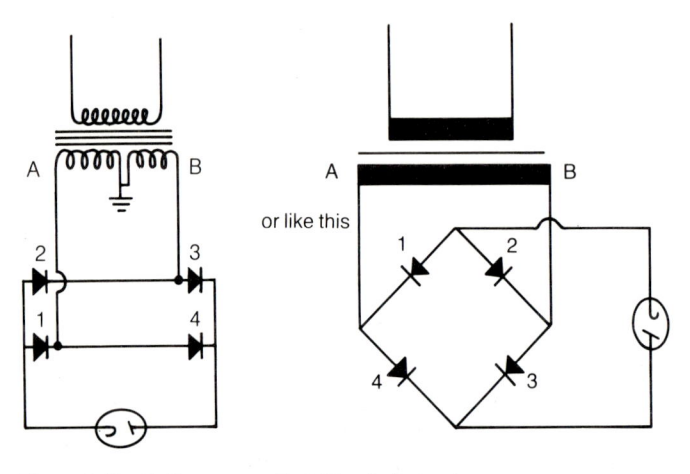

Figure 2.19 Full wave rectified (2 pulse) circuit

When 'A' is negative and 'B' positive electron current flows through rectifier 1 and if it were possible would return to 'B' via rectifier 2. However, rectifier 2 is non-conducting so the electrons pass through the X-ray tube to point 'C'. It would appear that electrons are free to pass through either rectifier 3 or 4 as both are conductive but in practice electrons flow through rectifier 3 to 'B'. This is because 'B' is positive and attracts the electrons whilst 'A' being negative repels them. During the next half cycle 'B' is negative and 'A' positive. Electrons now flow through rectifier 2; then as rectifier 1 is non-conductive the electrons pass through the X-ray tube from filament to anode, to point 'C', and on this occasion the electrons pass through rectifier 4 to 'A' which is positive.

Note that only two rectifiers are in circuit at any one time and that each half cycle of current flows through the X-ray tube in the same direction.

Single phase constant potential circuit using secondary switching

Constant potential units of modern design use a three phase supply, but for simplicity, the principle of operation is indicated here by using a single phase supply. This circuit (Figure 2.20), in addition to the components of a conventional four valve circuit, contains two capacitors and two high tension vacuum triode valves. The triode valves, as the name implies, consist of an evacuated glass envelope enclosing three electrodes, an anode, a cathode and a grid.

Preparing for an exposure

In this circuit (Figure 2.20), pressure on the exposure 'prepare' switch boosts the filaments of the X-ray tube and valves to their full working temperature, starts the anode rotating and *in addition* closes the primary contactor thus energizing the high tension transformer. When the capacitors C1 and C2 are fully charged (i.e. to the peak output voltage of the high tension transformer) current flow ceases, as the negative bias on the grids of the high tension triode valves render them non-conductive.

Making the exposure

The exposure is initiated by exerting full pressure on the exposure switch. This applies a *positive* voltage to the grids of the triode valves sufficiently high to neutralize the existing negative bias. The triodes are now fully conductive and current flows through the valves and the X-ray tube. At the end of an interval of time, determined by the timer, the positive voltage is removed from the grids of the triode valves, the negative voltage re-establishes itself on the grids, current flow ceases and the exposure is terminated.

DIAGNOSTIC X-RAY CIRCUITS

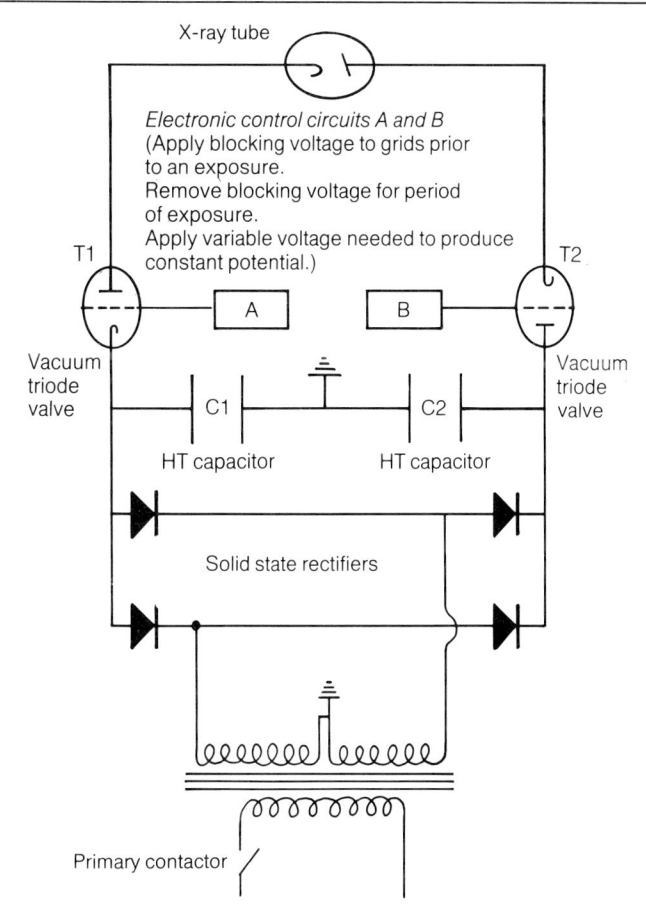

Figure 2.20 Diagrammatic representation of constant potential circuit

Functioning of the secondary circuit

Assume an exposure is to be made at 100 kV for 0.02 s. The rectified high tension transformer voltage is indicated by a dotted line in Figure 2.21. The continuous line indicates the smoothed rectified voltage from the capacitors.

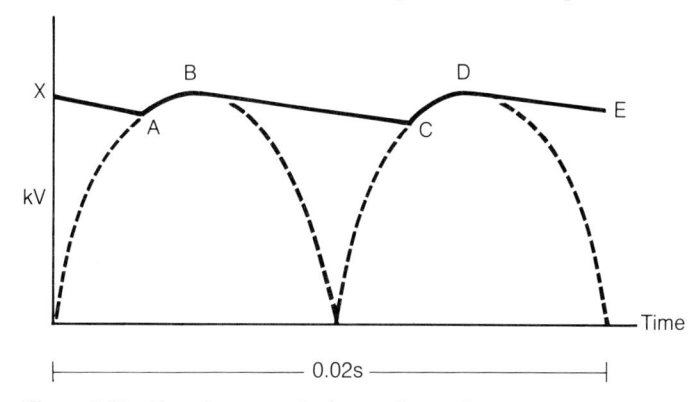

Figure 2.21 Capacitor smoothed secondary voltage

At the beginning of an exposure the negative bias is removed from the grids and the valves become conductive. The exposure commences at instant X. At this instant in time the rectified transformer voltage is at zero value whilst the capacitors, which have previously been charged to a potential of 100 kV, are free to discharge. The capacitors therefore begin to discharge through the triode valves and the X-ray tube (period X to A in the graph). As they discharge their voltage drops and after a brief period of time (at point A on the graph) the voltage of the partially discharged capacitors and the rectified voltage from the high tension transformer (which has been steadily rising since the beginning of the exposure) are of equal value. The high tension transformer voltage, however, continues to increase until it reaches peak value, at point B. During the period A to B the high tension transformer voltage is sustaining current flow through the X-ray tube and *also* recharging the capacitors to peak value. As the transformer output voltage drops the capacitors begin to discharge until at point C the rectified transformer voltage and the discharging capacitors are once again at the same voltage. The high tension transformer voltage now increases to a maximum at point D and the capacitor then discharges until point E when the exposure is terminated by reimposition of the negative bias on the grid of the valves. At this instant the output voltage of the high tension transformer is zero and the capacitors are partially discharged.

Constant potential across the X-ray tube is achieved in the following way. The output voltage from the capacitors is shown on the graph (Figure 2.22).

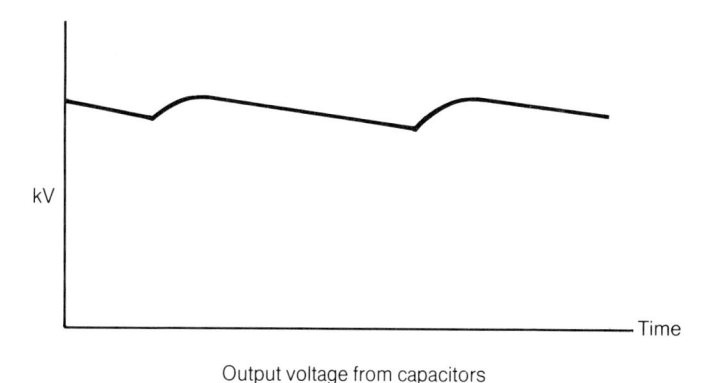

Figure 2.22 Capacitor smoothed voltage

Whilst this voltage varies less than the rectified transformer voltage it is still not constant. To achieve true constant potential it is necessary to remove the peaks of voltage 1, 2 and 3 on the graphs, which results in a constant potential as indicated by the thick black line in Figure 2.23.

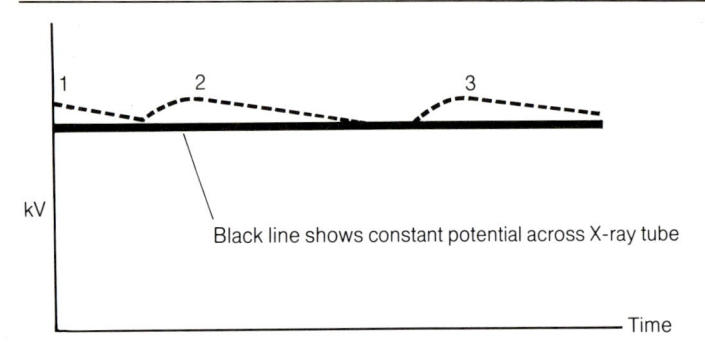

Figure 2.23 Constant potential

The peaks 1, 2 and 3 are removed by varying the negative bias on the grids of the triode valves (i.e. by applying a high negative voltage to the grids of the valves when the kV is at its peak and reducing the grid bias as the kV decreases). This variation of grid bias is, of course, automatic; the correct voltage being applied to the grid by an electronic control circuit.

The greatest advantage associated with constant potential generators is the very short exposure times it is possible to obtain and the high repetition rate (no mechanical contactor). This is of particular value in cine fluorography where exposure rates of 200 per second are not uncommon.

kV control – using high tension triodes

The kV across the X-ray tube, in addition to being made constant, may also be adjusted to any desired value by varying the voltage applied to the grids of the triode valves.

The triode valve may be considered as having an impedence, or internal resistance, which varies with grid bias, small variations in grid bias having a large effect on the internal resistance of the valve, the greater the negative bias of the grid the greater the impedence of the valve and the greater the voltage drop across the valve. By varying grid bias voltage to the valve it is therefore possible to vary the kV across the tube, any particular kV being obtained by applying the appropriate negative voltage to the grid.

In practice an autotransformer is used in the conventional way to produce a kV somewhat higher than that which is to be applied to the X-ray tube. The triode valve is then used in the manner described to reduce it to the required value.

Three-phase circuit six-pulse (six rectifiers)

Whilst single phase X-ray generators are connected to either a live phase and neutral, or two live phases of the a.c. mains supply, the three-phase (six-pulse) generator is connected to three live phases. The primary circuit is usually in triplicate, e.g. three autotransformers, three sets of primary contactors, three primary windings to the high tension transformer, etc. The circuit is drawn as in Figure 2.24. 'A' is the delta-connected triple primary winding of the high tension transformer whilst 'B' is the secondary winding, made up of three coils X, Y and Z in star connection. The midpoint of the star-connected secondary is at earth potential. The rectifiers are numbered 1–6.

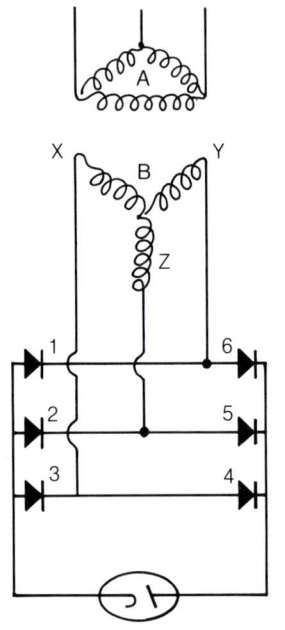

Figure 2.24 Rectified three phase (6 pulse) circuit

Functioning of the circuit

Current can flow in one way only through the X-ray tube irrespective of which end of the triple secondary winding is negative or positive with respect to the other windings. If, for example, Z is negative and X positive current can only flow through rectifier 2 to the X-ray tube then back to X via rectifier 4. By the same token if Y is negative with respect to Z current will flow through rectifier 1 through the X-ray tube and back to Z via rectifier 5. The current through the X-ray tube is always from filament to anode.

Some three phase circuits, particularly those to be used for techniques such as cine fluorography, where short exposures and fast repetition rates are needed, use capacitors and vacuum triodes to provide constant potential and secondary switching. The circuit functions in the same way as that described in the four-valve constant potential circuit but the use of a six-valve three-phase circuit ensures a greater source of power.

It is of interest to note that whilst a three-phase genera-

DIAGNOSTIC X-RAY CIRCUITS

tor is frequently described as having 'constant' potential (inverted commas indicating *almost* constant potential) the potential is not truly constant unless the secondary voltage is smoothed by means of capacitors and the remaining ripple removed by varying the negative voltage applied to the grid of a high tension vacuum triode valve.

Some manufacturers, however, accepting the ripple in the voltage waveform as being nearly constant, use (without capacitors) a *grid controlled X-ray tube* to function both as a producer of X-rays and a secondary switch. This provides the fast repetition rates needed for cine fluorography.

Advantages of the three-phase over single-phase circuits

From the diagrams in Figure 2.25 it will be appreciated that for a *given exposure time*, e.g. 0.01 s, the three-phase unit gives:

(1) more X-rays,
(2) X-rays of shorter average wavelength than the single-phase unit, even though kVp and mA are the same in each case.

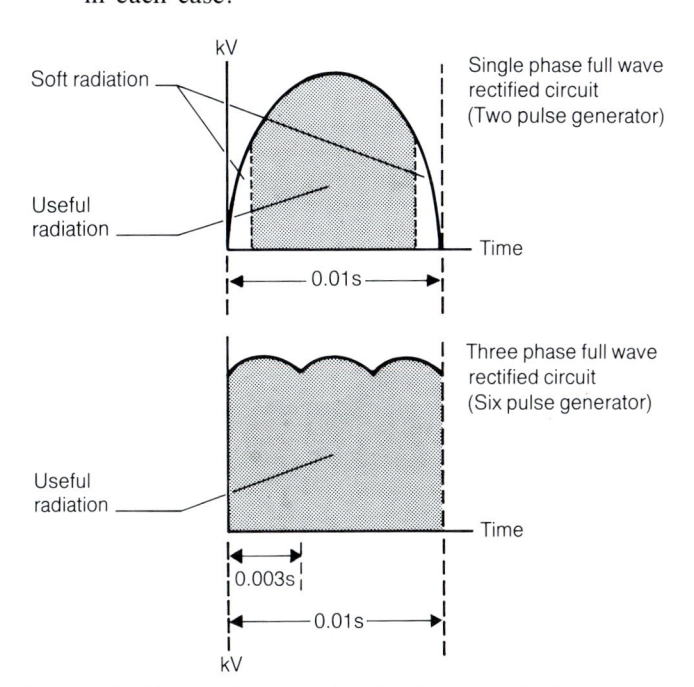

Figure 2.25 Useful radiation produced by 2 pulse and 6 pulse generators

This is due to the rectified three-phase voltage (and current) being closer to a constant value than single-phase voltage (and current) which is pulsating. This means that, whilst rectified single-phase voltage is at or near zero point at the beginning and end of each half cycle, the rectified three-phase voltage is close to peak value at all times and never drops to zero value.

It follows therefore, that if single-phase voltage (and current) is periodically at or near zero value during the exposure whilst three-phase voltage (and current) remains at or near peak value during the exposure, that the energy expended (X-rays produced) during the exposure is greater for the three-phase circuit than for that operating on single-phase although the kVp is the same in each case.

Radiographic advantages of three-phase X-ray generators compared to those operating on single-phase

As the kV remains constantly at a high value during the exposure:

(1) Less soft radiation is produced, resulting in a reduction in skin dose to the patient.
(2) More X-rays are produced for a given mA and kVp.
(3) Because of (2) the *same* film dose, e.g. radiographic exposure, can be achieved in a shorter time. Therefore reduction in exposure times is achieved.
(4) Improved tube rating is achieved at short exposure times (this will be discussed later in 'tube rating').
(5) The X-ray tube has a longer life due to more even thermal loading.

With reference to the third advantage above, it is important to remember that the amount of radiation needed to produce a particular film density (i.e. film dose) is constant for the particular film, screens, processing conditions, etc. being used, therefore the use of three-phase equipment does not reduce the amount of radiation needed, it only means that the same amount of radiation can be obtained in less time than is possible with single-phase generators.

Three-phase X-ray generators are of particular value when it is necessary to reduce exposure time to a minimum, e.g. paediatric, casualty, chest radiography, etc. or when heavy energy expenditure is required at a rapid rate, e.g. angiography, using film changers such as the AOT, etc.

The only real disadvantages that can be associated with three-phase equipment are not related so much to their use as their cost. Such equipment is extremely sophisticated and very expensive and on this account its use may be precluded.

12-pulse (12 rectifier) circuit

Whilst the three-phase (six pulse) circuit produces a voltage waveform which varies less than that of the single-phase circuit, the output voltage of the 12-pulse circuit varies even less and is *almost* constant in value. The circuit may be drawn as in Figure 2.26.

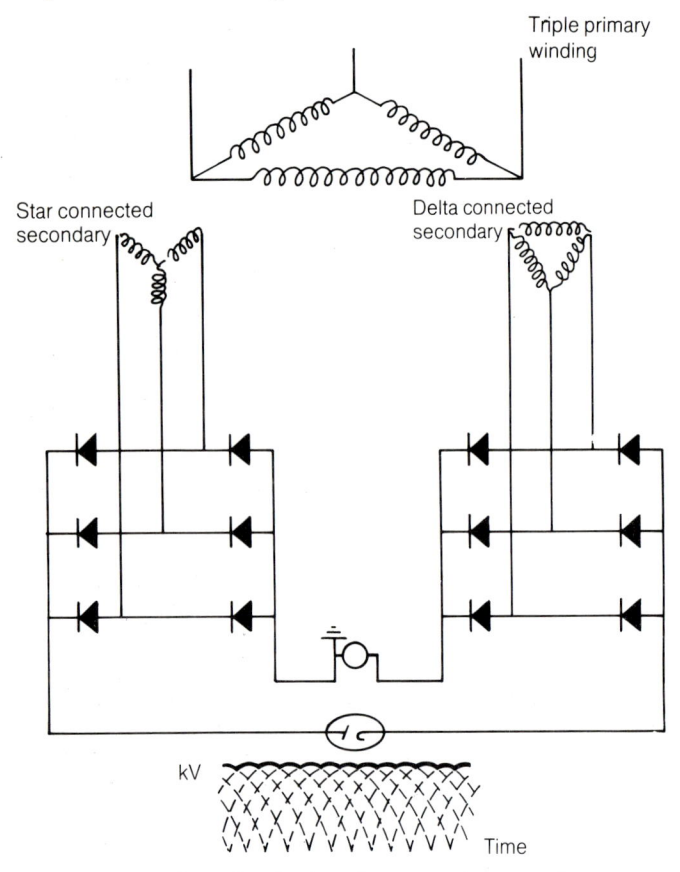

Figure 2.26 Twelve pulse circuit and output voltage waveform

The capacitor discharge unit is discussed on page 119.

POSITION OF METERS IN THE CIRCUIT

When a voltage is to be measured, using for example the prereading kV meter, the meter is connected *across* the circuit and when a current is to be measured, the meter is connected in *series* with the circuit. Examples of the latter are the mA and mA s meters which are connected in series with the secondary circuit at the midpoint of the high tension transformer (Figure 2.27).

As the measuring instrument in each case forms part of the circuit it is important that it should not significantly affect the value of the voltage or the current being measured. For this reason the voltmeter has a very high resistance in series with it whilst the mA meter has a very small internal resistance. From this it will be appreciated that the voltmeter with its high associated resistance allows

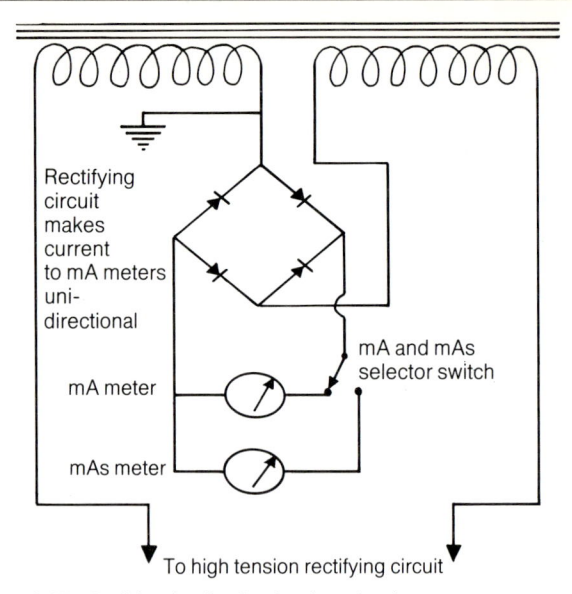

Figure 2.27 Position in circuit of mA and mA s meters

only a small proportion of current to flow through it and therefore causes only a very small change in the voltage drop across the resistor to be measured. The mA meter which is placed in series with the circuit, having very small resistance, interferes very little with the current flow.

Reading meters

Before reading a meter it is essential to check that it has been zeroed. To do this a small screw at the base of the meter is moved in a clockwise or anticlockwise direction until the needle is pointing to the zero point on the scale. Care should be taken that the glass covering of the meter is not damaged. A cracked glass may press on the needle resulting in a false reading, whilst a broken glass cover may cause glass fragments to fall into the moving part of the meter which may result in either a false reading or no reading at all.

In most circuits the mA meter is used to measure *rate* of current flow (exposures over 0.5 s) whilst the mA s meter, which reads the product of mA and time, is used for short exposures of less than 0.5 s. The mA s meter is similar in construction to the mA meter, but it has no return spring. Consequently the coil makes a continuous rotation during the exposure. When using the mA s meter, it is important to check that it has been zeroed. This is normally done by passing a reverse current through the coil. Zeroing is particularly important as the needle may creep across the scale between exposures due to the effects of electrostatic force. For example, friction on the glass front will cause the needle to move across the scale. This difficulty is overcome in some units where a reverse current

DIAGNOSTIC X-RAY CIRCUITS

is passed through the mAs meter when the unit is put into prep, thus ensuring that the meter is reading zero at the commencement of the exposure.

Let us now study the remaining parts of the primary circuit, e.g. filament circuit, timer circuit, compensating circuits, etc.

X-RAY TUBE FILAMENT HEATING CIRCUIT

The voltage for this circuit is obtained by tapping off an appropriate number of turns from the autotransformer. The block diagram shown in Figure 2.28 illustrates the layout of the principal components in the filament heating circuit.

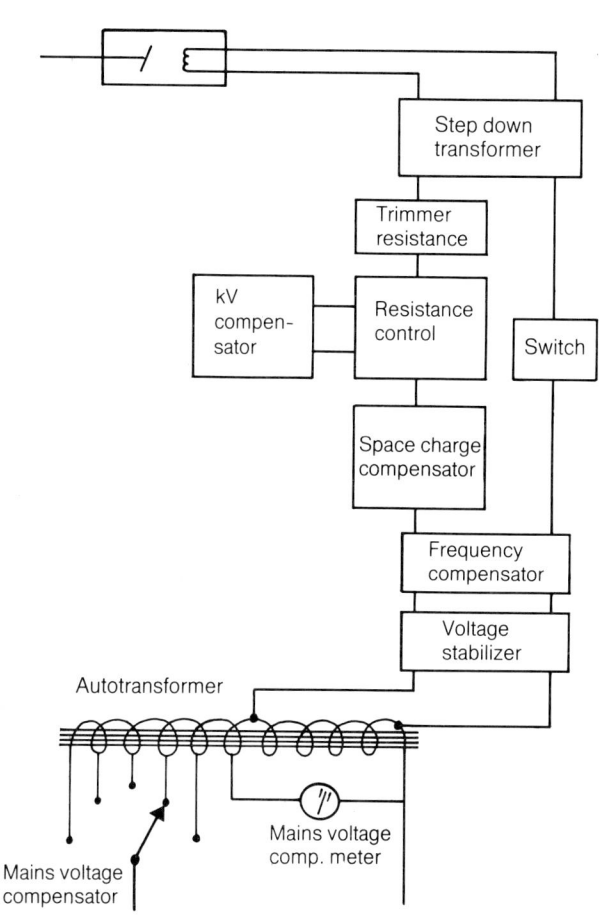

Figure 2.28 Block diagram of X-ray tube filament heating circuit

Longterm variations in the circuit supply voltage are compensated for by the mains voltage compensator which is part of the autotransformer. Minor variations, however, which occur during the actual exposure must be compensated for; this may be done by means of a static voltage stabilizer or an electronic voltage stabilizer.

The *static stabilizer*, so called because it has no moving parts, consists of a transformer and a capacitor connected in such a fashion that the effects of inductance and capacitance, at a particular frequency, ensure a stable output voltage. The static voltage stabilizer is frequency dependent, that is to say it only functions correctly with a mains frequency of 50 Hz. Any change in the mains frequency results in a variation in output voltage. Whilst the mains frequency itself cannot be adjusted, since this is determined by the speed at which the coils rotate at the electricity generator, the effect of such changes can be compensated for by increasing or decreasing the output voltage. This may be done manually or electronically.

The *electronic stabilizer* uses a transductor (an inductor which has its impedance varied by means of a separate d.c. winding). The electronic voltage stabilizer is *not* frequency dependent.

The *space charge compensator* compensates for the effects of space charge. Space charge is the collection of electrons around the filament and is greatest when there is no kV across the tube. As the voltage across the tube increases space charge decreases and maximum current (mA) flows when the kV is sufficiently high to pull all the electrons across to the anode as fast as they are emitted by the filament. This is called saturation current.

If the anode voltage is too low to produce saturation, electrons exist around the filament as a space charge and in these circumstances the filament heating current must be increased, if the mA is to be maintained at its original value, e.g. at 50 kV a certain filament heating current produces, say, 200 mA. When the anode voltage is reduced to, say, 40 kV the anode current (mA) drops to, let us say, 150 mA. To restore the current (reduced by the effects of space charge) to its original value of 200 mA, the anode voltage must be increased or, alternatively, the filament heating current increased. From the foregoing it can be appreciated that, because the anode current varies with anode voltage, the filament current must also be varied if the mA is to remain at a constant value when the kV is changed. This variation in filament heating current is achieved by means of a space charge compensator. From Figure 2.29 it can be seen that, as the kV control is moved to increase the voltage across the tube (anode voltage), the voltage applied to the space charge compensator transformer primary winding is in such a direction as to induce a voltage in the space charge compensator transformer secondary in such a direction as to oppose the voltage from the autotransformer, reducing current flow in the filament circuit. Conversely, when the kV control is adjusted so as to reduce the kVp across the tube, the voltage applied to the primary of the space charge compensator transformer is in such a direction that the voltage induced in the secondary is additive to the filament heating voltage, which results in an increase in filament temperature, In this way variation of kVp automatically adjusts the filament heating current to compensate for the effects of space charge.

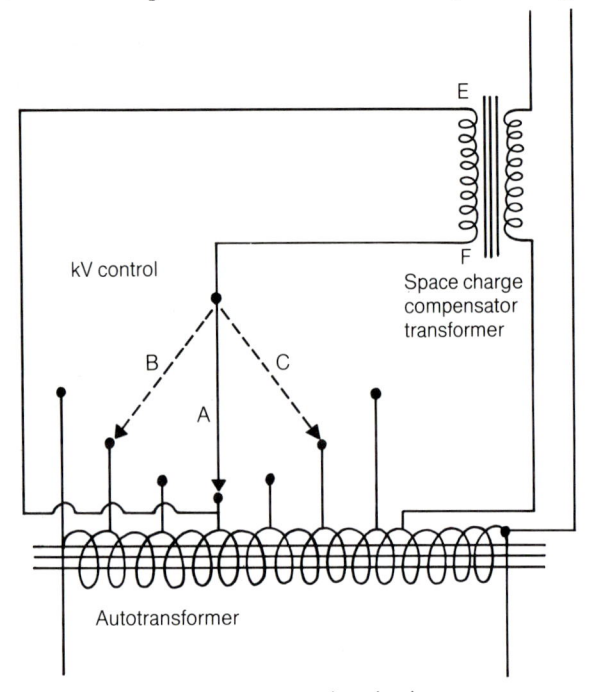

Figure 2.29 Space charge compensation circuit

Let us look again at Figure 2.29. When the kV control is in position A the voltage across EF is zero and the filament voltage is unaffected, so no compensation is needed at this particular kV. If, however, the kV control is moved to position B, i.e. kV is increased, or to a position C where the kV is reduced, a voltage is applied across EF, the value and direction of which is determined by the position of the kV selector arm. In Figure 2.30 end A of the autotransformer is at negative potential and end B is positive. In so far as the filament current is concerned, B is negative with respect to C and electron current flow is in the direction indicated by the arrows. The kV control is in position C and point Y is positive with respect to point X. Direction of electron current flow is indicated by the arrows. Current flow through winding G results in a voltage being induced in winding H which is additive to the filament circuit voltage and current flow in the filament circuit is increased. From this it can be appreciated that reduction in kV results in an automatic increase in filament heating current.

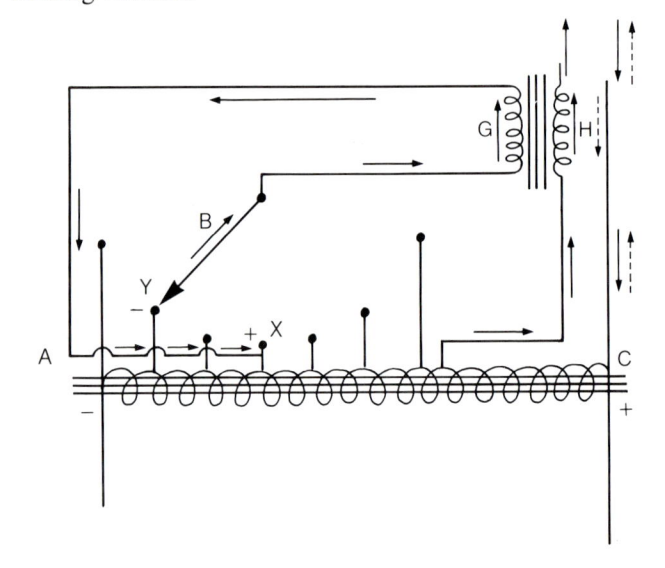

Figure 2.31 Direction of voltage induced into secondary of space charge transformer (H) indicated by dotted arrows (this time subtractive)

In Figure 2.31 the kV control is now in position B, i.e. kV has been increased. It can be seen that Y is now negative with respect to X and electron current is now in the opposite direction to that shown in Figure 2.30.

In these circumstances the voltage induced into the winding H is in opposition to the filament voltage and in consequence the filament heating current is reduced. From this it can be seen that increase in kV results in an automatic reduction in filament heating current.

kV COMPENSATOR

Ganged to the mA control is the kV compensator. This ensures that as the mA is increased the resultant drop in

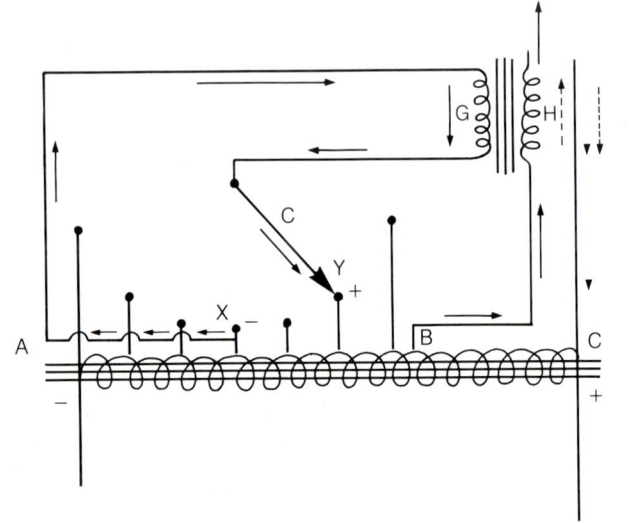

Figure 2.30 Direction of voltage induced into secondary of space charge transformer (H) indicated by dotted arrows (induced voltage in this case is additive)

DIAGNOSTIC X-RAY CIRCUITS

kV from the high tension transformer is automatically compensated for. This is achieved in slightly different ways depending on whether the unit uses a prereading kV meter to indicate kV as found in some older major units and on some mobile equipment, or, as in the case of more modern equipment, the kV is indicated on a scale or indeed by means of a digital readout. Let us first of all consider what happens when a prereading kV meter is used.

Such a meter measures the output voltage of the autotransformer, previously selected by means of the kV control, which is to be applied to the primary winding of the high tension transformer during an X-ray exposure. As the high tension transformer has a fixed ratio of secondary to primary turns, say 300:1, it follows that the application of say 200 V to the primary winding of the high tension transformer will result in a secondary voltage of 200 × 300 or 60 kV. The prereading kV meter is therefore measuring the primary voltage, in this case 200 V, which will result during the X-ray exposure, in a secondary voltage of 60 kV. If the meter which is measuring 200 V is therefore calibrated not in terms of the primary voltage of 200 V it is *actually* measuring, but the 60 kV that will be delivered by the secondary of the high tension transformer *during* the actual exposure, we have a means of predicting the kV before an exposure is made. This is the reason for it being called a prereading kV meter.

The voltage applied to the X-ray tube is always expressed as a *peak* value whilst primary voltage is measured as an r.m.s. value (see footnote). In our previous example an applied potential difference of 200 V r.m.s. resulted in an output at the secondary of 60 kV r.m.s. However,

peak value = 1.414 × r.m.s. value.

Therefore

60 kV × 1.414 = 85 kVp (approx.)

The meter would, therefore, be calibrated to read 85 kVp. Because the prereading kVp meter is in the primary circuit, and therefore at low tension, it may be located on the control panel and by calibrating it in terms of the *anticipated* kVp we are able to set a particular kVp value before the high tension transformer is even energized. It must be emphasized once again, however, that the prereading kVp meter does *not* measure the kVp obtained from the secondary winding of the high tension transformer during the exposure but the voltage to be applied to the primary of the high tension transformer and which will *result* in that particular kVp.

Peak value of voltage (or current) is the maximum value reached in a sinusoidal waveform.
For a constant potential generator peak value and r.m.s value are equal but for a 6 pulse generator peak value is 1.048 × r.m.s. value whilst r.m.s. value is 0.94 × peak value.
For a 2 pulse generator peak value is 1.414 × r.m.s. value and r.m.s. value is 0.707 × peak value.
See also appendix.

It will be recalled that when an exposure is made the secondary voltage is reduced to an extent which is dependent on the value of the current flowing in the secondary circuit, i.e. the greater the secondary current (mA) the greater is the reduction in kVp. Relating this to the example used previously, let us say that the application of 200 V r.m.s. to the primary of the high tension transformer results in an output from the secondary of 85 kVp when the secondary current is 100 mA.

If however, the secondary current is increased to say 500 mA we will get less than 85 kVp at the secondary of the high tension transformer; let us say that in fact we get 80 kVp. To maintain the secondary voltage at the correct value (85 kVp), when the secondary current is increased to 500 mA, we must increase the primary voltage by about 12 V r.m.s. In practice it is arranged that, in the above case, the prereading kVp meter reads 85 kVp when 100 mA is selected but the selection of 500 mA automatically reduces the meter reading to 80 kVp. To restore the meter reading to 85 kVp necessitates the selection of sufficient extra tappings by the kV selector to provide an extra 12 V to the primary of the high tension transformer. This is called prereading kVp meter compensation and may be achieved in the following way.

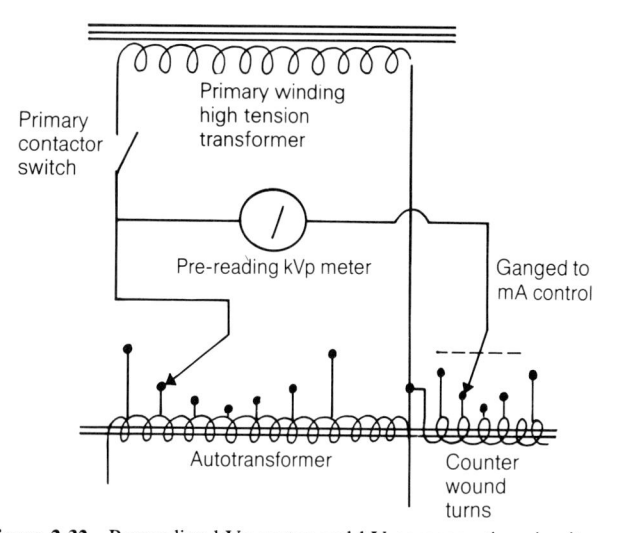

Figure 2.32 Prereading kVp meter and kV compensation circuit

One end of the autotransformer winding has a number of extra turns which are counterwound, i.e. wound in the opposite way to those of the main winding (see Figure 2.32). The kVp meter is connected to the tapped output of the autotransformer (via kVp control) at one end, and to a number of counterwound turns at the other, the precise number being determined by the value of the mA selected. (See Figure 2.33 for the way in which this is done.) Selection of the appropriate number of counterwound turns is automatic, as the control is ganged to the mA selector switch, i.e. the mA selector arm and the counterwound turns selector arm are physically linked, therefore movement of one automatically causes movement of the other. Consequently, movement of the mA selector arm, i.e. selection of a particular mA value, results in the automatic selection of an appropriate number of counterwound turns by the prereading kVp meter compensator control. The kVp meter reading is therefore reduced by an amount which is dependent on the number of counterwound turns selected, and this in turn is determined by the mA value selected.

Movement of the mA selector arm also moves the arm which selects a number of counterwound turns appropriate to that particular voltage drop. kVp meter reading *reduces*, as mA *increases*.

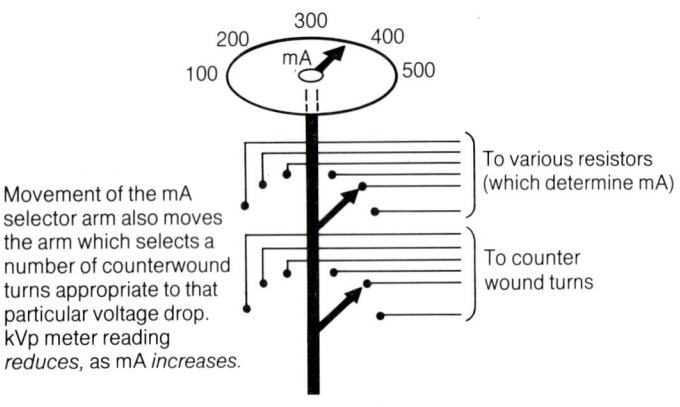

Figure 2.33 Prereading kV compensation

The effect of the counterwound turns is to induce a voltage acting in an opposite direction to that of the main winding. As the voltage induced into the counterwound turns is of smaller value than the voltage induced into the main autotransformer winding, and is acting in an opposite direction, it has a subtracting effect and reduces the value of the main voltage. If, for instance, 200 V is induced into the turns selected from the autotransformer, by means of the kV control and 15 V is selected from the counterwound turns, the voltage across the meter is 200 − 15 = 185 V. As the number of selected counterwound turns increases with increase in mA selected it can be appreciated that increase in mA causes a reduction in the voltage indicated on the prereading kVp meter. To restore the voltage to its original value the number of turns selected by the kV control must be increased or, of course, the mA value reduced.

An example might make this clearer. We will use the same values as before. Assume that an exposure of 85 kVp and 100 mA is to be made and that this necessitates the kV and prereading kVp compensation controls being set as shown in Figure 2.34.

The prereading kVp meter gives a reading of 85 kVp. Imagine the secondary current is now to be increased to 500 mA whilst the secondary voltage remains unchanged at 85 kVp. Rotating the mA selector control to increase

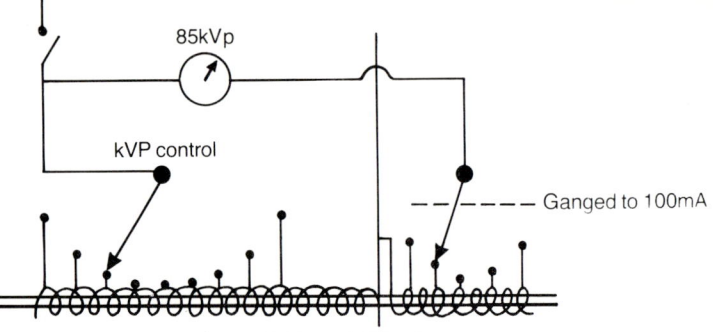

Figure 2.34 Setting for 85 kVp and 100 mA

the current in the secondary circuit to 500 mA also increases the number of counterwound turns to which the kVp meter is connected and in consequence increases the opposing voltage. The kV control has not been moved so the main voltage from the autotransformer is unchanged. In these circumstances it can be appreciated that, the voltage induced into the main autotransformer winding being constant whilst the opposing voltage obtained from an increased number of counterwound turns is increased, the voltage now registered on the prereading kVp meter is reduced (Figure 2.35).

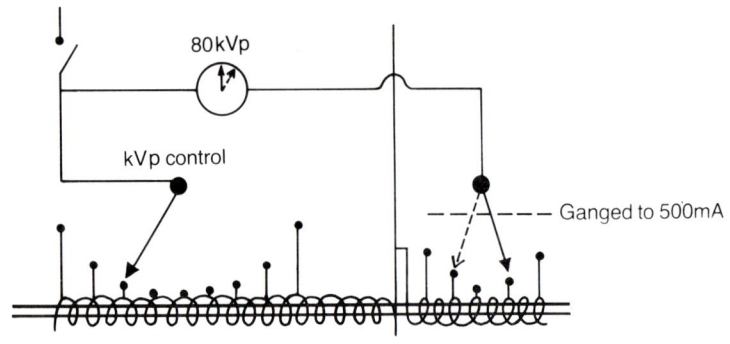

Figure 2.35 mA increased to 500, meter now reads 80 kVp

To restore the kVp meter reading to its original value we must *either* reduce the mA value and thereby reduce the number of selected counterwound turns, *or* increase the number of turns selected by the kV control and thereby increase the voltage from the main autotransformer winding (Figure 2.36).

Increase in the voltage applied to the primary winding of the high tension transformer when the secondary current (mA) is increased and reduction of the primary voltage when the mA is reduced provides the necessary compensation for variation in kVp due to changes in mA, thus ensuring a constant kVp at different mA values.

Before leaving the subject of kVp meter compensation certain important facts should be re-emphasized:

DIAGNOSTIC X-RAY CIRCUITS

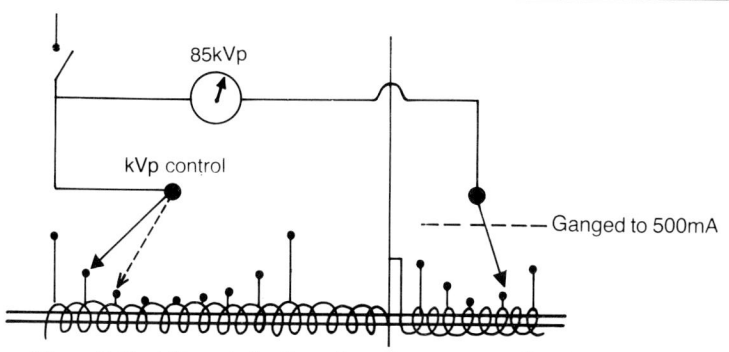

Figure 2.36 kV control adjusted so that meter reading is restored to 85 kVp

(1) The prereading kVp meter does *not* measure kVp. It measures *primary* voltage.

(2) The fact that the prereading kVp meter is connected across a number of turns of the autotransformer winding *plus* a number of counterwound turns affects the meter reading *only*. It does *not* directly affect the voltage applied to the primary winding of a high tension transformer. This voltage is determined *only* by the number of autotransformer turns selected by the kV control. Study Figure 2.37 carefully. The connections of the prereading kVp meter to the autotransformer winding via the kV control and to the counterwound turns are shown as dotted lines whilst the connections of the primary winding of the high tension transformer to the autotransformer winding, via the kV control, are shown in heavy lines. This should demonstrate that the meter circuit has no *direct* influence on the voltage applied to the primary winding of the high tension transformer. This can only be influenced by selecting a greater or lesser number of turns from the autotransformer.

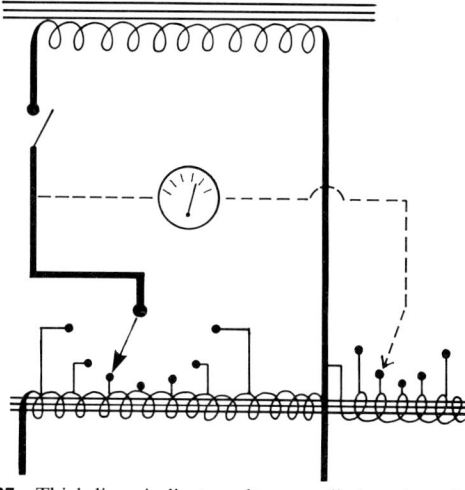

Figure 2.37 Thick lines indicate voltage applied to the primary of the high tension transformer and show that it is not affected by changes in voltage across the meter

kV compensation when there is no prereading kV meter

As stated previously, kV meters are used mainly with mobile units. Most modern units indicate kV by means of a digital readout. Where there is no prereading kV meter, compensation for kV drop on load may be achieved in the following way (Figure 2.38).

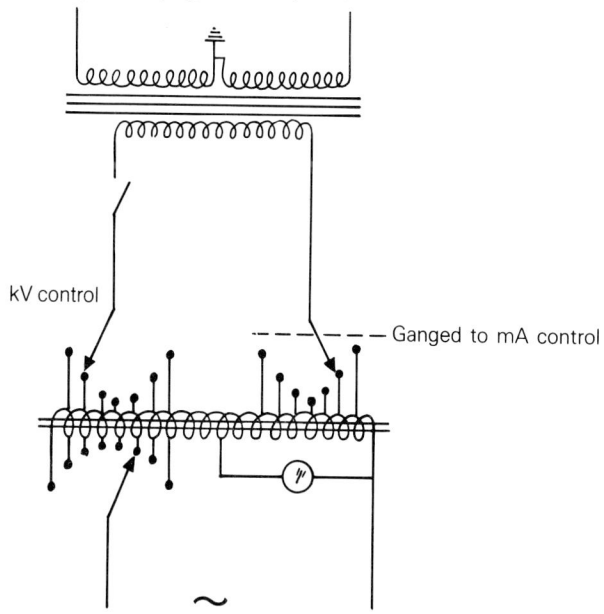

Figure 2.38 kV compensation circuit

It will be noted that once again there is a selector which is ganged to the mA control. This time, however, there are no counterwound turns. The operation of the circuit is simple in that increase in mA (which would lead to reduction in the kV applied to the tube) automatically increases the number of turns tapped from the autotransformer whilst a reduction in mA reduces the number of tapped turns. In this way the kV is maintained at the selected value despite changes in mA. *Note*: In each case the *primary* voltage is being changed when mA is changed to make up for the energy lost as heat in the secondary winding of the high tension transformer.

THE mA CONTROL

This consists of a number of resistors as shown in Figure 2.39, any one of which may be selected at will to provide the necessary voltage across the filament of the tube and therefore produce the desired mA. (R1–R6 represent different values of resistance, each resistor corresponding to a particular mA value.) Each mA can be adjusted in value by altering the value of the controlling resistor, i.e. R1–R6. This is normally done by the Engineer.

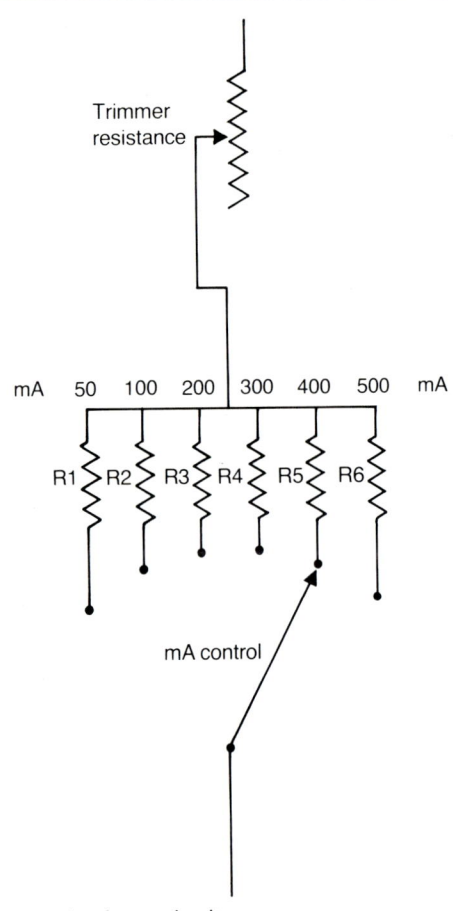

Figure 2.39 mA selector circuit

TRIMMER RESISTANCE

This a variable resistor which is used to alter the value of all mA readings. Thus if all mA values are less than they should be, as occurs for instance when the filament wears thin due to age and consequently has increased resistance, the trimmer resistance can be reduced, restoring all mAs to their original value.

FILAMENT STEP-DOWN TRANSFORMER

The next component is the filament step-down transformer. This consists of two primary and two secondary windings, one for the broad focus and one for the fine focus. The filament supply voltage may be applied to *either* of the primary windings. The switching is arranged in such a fashion that only one primary winding can be energized at any one time. It will be noted that the negative side of the high tension transformer is connected to the conductor which is common to both filaments (Figure 2.40).

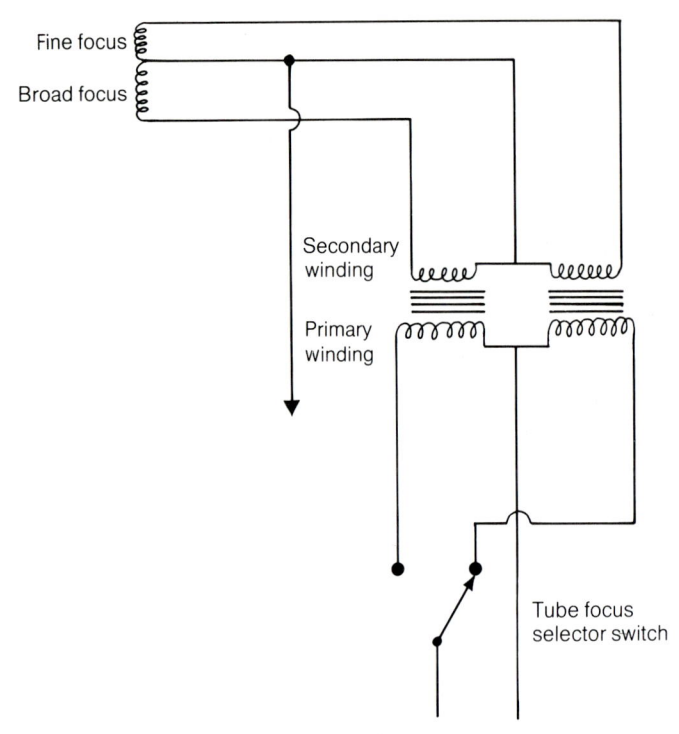

Figure 2.40 Tube focus selector circuit

The filament heating transformer reduces the primary voltage of, say 200 V, to approximately 10 V. It must be clearly appreciated, however, that when an exposure is being made this potential difference (10 V) is applied to conductors which are already at a high potential difference with respect to earth. An example might help to make this clear.

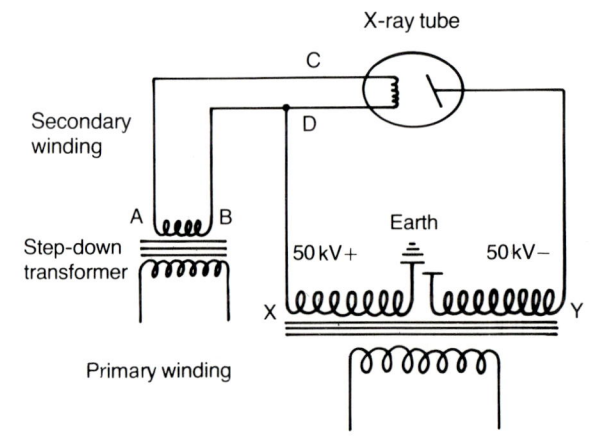

Figure 2.41 Self rectified circuit

DIAGNOSTIC X-RAY CIRCUITS

In the circuit diagram (Figure 2.41) X and Y are the ends of a high tension transformer secondary winding. It should be noted that end X of the winding is 50 kV positive to earth (during an exposure) and that points A, B, C and D are at the *same* potential. If the step-down transformer is not energized no voltage is induced into its secondary winding and points C, D remain at 50 kV. As there is no potential *difference* across the filament no current flows through it. If, however, the step-down transformer is energized and a potential difference of 10 V is induced across its secondary winding one end of the winding is 10 V higher than the other, i.e. A is now 10 V higher than B. This means that B is at a potential of 50 000 V (50 kV) to earth and A at 50 010 V which means a potential difference of 10 V across A–B, C–D and of course, the filament itself.

The important thing to remember is that, although the voltage induced into the secondary winding of the step-down transformer is small it is being *added* during the exposure to an existing voltage of very high value. It is necessary therefore to provide electrical insulation between the secondary and primary windings of the step-down transformer sufficient to withstand the full value of the secondary voltage on that side of the circuit, in this case 50 kV with respect to earth.

EXPOSURE SWITCHING (PRIMARY CIRCUIT)

Pressing the X-ray exposure button energizes the timer circuit, which in turn energizes the solenoid of an electromagnet, causing a switch in the primary circuit to be closed. The current which now flows in the primary and secondary circuits results in the production of X-rays at the target of the X-ray tube. At the end of a period of time, determined by the timer mechanism, current stops flowing in the timer circuit, the solenoid of the electromagnet ceases to be energized and the switch in the primary circuit opens, terminating the exposure.

The primary switch may be mechanical (electromagnetic) or electronic in operation. The electronic type will be considered in detail in the next chapter. (*Note*, electronic switching is also employed in the secondary circuit – this will also be considered later.)

The mechanical (electromagnetic) contactor switch

Study the diagrammatic representation of the primary switch in Figure 2.42. Note especially the following points, which should help you understand the basic principles underlying the structure and operation of such a switch.

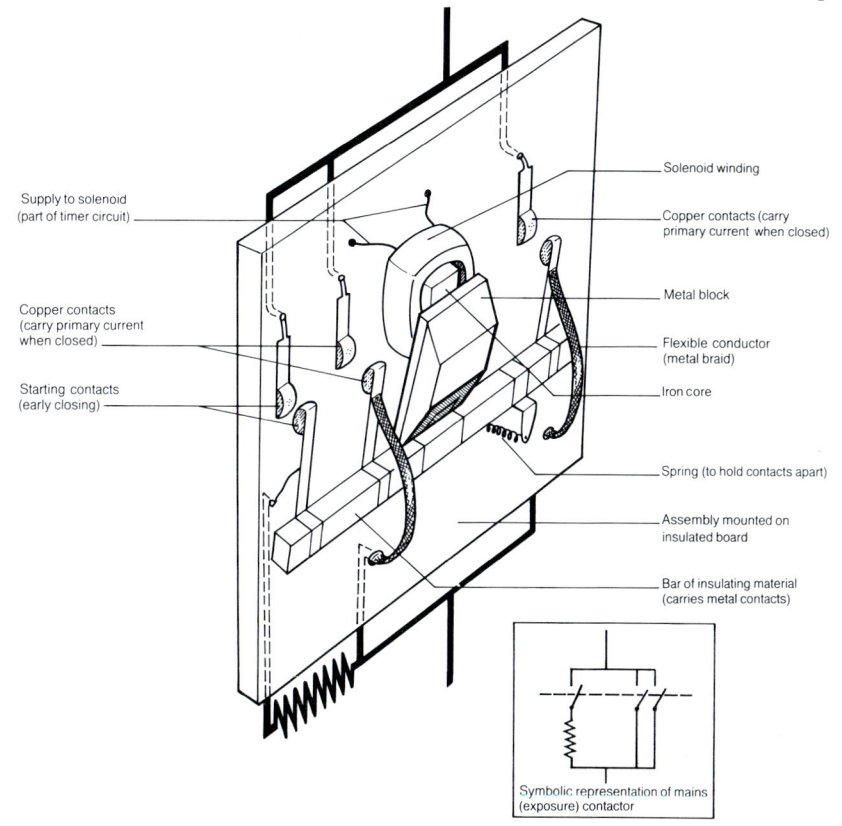

Figure 2.42 Diagrammatic representation of mechanical switch and inset symbolic representation

(1) *Fixed components*, secured to a base board of insulating material, include:

    (a) A solenoid whose winding is in series with the timer circuit.

    (b) The core, which is magnetized when current flows through the solenoid.

} Functions as an electromagnet when current flows in the timer circuit

    (c) A number of copper contacts (in this case three).

(2) *Moveable components* consist of an insulated bar free to rock through a small angle and attached to it:

    (a) Copper contacts (in this case three) held on arms which are firmly secured to the rocker bar and which therefore move, or rock, with it.

    (b) A large piece of metal which is attracted to the core when the solenoid has current flowing through it.

The insulated rocker bar is spring-loaded to ensure that the contacts open at the end of an exposure.

Note also the symbolic representation of the switch, which is frequently drawn thus and is connected in the circuit as shown in Figure 2.43. It is necessary to absorb initial current flow as there is a momentary surge of current at the beginning of the exposure. This initial surge is absorbed by the resistor (R) which is of high resistance. Contact A closes before contact B. Primary current therefore flows through resistance (R) for a fraction of time before contact B closes. As soon as contact B closes resistance (R) is bypassed.

In major units a phasing circuit is used to ensure that the contacts close and open when voltage is at or near zero point, i.e. whilst little or no current is flowing. This minimizes arcing which would otherwise cause damage to the copper contacts. It must be remembered that the primary current is of very high value in a diagnostic circuit, currents of 100–300 A being fairly representative.

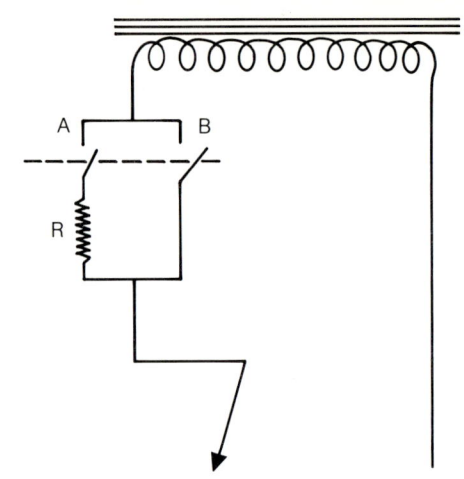

Figure 2.43 Primary switch and surge resistor

Sheets of asbestos on either side of each set of contacts give protection against the heat generated by the spark which occurs at 'make' and 'break' of current flow. An asbestos-lined box fitted over the contactor fulfils a similar function and also deadens the noise made by the switch when the contacts close.

Not all contactor switches function in air, some are oil-immersed, the oil quenching the spark generated at 'make' and 'break'. Contactors operating in oil need to be bigger and more powerful than those operated in air because of the resistance to movement offered by the oil.

Because the contactor closes with considerable force, the board to which it is attached may be mounted on strong springs to avoid mechanical damage. As there are obvious limitations to the speed with which mechanical switches can be opened and closed and to the rapidity with which they can be operated most modern high powered units use electronic switching in either the primary or secondary circuits. Electronic switching is discussed in the next chapter.

Note: Until now we have considered primary switching in terms of a single switch. It should be noted however that some equipment has not one but two switches, one to 'make' the circuit and the other to 'break' it.

3
Electronic devices

THE THERMIONIC DIODE VALVE	35
Operation of the valve	35
Thermionic emission	36
ELECTRONIC SWITCHING (primary circuit)	36
The thyratron valve	36
SOLID STATE DEVICES	37
THE SOLID STATE RECTIFIER	37
Conduction band theory	38
Conductors	38
Insulators	38
Semiconductors	38
Improving the conduction characteristics of a semiconductor	38
AVALANCHE DIODE	40
Zener diode	40
Light emitting diode (LED)	40
THE TRANSISTOR	41
Mode of operation	41
THE THYRISTOR (SCR)	41
The triac	42
The diac	42
FIELD EFFECT TRANSISTOR (FET)	42

Before considering electronic switching in the primary circuit we should perhaps look at the word electronic and consider its meaning. The term 'electronic' means the control of electron motion in a circuit by means of thermionic valves (or solid state devices). Until recently thermionic diode valves were used for high tension rectification and thermionic triode valves (thyratrons) for primary switching. However, these devices are now rarely, if ever, used in modern X-ray circuits. In each case they have been superseded by solid state devices which have numerous advantages. However, an understanding of *some* thermionic devices is still essential, i.e. the X-ray tube itself, the grid controlled X-ray tube, vacuum triodes in the high tension circuit, etc. In addition to these an understanding of the way in which other now obsolete thermionic devices work should make it easier to understand the working of solid state equivalents which have replaced them. To avoid any confusion to the reader it will be clearly stated when the device being described is obsolete and is being described for purposes of understanding only.

THE THERMIONIC DIODE VALVE (now obsolete)

The thermionic diode valve consists essentially of two electrodes in an evacuated glass envelope (Figure 3.1). One electrode, the filament, is made of thoriated tungsten wire, and is heated, whilst the other, a cup-shaped cylinder made of nickel, remains cold.

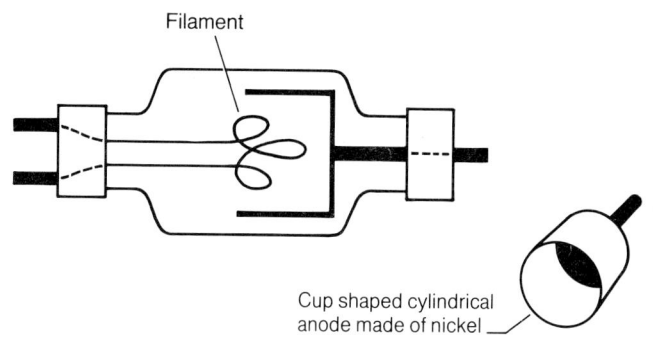

Figure 3.1 High tension thermionic diode rectifying valve

Operation of the valve

When the thoriated tungsten filament is heated, electrons are emitted by the process of *thermionic emission* (see following note on thermionic emission). If the cylindrical electrode is positive with respect to the filament, electrons are attracted to it (Figure 3.2). If, however, the filament is positive and the cup-shaped electrode negative, i.e. during the inverse half cycle, no current flows, as the cylindrical electrode is cold and does not emit electrons. If the cylindrical electrode were to become heated to such a temperature as would allow the emission of electrons,

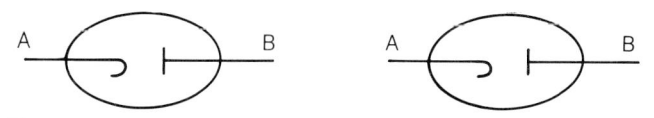

Figure 3.2 When A is negative and B is positive electron current flows, but when A is positive and B is negative *no* current flows

then the diode would stop functioning as a valve, as current flow would be possible in both directions. It is essential therefore, if the valve is to function correctly, to ensure that the cylindrical electrode never reaches the critical temperature at which electrons would be emitted.

Thermionic emission

This is the emission of electrons from a body by the application of heat energy. Consider a piece of metal such as tungsten. It is rich in 'free' electrons which are able to move freely within the metal. They do not, however, under normal circumstances (i.e. low temperature) have sufficient energy to leave the surface of the metal. This is due to the cumulative force exerted by the metal's positive nuclei which tend to keep the electrons within the confines of the metal. If, however, the energy of the electrons is increased, by heating the metal, the free electrons nearest the surface of the metal are able to overcome the attractive force of the nuclei and leave the confines of the metal. The additional energy needed by the electrons to overcome the force of attraction exerted by the atomic nuclei of a metal is called the work function of that particular metal. Different metals have different work functions.

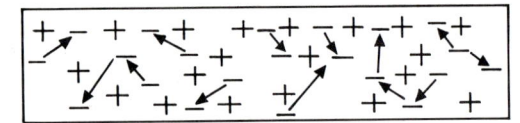

Figure 3.3 Tungsten at low temperature

'Free' electrons move in a haphazard fashion *within* the metal at low temperature (Figure 3.3). They do not possess the necessary energy to leave the surface of the metal.

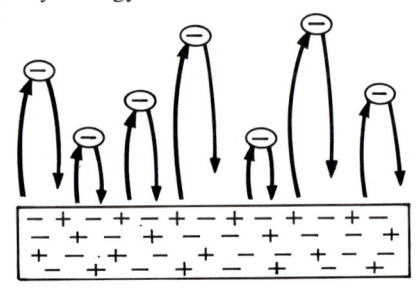

Figure 3.4 Tungsten at high temperature

When the tungsten is heated to a sufficiently high temperature, some of the electrons nearest the surface acquire the extra energy needed to lift them from the surface of the metal (Figure 3.4). If the heated metal is contained within a vacuum, the electrons are able to move some distance from the surface before they are attracted back. The reason they are attracted back is that those atoms which lost electrons are now positive and exert a force of attraction on the liberated electrons. If there is another force in the vicinity of the liberated electrons, such as a positive electrode, then it also exerts a force of attraction on the liberated electrons and attracts some or all (depending on its strength) of them towards it.

ELECTRONIC SWITCHING (Primary Circuit)

Switching of the primary current may be achieved by the use of triode valves, called thyratrons, now obsolete, or by solid state devices called thyristors. Let us consider first the way in which the thyratron works.

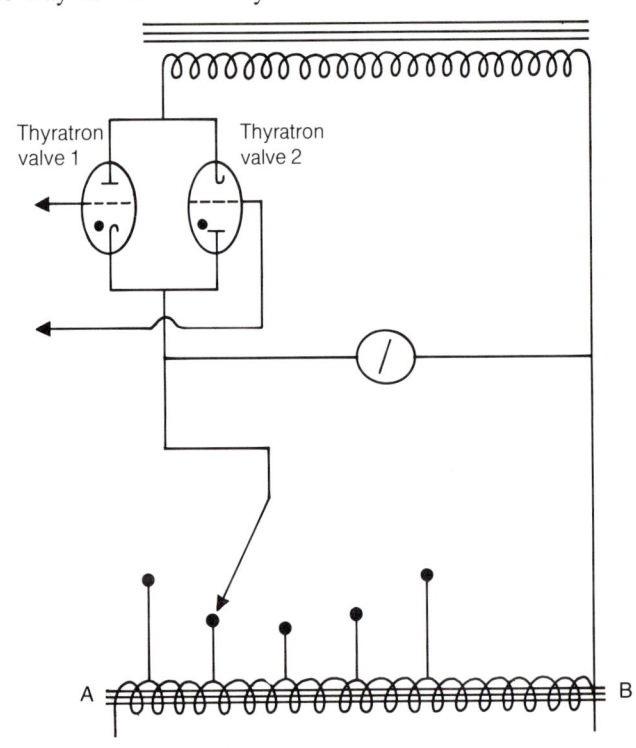

Figure 3.5 Primary switching using thyratron valves

The thyratron valve (*now obsolete*)

This consists of a gas-filled glass envelope which encloses a cathode, a grid and an anode. The presence of gas ensures a rapid and large flow of electrons (by ionization) when the valve is conducting.

Electronic switching in the primary circuit of a single-phase generator operates in the following manner. Two thyratrons in inverse parallel connection are connected in series with the primary circuit as shown in Figure 3.5. When 'A' is negative and 'B' positive, electron current flows from 'A' through valve 1 to 'B' via the primary winding of the high tension transformer. When 'B' is negative and 'A' positive, electrons flow from 'B' through valve 2 via the primary winding of the high tension transformer to 'A'.

Prior to an X-ray exposure the timer circuit maintains the grid of each thyratron at negative potential with respect to the filament. Because the grid is close to the filament the repelling effect on filament electrons is very much greater than the force of attraction exerted by the anode (Figure 3.6). Under these circumstances no electron current flow is possible.

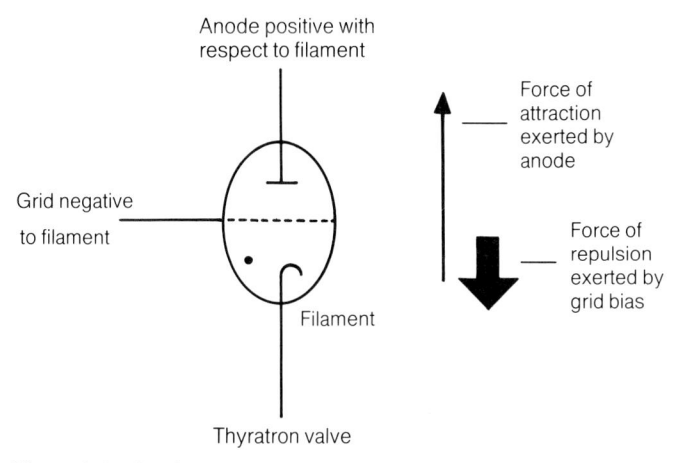

Figure 3.6 Gas-filled triode valve (thyratron)

At the beginning of an exposure the timer circuit removes the negative bias from the grids of the thyratrons. Current is now able to flow in the primary and secondary circuits. At the end of the exposure the negative voltage is re-applied to the grids, by the timer circuit. This does not stop current flow instantaneously, unless the mains voltage is at zero when the voltage is applied to the grids. If the mains voltage is of sufficient value to maintain ionization (between A and B or C and D in Figure 3.7), current continues to flow until the mains voltage next reaches zero value, after A–B at X, after C–D at Y, etc.

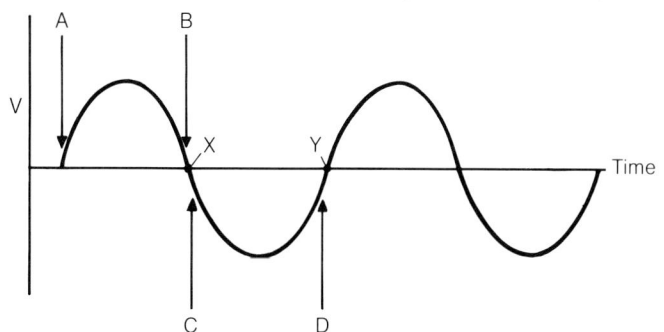

Figure 3.7 Current flow can be stopped only when voltage is at or near zero valve

SOLID STATE DEVICES

So far we have seen that *gas-filled* triodes (thyratrons) may be used in the primary circuit as switches whilst *vacuum* triodes (Figure 2.20) are used for switching in the secondary circuit. We will also see that the vacuum triode in the form of a grid controlled X-ray tube can combine the functions of an X-ray tube with that of a switch (Figure 5.19).

All these devices require, of course, a heated filament, a cathode, an anode and a glass envelope to contain either a vacuum or a gas. Note that *vacuum* devices are used in the secondary circuit whilst gas-filled devices are used in the primary. The reason for this will become apparent later.

Solid state devices have no filaments, no glass envelope and no associated components such as step-down transformers to heat the filaments, etc. Their use, therefore, in the X-ray equipment offers obvious advantages in terms of space, reliability, etc.

Solid state devices tend to be used mainly in the primary circuit. The *only* solid state device to be used in the secondary circuit is the solid state rectifier, so let us look at that first and then go on and see how it works.

THE SOLID STATE RECTIFIER

In each of the high tension circuits so far described, rectification has been achieved with the use of solid state rectifiers. Such devices have the same function as thermionic diodes in that they allow current to flow in one direction only, current flow in the inverse half cycle being suppressed. At this point, however, their similarity ends as they achieve their objective in completely different ways. Whereas the thermionic diode needs a step-down transformer to provide its filament with the necessary heating current, the solid state rectifier has no need for such associated devices.

This means that solid state rectifiers take up less space which means that they can be built into a single structure tube head, for instance, to provide full-wave rectification for high powered mobile units. They are also more reliable, have longer life, etc., all good reasons why the manufacturer of modern X-ray equipment now uses them in preference to thermionic diode valves.

The circuit symbol for a solid state rectifier is shown in Figure 3.8. Note that the black arrow head in the symbol points in the direction of conventional current flow. *Electron* current is in the *opposite* direction as indicated by the dotted arrow (which does not of course form part of the circuit symbol).

To understand how such a device works requires that we first of all understand how and why electrical conduction takes place easily in some substances and much less easily in others.

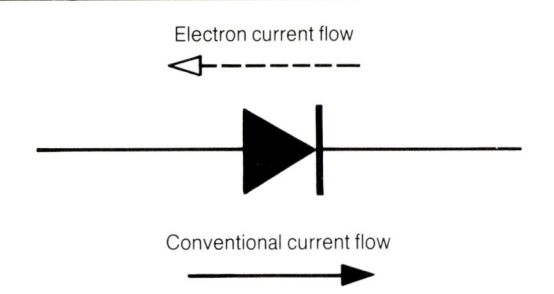

Figure 3.8 Circuit symbol for the solid state rectifier

Conduction band theory

Conductors

An electrical conductor, such as a metal, allows a steady drift of electrons through the conduction band when a potential difference is applied across its ends. This is due to the fact that the valence and conduction bands overlap as shown in Figure 3.9.

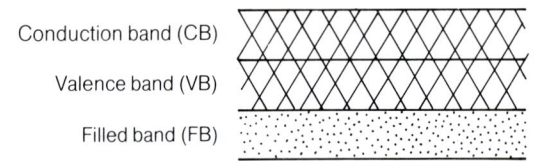

Figure 3.9 Conduction band diagram for a conductor

Insulators

On the other hand insulators have a large gap between the valence and conduction band such that in normal circumstances (i.e. when the temperature of the material is not too high and when the potential difference is not excessive) there is insufficient energy in the electric field to raise electrons from the valence band to the conduction band. This is illustrated in Figure 3.10.

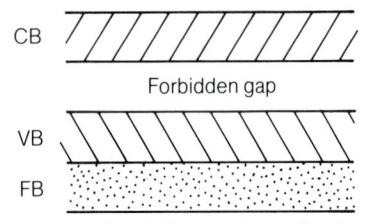

Figure 3.10 Conduction band diagram for an insulator

Semiconductors

As its name implies a semiconductor falls midway between a good conductor and a bad conductor (insulator) so far as its conduction characteristics are concerned. This is illustrated in Figure 3.11. It will be noted that the gap between the valence band and the conduction band is much less than that of the insulator. The energy differences between the bands of three different materials are illustrated in Figure 3.12.

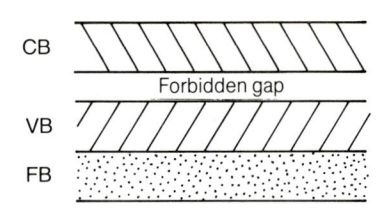

Figure 3.11 Conduction band diagram for a semiconductor

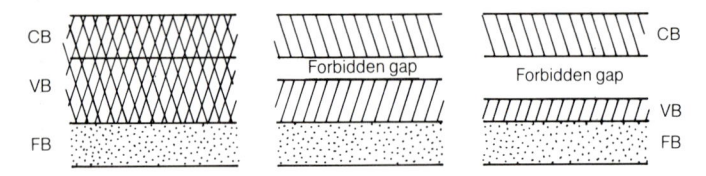

Figure 3.12 Conduction band diagrams for a conductor, semiconductor and insulator

Improving the conduction characteristics of a semiconductor

Under normal circumstances a pure semiconductor such as silicon will not easily conduct. If, however, its temperature is raised, some of the electrons in the valence band may gain sufficient energy to bridge the energy gap and become carriers in the conduction band. *A semiconductor, therefore, has its conductivity increased by heating.* Its conductivity may also be increased by fusing into the semiconductor an impurity which will provide electrons at an energy level only slightly less than the conduction band as shown by the dotted line in Figure 3.13. When a potential difference is applied across the material the electrons in the energy band lying just below the conduction band gain energy from the electric field which enables them to pass into the conduction band and thus current is able to flow. Such carriers are called 'n' type carriers as they are electrons and thus negative carriers, and the material is called an 'n' type material. The added impurity in this case would be phosphorus or arsenic.

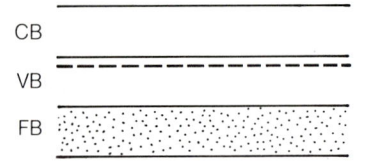

Figure 3.13 Semiconductor material with 'n' type impurity

ELECTRONIC DEVICES

If, however, an impurity is added to a semiconductor which provides an energy level just higher than the valence band, e.g. boron or indium, and a potential difference is applied, electrons are given sufficient energy to move out of the filled band but *not* into the conduction band (Figure 3.14).

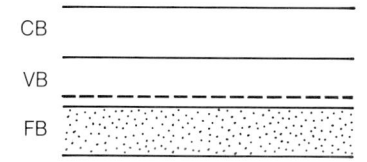

Figure 3.14 Semiconductor with 'p' type impurity. Energy level indicated by dotted line

As the electron is raised out of the filled band, however, it leaves behind a 'hole' and these 'holes' appear to move in the opposite direction to electron current (Figure 3.15). They are said to be positive or 'p' type carriers.

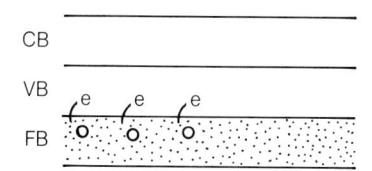

Figure 3.15 Conduction by holes

Now, just as a piece of copper has lots of 'free' electrons and yet remains electrically neutral (unless a potential difference is applied across it), so a piece of 'n' type semiconductor and a piece of 'p' type semiconductor also remain electrically neutral unless connected in a circuit and a potential difference applied. If, however, a piece of 'n' type material has a 'p' type impurity fused into it, it would seem that the electrons and holes would arrange themselves as shown in Figure 3.16. This, however, is not the complete picture as some of the electrons from the 'n' type material move across the boundary to the 'p' type material as shown in Figure 3.17. After the initial movement, however, no more electrons move across. This is because movement of electrons from 'a' to 'b' gives 'b' a small negative charge which repels further migration of electrons from 'a'. At the same time the electrons lost from 'a' give 'a' a small positive charge and the material now looks as shown in Figure 3.18. There is thus a small potential difference of about 0.1 V developed across the junction at 'b' due to the migration of electrons. The layer which has lost electrons is therefore called the depletion layer. Such a device is called a solid state rectifier.

Let us now see what happens if we apply a potential difference across its ends, as shown in Figure 3.19. There is a movement of electrons through the material towards

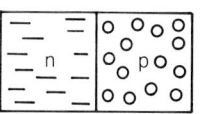

Figure 3.16 Electrons and holes are not equally distributed

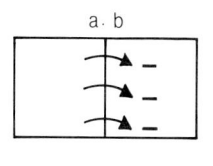

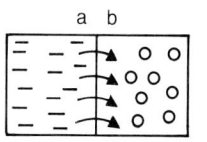

Figure 3.17 Migration of electrons to the 'p' type material

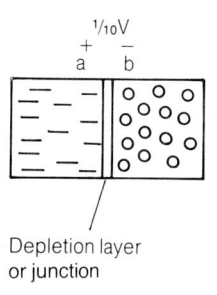

Figure 3.18 Solid state rectifier

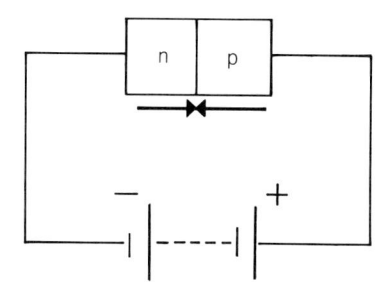

Figure 3.19 Solid state rectifier forward biased (current flows)

the junction in one direction and a movement of 'holes' towards the junction in the other. The small potential difference of 0.1 V at the junction is overcome and the electrons and holes neutralize one another as fast as they recombine at the junction. However, fresh electrons are introduced at the 'n' side of the material and fresh holes are created at the 'p' side by movement of electrons to the positive pole of the battery.

Now let us connect the battery in the opposite sense, i.e. in the reverse direction as in Figure 3.20. Electrons are now swept back from the junction, the original 0.1 V potential barrier is reinforced, thus offering great opposition to current flow. The device thus acts as a rectifier allowing current to flow easily in one direction but not in the other. If an alternating voltage is applied it will be found that the inverse half cycle of current will be suppressed (except for a very small reverse current due to minority carriers).

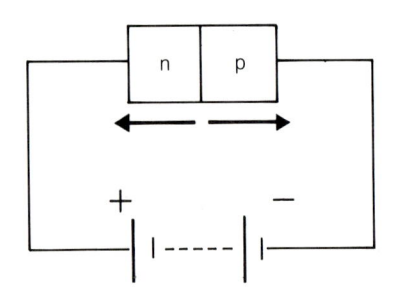

Figure 3.20 Solid state rectifier reverse biased (only negligible current flows)

Unlike the vacuum diode, the solid state rectifier has no need for a step-down transformer, has no filament to wear out and therefore has a much longer life. Its characteristics remain constant over a long period of time and a full-wave rectifier system takes up much less room.

When used for high tension rectification one such rectifier would be unable to withstand the high voltage applied across it during an exposure so a large number of individual rectifiers are connected in series within a tube some 25 cm long and 2.5 cm in diameter. There is a protective plastic covering over the tube excepting at its ends which have metal caps for connection into the circuit (Figure 3.21).

Rectifiers are the only solid state devices used in the secondary circuit. All other components such as switching triodes, X-ray tube, etc. are thermionic vacuum devices.

AVALANCHE DIODE

When a p n junction is reverse biased a negligibly small current flows, due to minority carriers, i.e. electrons from the 'p' region and holes from the 'n' region. The number of such reverse carriers is limited and the reverse current is usually sufficiently small as to be ignored. If, however, the reverse voltage in an avalanche diode is raised to a sufficiently high value, at a certain critical voltage, the internal resistance of the device drops to a low value, breakdown occurs and a high current flows. This surge of current is due to the electrons from the 'p' region gaining sufficient energy from the electric field to ionize atoms within the crystal lattice and so produce an ever increasing number of electrons and holes once breakdown occurs. Such a device is used in voltage stabilizer and voltage reference circuits. See Figure 3.22 for its symbol.

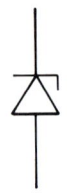

Figure 3.22 Circuit symbol for avalanche and zener diodes

Zener diode

This diode exhibits breakdown at a lower voltage than the avalanche diode. Breakdown is due this time not to the avalanche effect but to the zener effect. This effect is thought to be due to spontaneous generation of electron hole pairs from the inner shells of atoms in the junction region. Whilst this region is usually carrier free, the intense electric field across the junction provides the necessary energy to produce the current carriers.

Light emitting diode (LED)

We have seen that when a p n junction is forward biased electrons and holes flow towards the junction where they recombine. In light emitting diodes this recombination results in the release of energy, in the form of light. LEDs may be used in digital displays.

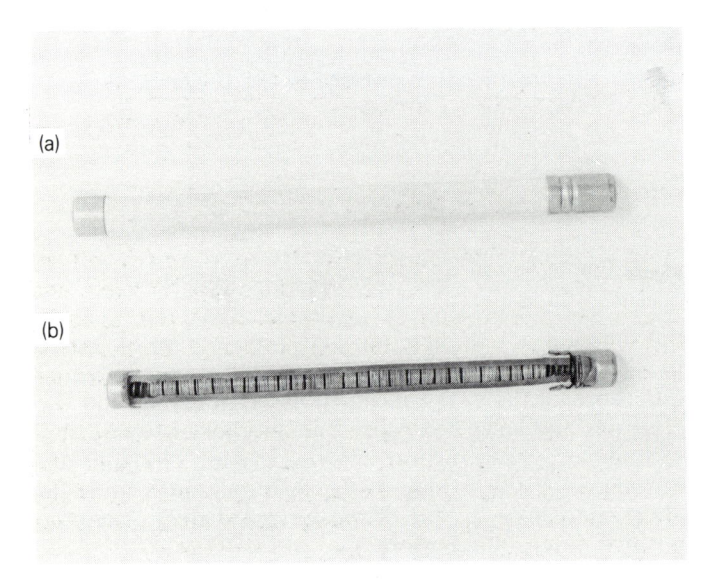

Figure 3.21 (a) Solid state rectifier as used in high tension circuit. (b) Cut away section of high tension rectifier showing numerous individual rectifiers in series connection

THE TRANSISTOR

We have seen that the vacuum triode valve can be made conductive or non-conductive depending on whether or not its grid is biased sufficiently with respect to its filament and that such a device may be used as a secondary switch or as a means of controlling kV. We will also see that an X-ray tube may function as a switch as well as a producer of X-rays. These are all examples of thermionic vacuum triodes used in the secondary circuit of X-ray equipment.

The solid state equivalent of the triode valve is the transistor. It may be drawn schematically as in Figure 3.23 as an n p n transistor, or in Figure 3.24 as a p n p transistor. The circuit symbol is drawn as in Figure 3.25. Unlike the vacuum triode it has no need for a glass envelope, filament or step-down transformer. Note that the transistor is *never* used in the high tension circuit as it could not withstand the high tension needed to produce X-rays.

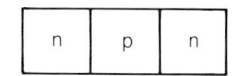

Figure 3.23 n p n transistor

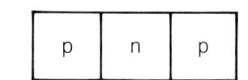

Figure 3.24 p n p transistor

Figure 3.25 Circuit symbols for n p n and p n p transistors

Mode of operation

The transistor may be used as a power, current or voltage amplifier, or as an electronic switch. It has three connections called the emitter, base and collector which might be connected as in Figure 3.26. The n p (emitter base) part of the transistor is forward biased with respect to battery A, i.e. electrons act as majority carriers which flow through the n (emitter) part of the transistor whilst 'holes' acting as majority carriers pass through the p (base) part of the transistor to neutralize electrons at the n p junction. The n p (emitter base) part of the transistor is therefore acting in a manner similar to the n p rectifier previously described. Because the emitter base junction is forward biased, a lot of electrons are injected into the base where they become minority carriers; some recombine with 'holes' in the base but a large number are swept across the p n (base collector) junction attracted by the large potential of battery B which, in the presence of these minority carriers, overcomes the negative biasing of the p n junction.

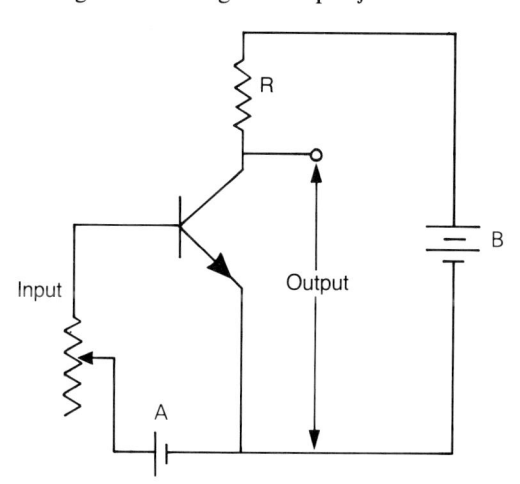

Figure 3.26 The transistor as a current amplifier

The transistor is only conductive when a base current flows and the greater the base current the greater is the collector current. As the collector current (ic) is large compared to the base current (ib) the transistor is a current amplifier. In the case of a d.c. input the amplification factor = ic/ib.

If an a.c. input signal is superimposed on a d.c. supply the amplification factor = change in ic/change in ib.

When there is a resistor in the collector circuit, (R in Figure 3.26) voltage amplification can be obtained. Variation in collector current causes a varying voltage drop across the resistor.

$$\text{Voltage gain} = \frac{\text{change in output volts}}{\text{change in input volts}}$$

THE THYRISTOR (SCR)

You will recall that the gas-filled triode valve (thyratron) can be used as an electronic switch to rapidly make and break the high primary current which flows during an X-ray exposure. The solid state equivalent of the thyratron is the thyristor or more correctly the silicon-controlled rectifier (SCR).

It may be drawn schematically, or as a circuit symbol as in Figure 3.27. It has three connections, a cathode, an anode, a gate and three junctions, J_1, J_2 and J_3. If the thyristor is connected to a source of potential difference so that the anode end (p) is negative and the cathode end (n) positive no current flows through the device as the two p n junctions, J_1 and J_3, are reverse biased. Even if the potential difference is reversed so that the cathode end (n) is negative and the anode end (p) is positive current will still not flow because the p n junction J_2 is reverse biased. So, in the absence of any current to or from the gate, the thyristor is non-conducting in either direction. If, however, a positive pulse is applied to the gate, current flows from cathode to gate, minority carriers (electrons) are produced in the p part of the thyristor, the negative bias is overcome and a surge of electrons pass through the thyristor.

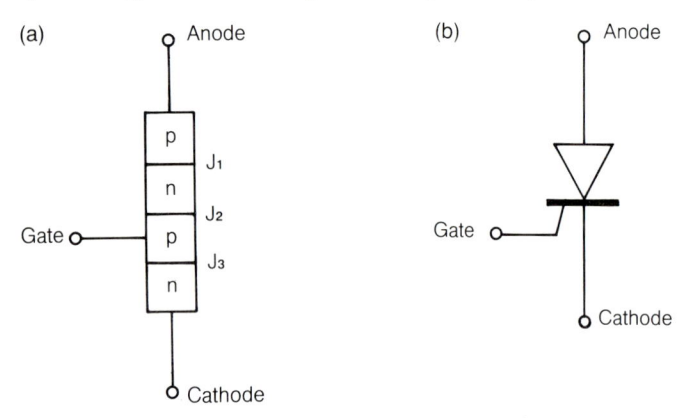

Figure 3.27 The thyristor drawn (a) schematically and (b) as a circuit symbol

In effect, a small positive pulse to the gate causes a large current to flow through the thyristor. Because the thyristor is also a rectifier it is necessary to have two in opposed parallel connection, in series with the primary circuit (Figure 3.28).

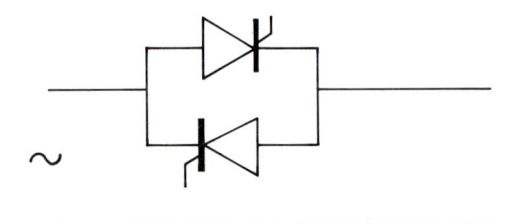

Figure 3.28 Thyristors in opposed parallel connection

Silicon-controlled rectifiers can handle up to 200 A at mains voltage, they are fast acting and have a relatively small power consumption. They can be switched on with a gate voltage of about 1.0 V. They are now used in most modern X-ray equipment for switching the primary current.

The Triac

This is a single three-terminal device which can conduct or block in either direction and can be triggered on with a gate signal of either polarity. It is the equivalent of two SCRs in inverse parallel connection as shown in Figure 3.29.

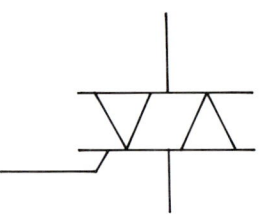

Figure 3.29 Circuit symbol of the triac

The diac

This is a single two-terminal device which has a breakdown voltage of about 32 V. When this voltage is reached, in either direction, the internal resistance of the device falls and current flows. The diac is used mainly as a trigger device for SCRs. Its symbol is shown in Figure 3.30.

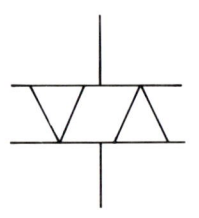

Figure 3.30 Circuit symbol of the diac

FIELD EFFECT TRANSISTOR (FET)

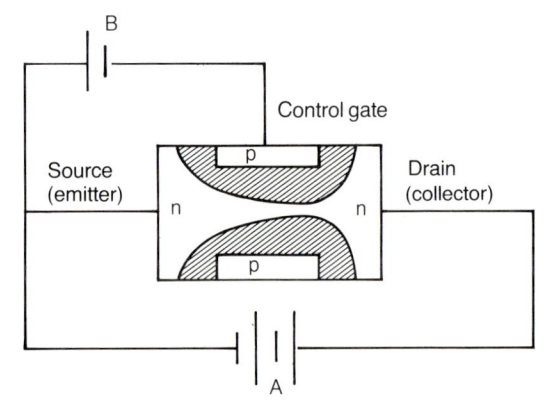

Figure 3.31 Field effect transistor

In Figure 3.31 note that the device is forward biased by battery A but reverse biased by battery B. We have previously seen that the greater the reverse bias across a p n junction the wider is the depletion layer and, conversely, the smaller the biasing voltage the thinner is the depletion layer. The FET therefore has its current carrying ability influenced by the gate voltage. The FET functions in a similar manner to the triode valve, the source corresponding to the cathode, the gate to the grid and the drain to the anode. The symbols of the FET are shown in Figure 3.32.

Other types of FETs include MOSFETs (metal oxide semiconductor FET) which are used mainly in integrated circuits, particularly digital memory chips.

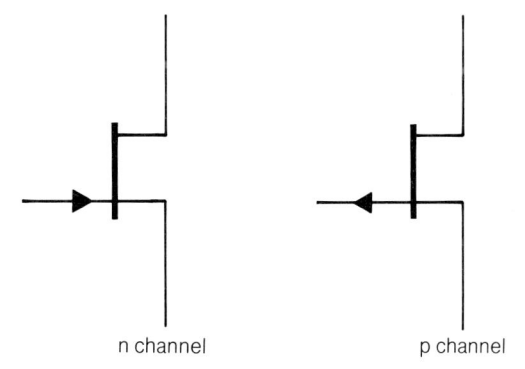

n channel   p channel

Figure 3.32 Symbols for FET

4
Exposure timers and specialized X-ray generators

CLOCKWORK TIMER	44
THE ELECTRONIC TIMER	45
AUTOMATIC EXPOSURE CONTROL	46
Phototimer	46
The iontomat	46
Density control	47
The response or reaction time	47
mAs CONTROL (TIMER)	47
GUARD TIMER	47
PRIMARY CONTACTOR EXPOSURE SWITCHING CIRCUIT	48
INTERLOCKED CIRCUITS	48
Initial delay circuit	48
Tube filament interlock	49
Tube filament boost	49
Anode delay circuit	49
X-ray tube overload protection circuits	49
X-ray tube overload circuit (protection against single exposure)	50
Percentage tube load indication	51
Tube overload circuit (protection against multiple exposures)	51
'Loadix'	52
THE FALLING LOAD GENERATOR	52
HIGH TENSION CHANGEOVER SWITCH	53
SHARED GENERATORS	53
HIGH FREQUENCY GENERATORS	54
THE CONTROL PANEL OR CONSOLE	55

We have seen that the primary current in an X-ray unit may be switched on or off by means of electromechanical contactors, thyratrons or thyristors. As the length of time for which the switching device is closed is one of the factors which determines film blackening, some means of accurately measuring and reproducing the time of exposure is essential. One or other of a number of different types of timer may be used for this purpose, the simplest of which is the clockwork timer.

CLOCKWORK TIMER

The principle of operation is that a tensioned spring takes a certain length of time to unwind (usually through a system of gears). From Figure 4.1 it can be seen that a spring is tensioned when the pointer is moved over the scale which is graduated, usually from 0 to, say, 10 seconds. Tensioning of the spring, i.e. setting of the timer, closes contacts A and B. Pressure on the exposure button releases the spring (the pointer begins its movement towards zero) and simultaneously closes contacts C–D. Closure of these contacts (a) completes the primary circuit and initiates the exposure, i.e. C–D functions as a primary

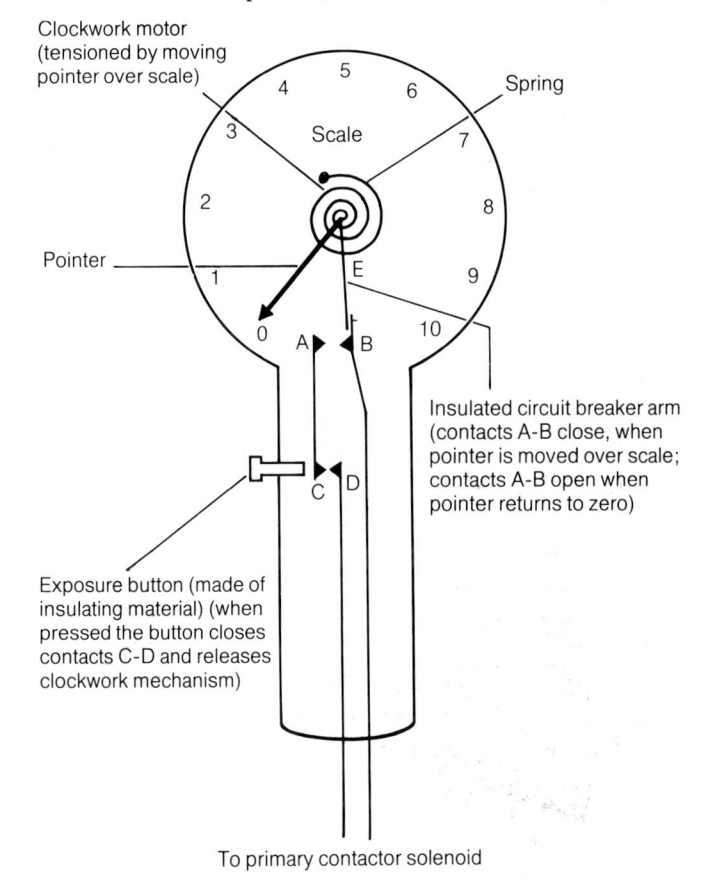

Figure 4.1 Clockwork timer

EXPOSURE TIMERS AND SPECIALIZED X-RAY GENERATORS

contactor switch, or, (b) causes current to flow through a solenoid which closes the primary contactor and initiates the exposure. When the pointer reaches zero position, contacts A–B are opened by the insulated arm E and the exposure is terminated.

Whether a clockwork timer is used in an X-ray circuit to function as a primary switch in addition to its timing function or whether the clockwork timer is used to operate a relay is determined by the value of current flow in the primary, i.e. whether it is a portable unit (low power) or a mobile unit (higher power). Clockwork timers are simple, strong and robust and are used on most portable and some mobile units. They are not accurate for short exposure times and must be reset after each exposure.

Note: Clockwork timers are *never* used on major units and even mobile units now use a more sophisticated kind of timer. It should be noted that some equipment is provided with two primary switches connected in series with one another. One is the "make" switch, normally open, which is closed at the start of the exposure and the other is the "break" switch, normally closed which opens to terminate the exposure.

THE ELECTRONIC TIMER

This timer operates on the principle that it takes a specific length of time to charge a given capacitor to a given voltage through a given resistor. From Figure 4.2 it can be seen that closure of the exposure switch completes the circuit through the solenoid of the primary 'make' contactor switch. Current now flows through the primary circuit and the X-ray exposure commences. At the same instant current begins to flow through the timer circuit and the capacitor begins to charge. When the voltage across the plates of the capacitor reaches a specified value, determined by the value of resistor selected, current to the base of the transistor initiates current flow in the collector circuit; this then triggers the thyristor which allows current to flow through the solenoid of the primary 'break' contactor. Current flow in the primary circuit is therefore stopped and the exposure is terminated. A switch shorts out the capacitor after the exposure and it remains closed until the unit is put into 'prep' ready for the next exposure. This ensures that the capacitor is always completely discharged at the beginning of an exposure.

The length of exposure is determined by the value of resistor selected as this controls the time it takes for the capacitor to reach the critical stage at which it will switch 'on' the transistor.

When equipment uses only one primary contactor switch to "make" and "break" the primary current the solenoid Sc in Figure 4.2 is used to open an interlock switch in the primary contactor circuit and thus terminate the exposure.

Note: All primary switches used with major units are phased, that is to say they can only close and open when the primary voltage is passing through zero value. This is to prevent damage to contactors which would otherwise occur if they were opened or closed when the voltage was at high value due to the dissipation of large amounts of power by the switch.

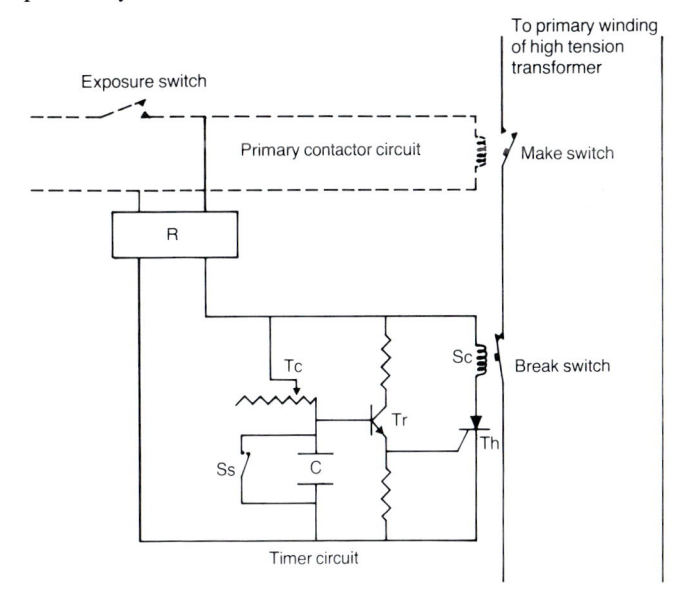

Tc – Timer control
Ss – Shorting switch (open when unit is put into 'prep')
C – Capacitor
Tr – Transistor
Th – Thyristor
R – Rectified and smoothed d.c. input
Sc – Solenoid coil of primary 'break' contactor switch

Figure 4.2 Simple circuit to illustrate principle of electronic timer

Capacitor begins to charge, through a resistor at the same instant that current flows through the 'make' primary contactor (exposure starts)

Transistor passes a trigger pulse to the thyristor when the capacitor reaches a critical voltage (time to reach this voltage is determined by the value of selected resistance)

Thyristor switches current to 'break' contactor (exposure ends)

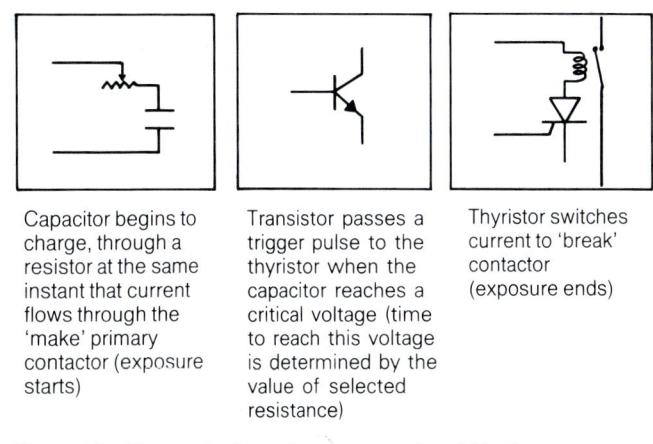

Figure 4.3 Electronic timer drawn as a series of blocks

It should also be borne in mind that this description of an electronic timer is extremely simple and, although it adequately describes the basic principle of operation, the circuits used in modern X-ray timer circuits are, of course, much more complex and a thyristor would act as the primary switch rather than a mechanical switch as shown in Figure 4.2. After studying Figure 4.2 consider, for the sake of simplicity, the timer in terms of a series of blocks as shown in Figure 4.3.

AUTOMATIC EXPOSURE CONTROL

A given amount of radiation is needed to produce a given density on a radiograph. Automatic exposure control ensures that the film always receives this fixed amount of radiation despite changes in kV, mA, focus film distance (FFD) or patient thickness, etc. There are two main types of autotimer, namely the phototimer and the iontomat.

Phototimer

A phototimer such as the CGR Luminex device consists essentially of a luminescent sheet (i.e. lucite sheet which transmits light in a similar fashion to glass fibres) onto which is coated a thin photoemissive layer (Figure 4.4). This luminescent sheet is situated between the grid and cassette when used with a moving grid mechanism or directly in front of the cassette when used with a chest stand. It is, of course, within a light tight container, the side of the sheet presenting to the radiation being masked with the exception of three windows, any one or all of which may be selected by the operator.

When an exposure is made radiation passes through the patient and the grid to the luminescent sheet and then to the cassette. Light is produced at one, or all, of the windows which is then transmitted through the sheet to a series of photomultiplier tubes. A current proportional to the intensity of the light is amplified and used to charge a capacitor. On reaching a critical voltage the capacitor discharges to the base of a transistor which then produces a pulse of current to the gate of the thyristor, thereby allowing current to flow through the solenoid of the 'break' contactor terminating the exposure. The time taken for a given amount of radiation to reach the cassette and for a given amount of luminescence to be produced is, of course, governed by the intensity of the X-ray beam (mA), its quality (kV), the FFD and the thickness of the patient part.

Note: The luminescent sheet tends to absorb more radiation at low kV than it does at high kV values. A compensation circuit must therefore be provided to compensate for this effect.

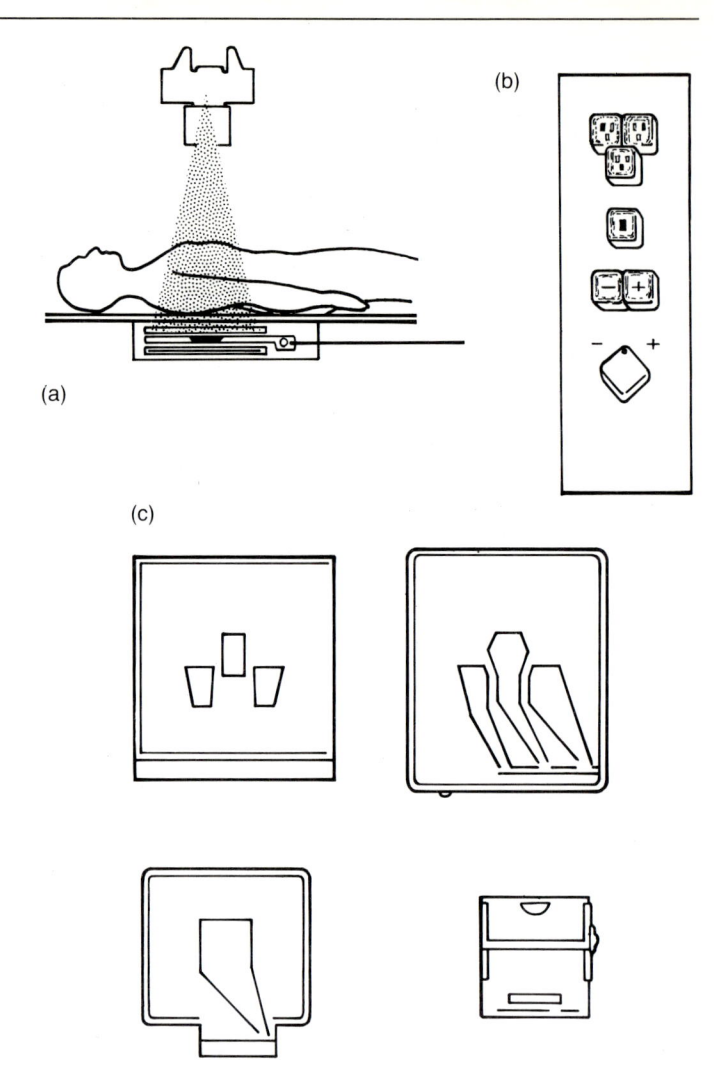

Figure 4.4 (a) Luminex system used in bucky. (b) Controls on operating console. (c) A series of different shaped sensing heads are available for different situations

Automatic brilliance control for fluoroscopy is described on page 114.

The iontomat

Automatic exposure control using ionization chambers rather than photomultiplier tubes is the system used in the majority of X-ray units. A panel containing three ionization chambers, as shown in Figure 4.5 is situated between the grid and front of the cassette. The ionization chamber panel is quite radiolucent and in normal radiography no pattern of the chambers can be detected.

The principle of operation of the iontomat circuit is similar to that of the phototimer. The capacitor is charged at a rate which is determined by the amount of ionization taking place and when it is charged to a given voltage it initiates current flow through the transistor which in turn energizes the thyristor. Current then flows through the coil of the 'break' contactor and the exposure is terminated. In the case of both the phototimer and the iontomat the exposure is terminated when a fixed amount of radiation has reached the face of the cassette (or other recording medium). The time taken for this fixed amount of radiation to reach the cassette is determined by the selected kVp and mA, the FFD, thickness of patient, etc.

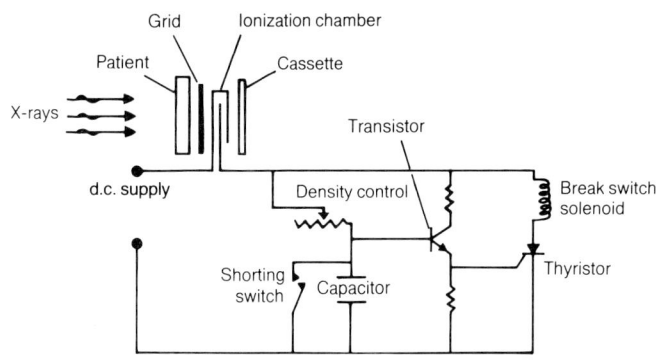

Figure 4.5 Automatic exposure control using an ionization chamber

Density control

By altering the value of a series resistor in the capacitor charging circuit, the amount of radiation and consequently the density of the film may be adjusted to suit individual requirements or to match different speed screens, etc.

Note: That in this case the time taken to charge the capacitor is determined by the resistor (density control) *and* the ionization chamber. In the case of the phototimer a photocell is used instead of an ionization chamber.

Most automatic exposure control devices have three ionization chambers for general radiography, one or more being selected at will to suit the particular requirements of the examination. Particular shapes are available for different purposes as indicated in Figure 4.6.

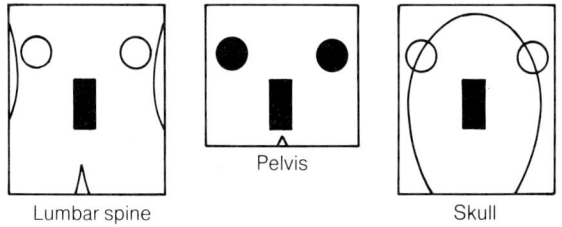

Figure 4.6 The diagrams illustrate the most appropriate selection of ionization chambers for different examinations. The selected chambers are shown in black

Care must be taken in the use of automatic exposure control devices. For instance, it is important to ensure that an ionization chamber is in the field of radiation when an exposure is made. It is also important to ensure that the correct chamber is used for a particular examination and that scatter is reduced to a minimum by careful restriction of beam size etc.

The speed of intensifying screens and the type of cassette used in the department should be standardized or, if different speed screens are used, they should be clearly marked so that the density control can be used to compensate for difference in speed.

The response or reaction time

The reaction time for any system is the time taken for the system itself to respond to a signal. In the case of the automatic exposure control it is the time it takes the circuit and the switches to respond. This time is to a large extent determined by the type of primary (exposure) switching being employed, being much longer for mechanical switches than it is for thyristors, for example. Secondary switching using a grid controlled X-ray tube or vacuum triode valves may have a response time as short as 1 ms, whilst primary mechanical contactors may have a response time of up to 30 ms. If an exposure is to be made of less than 20 ms (0.02 s) it is probably wiser to use a lower mA or slower speed screens to ensure that the exposure time is longer than 20 ms if older equipment using mechanical switching is being used.

mAs CONTROL (TIMER)

The mAs control rather than measuring a fixed period of time measures a quantity of charge, i.e. mA × time. It will be recalled that the midpoint of the high tension transformer is at earth potential and that the mA meter is connected at this point in series with the secondary winding. Because the same current flows through all parts of a series circuit it will be appreciated that current flowing through the midpoint of the secondary winding is of the same value as that flowing through the X-ray tube and it is at or near earth potential. If this low tension secondary current is fed to a capacitor, it can be arranged to initiate current flow to the primary 'break' contactor coil and terminate the exposure when a selected value of mAs has built up on its plates. When such a timer is used to control secondary switching values down to 1.0 mAs can be achieved.

GUARD TIMER

Should there be a breakdown in any of the timers previously described there would be an obvious risk of continuous emission of radiation from the X-ray tube with consequent risk of overexposure of the patient and/or damage to the X-ray equipment. To obviate this problem a guard timer is incorporated into the circuit. This timer comes into operation and terminates the exposure if the main timer fails. Once the guard timer is activated it cuts off power to the equipment which cannot be restored until the equipment has been checked by the service engineer.

PRIMARY CONTACTOR EXPOSURE SWITCHING CIRCUIT

The primary contactor circuit is interconnected with the timing circuit as shown in Figure 4.7, the voltage for these circuits being obtained from the autotransformer. The voltage must, of course, be rectified before being used to charge the capacitor. It will be noted that there are a number of switches in series with the primary contactor circuit and that the circuit cannot be completed, i.e. current cannot flow through the make solenoid and close the primary contactor switch, until each set of contacts has been closed.

From Figure 4.7 it will be noted that there are a number of switches in series connection with the primary contactor circuit and that each of these switches is controlled by a solenoid. Each of the solenoids is in series connection with a specific circuit, e.g. filament heating circuit, etc. and in consequence, each of the interlock switches A, B, C and D, will be closed only when the particular circuit with which it is connected is energized. Unless all switches are closed, the primary contactor circuit cannot be completed.

Note: We will see later in Chapter 13 that a logic control circuit may be used in modern equipment rather than a series of mechanical switches.

INTERLOCKED CIRCUITS

Some of the more important circuits interlocked with the primary contactor circuit are:

the initial delay circuit (A),
X-ray tube filament circuit (B),
anode stator supply circuit (C),
X-ray tube overload circuit (D).

Other examples of switches interlocked with the primary contactor circuit include the tomography switch which prevents an exposure being made unless the tomographic attachment is connected and 'set', and the screening interlock switch which prevents the screening circuit being energized on 'radiography' mA values, etc.

Let us consider some of these circuits in greater detail.

Initial delay circuit

When the unit is switched on at the mains and the primary circuit is energized, a time delay (sometimes indicated by a red light on the control panel) is imposed, before an exposure can be made. The necessary delay may be achieved by means of a delay tube as shown in Figure 4.8. This consists essentially of a bimetal strip heated by means of a small coil which is energized when the mains supply is switched on. The primary contactor circuit cannot be completed as switch A is open. After a fixed period of time the bimetal strip bends and contacts B–C are closed. Relay D is then energized and closes initial delay interlock switch A. At the same time switch E is opened (A and E are ganged) and the red delay light switches off indicating that the initial delay period has been completed.

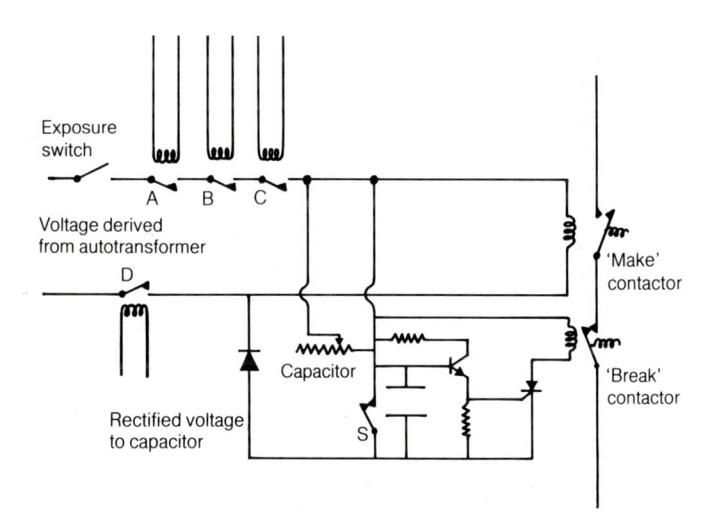

Figure 4.7 Primary contactor exposure and timing circuit

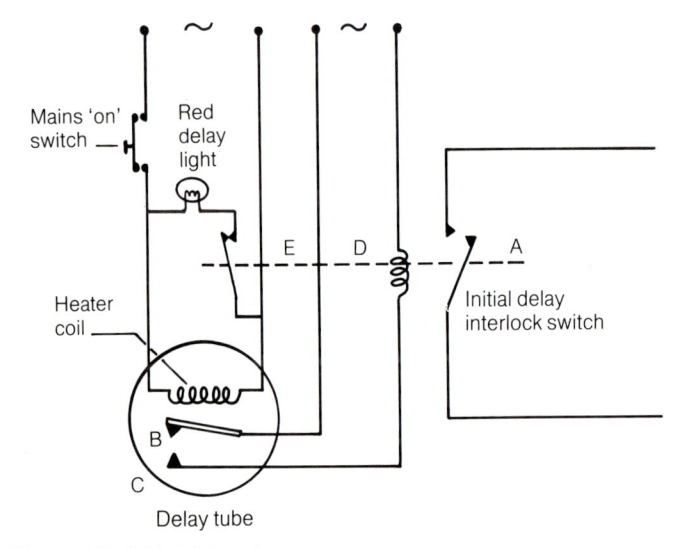

Figure 4.8 Initial delay circuit

EXPOSURE TIMERS AND SPECIALIZED X-RAY GENERATORS

Alternatively, an electronic circuit similar to the one described later for the anode delay circuit can be used.

Tube filament interlock

In series with the primary of the tube filament circuit there is an interlock switch which ensures that an exposure cannot be made until the filament circuit has been switched on. Not only must the filament circuit be completed before an exposure is made, but the filaments of the X-ray tube (and valves) must be brought up to full working temperature. This is achieved in the following way.

Tube filament boost

When the unit is put into 'prep' ready for an exposure, a delay is introduced which allows time for the filament of the X-ray tube to reach full rotational speed before an exposure is made. The X-ray tube and high tension valve filaments are brought to full working temperature by shorting out a resistance as shown in Figure 4.9.

As the filament is boosted to full working temperature when the unit is put into 'prep' it will be appreciated that the unit must be held in 'prep' for as short a time as possible. Keeping the 'prep' time as short as possible prolongs the life of the filament and thus extends its working life. As the anode is also rotated when the unit is put into 'prep' tube life is extended by minimizing the 'prep' time and thereby reducing wear on the bearings.

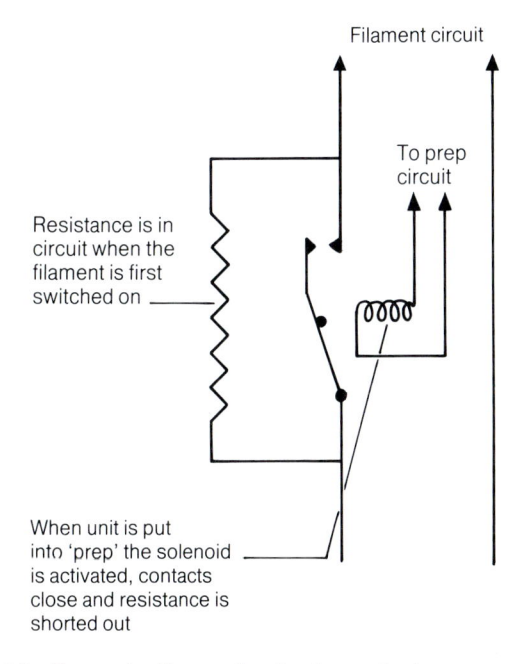

Figure 4.9 X-ray tube filament heating boost circuit

The necessary delay period during which the filaments of the valves and X-ray tube reach full working temperature and the anode reaches full rotational speed is imposed by the anode delay circuit.

Anode delay circuit

The necessary delay of approximately 2.0 s for anodes rotating at conventional speed (3000 rev/min) and up to 6.0 s for anodes rotating at high speed (up to 12 000 rev/min) may be achieved by having a capacitor and resistor connected in parallel with the supply to the coil of the interlock switch (Figure 4.10).

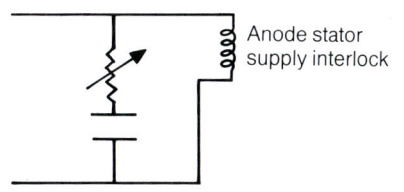

Figure 4.10 Anode delay circuit

When the unit is put into 'prep' current flows through the stator windings and also to the coil of the interlock switch; it does not, however, immediately close the switch as the current flows initially to the capacitor which it begins to charge. Only after a period of time which is determined by the value of resistance and the capacitance of the capacitor will current flow through the coil and close the interlock switch. The time delay is set by the manufacturers and depends, of course, on the time needed for the anode to reach a given rotational speed. It thus becomes impossible to make an exposure until the anode has reached full rotational speed.

X-ray tube overload protection circuits

Protection of the X-ray tube against the effects of electrical overload may be achieved in a number of ways. Most systems protect the tube against the effects of a single exposure and the anode should be given time to cool before an exposure is repeated. The length of time needed for the anode to lose all or some of its heat may be calculated from an anode cooling chart (see Figure 6.24 in Chapter 6). As the tube may not be protected against a series of repeat exposures, as would occur in angiography or cineradiography examinations, it is essential that the appropriate rating chart be consulted if the tube is not to be subjected to thermal damage (see Chapter 6).

Overload systems protecting the tube against single exposures and those protecting the tube against multiple exposures will now be considered separately.

X-ray tube overload circuit (protection against single exposure)

The interlock system described is an example of a very simple type and it ensures that an exposure cannot be made if the exposure time associated with a particular mA would result in overload conditions for the X-ray tube. From the appropriate tube rating chart it is noted that the following exposure times must not be exceeded at the mA values quoted when maximum kVp, say 90, is applied to the tube.

$$0.1 \text{ s at } 400 \text{ mA}$$
$$0.5 \text{ s at } 300 \text{ mA}$$
$$2.5 \text{ s at } 200 \text{ mA}$$

From Figure 4.11 it will be noted that circuit A, B or C corresponding to 200 mA, 300 mA and 400 mA respectively may be brought into circuit by means of the rotary switch S which is ganged to the mA control.

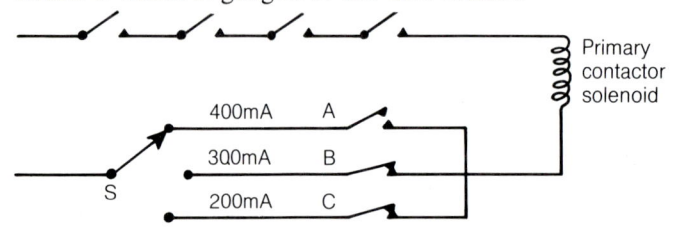

Figure 4.11 Overload protection circuit. Exposure cannot be made unless mA is reduced

From Figure 4.11 it will be noted that 400 mA has been selected and in consequence the rotating switch S to which the mA control is ganged (connected) has selected circuit A. As the interlock switch in this circuit is open it follows that an exposure cannot be made until such time as

(a) the mA is reduced thereby selecting circuit B or C where the interlock switches are closed, or

(b) the interlock switch in circuit A is closed and this, as we shall see in a moment, can only be done by selecting a shorter exposure time.

The interlock contacts in circuits A, B and C are opened or closed by means of plastic discs shaped as shown in Figure 4.12, which are connected to the spindle of the timer control. As the timer control knob is rotated in a clockwise direction to increase exposure time, a disc also rotates and at a certain position determined by the degree of rotation, the contacts spring apart opening the circuit.

Whilst the tube overload system just described is simple and effective, it is nevertheless restrictive in that a reduction in kV does not close the interlock switch and make an exposure possible, and it does not protect the tube against a series of exposures made rapidly one after the other.

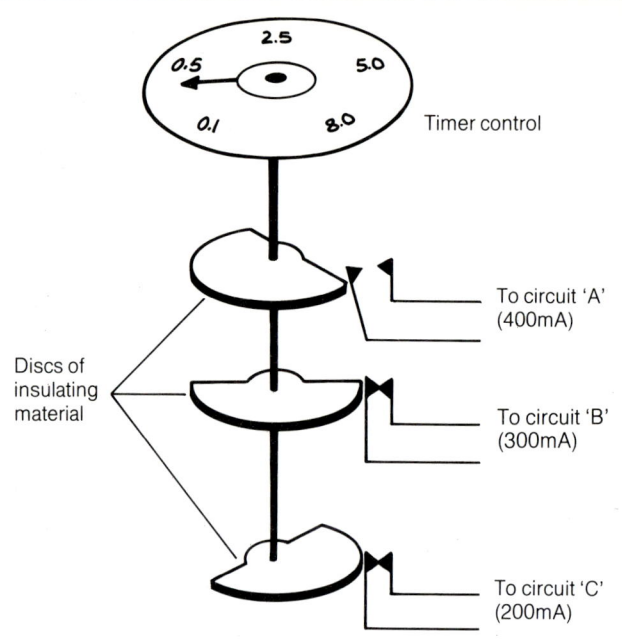

Figure 4.12 Overload protection circuit. Exposure cannot be made at 400 mA

An overload system providing an increased degree of flexibility, i.e. where kV, mA and time each have an effect on the operation of the interlock switch will now be discussed.

From Figure 4.13 it will be noted that the voltage tapped from the autotransformer which results in a particular kVp across the X-ray tube during an exposure is also applied to a transformer T1. The output voltage of T1 is proportional to the logarithmic value of kVp. Another voltage proportional to the logarithm of the selected mA T2 is added to this and finally a voltage proportional to the logarithm of the selected exposure time T3 is added to the other two.

As the three voltages being added together are logarithmic values the final voltage is proportional to the antilog value of the product of kV, mA and time. This voltage when rectified is used to charge a capacitor which, on reaching a critical voltage, operates a relay opening the tube overload interlock switch in the primary contactor circuit. It is not possible to make an exposure until such time as the product of kV, mA and time has been reduced to such a value as to be within the rating of the X-ray tube. This may be achieved by reducing the kV, mA or time factors to such an extent that the tube overload interlock switch closes and an exposure can then be made.

It must be emphasized that this system also gives protection against a single exposure only and that a proper interval of time must elapse before the exposure can be safely repeated.

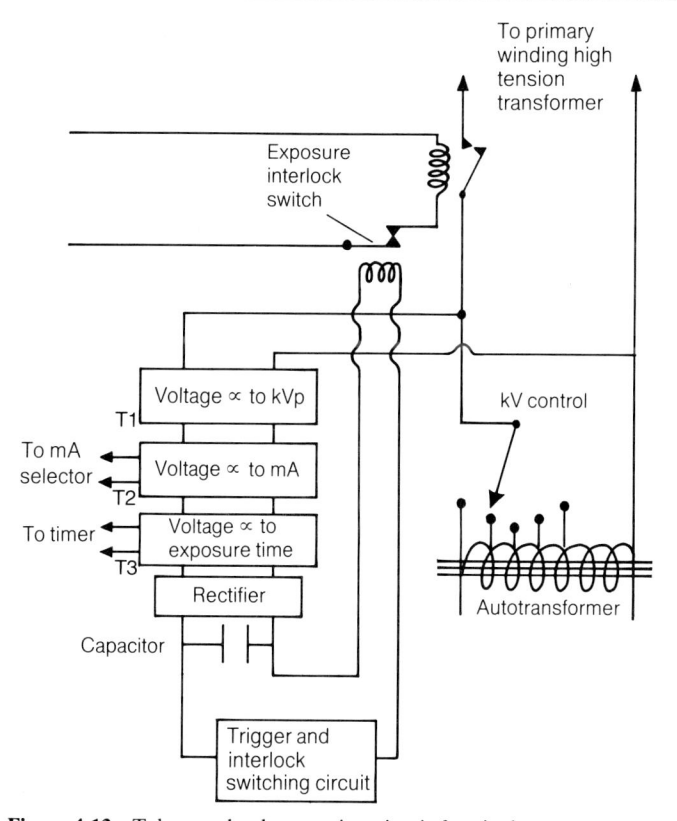

EXPOSURE TIMERS AND SPECIALIZED X-RAY GENERATORS

Figure 4.13 Tube overload protection circuit for single exposure

Percentage tube load indication

The fully charged capacitor is analogous to the fully loaded tube. Maximum product of kV, mA and time, i.e. heat units, is equated to a given charge on the plates of the capacitor. The charge acquired by the capacitor is thus proportional to the number of heat units put into the anode during an exposure. If, for example, a particular exposure represents 75% of the maximum heat units, i.e. 75% maximum permissible kV, mA and time, then the capacitor would be holding 75% of its maximum charge. The meter, although measuring charge on the capacitor, may be calibrated in terms of percentage tube loading.

Tube overload circuit (protection against multiple exposures)

An overload system which protects the tube against the effects of repeated exposures will now be discussed. This system terminates the exposure when the heating effects associated with a series of exposures reach maximum safe value.

The three critical parts of the heat path through the X-ray tube, i.e. the target, anode and the oil surrounding the tube insert are represented by three capacitors (Figure 4.14). One capacitor represents the target and when fully charged is analogous to the target of the tube at maximum safe temperature. We know that heat is conducted from the target to the mass of the anode and, similarly, the first capacitor leaks its charge through a resistor to a second capacitor which represents the mass of the anode. Thus, just as heat builds up at the target and is then conducted to the mass of the anode, so charge builds up on the first capacitor and then discharges through a resistor to a second capacitor at a similar rate. In a similar fashion as heat is transferred from the anode through the molybdenum stem by conduction and from the anode to the oil surrounding the insert by radiation, so charge is lost from the second capacitor through a resistor to a third capacitor which represents the temperature of the oil. Finally, heat transfer from the oil through the casing to the outside air is represented by the discharge of the third capacitor through a resistor.

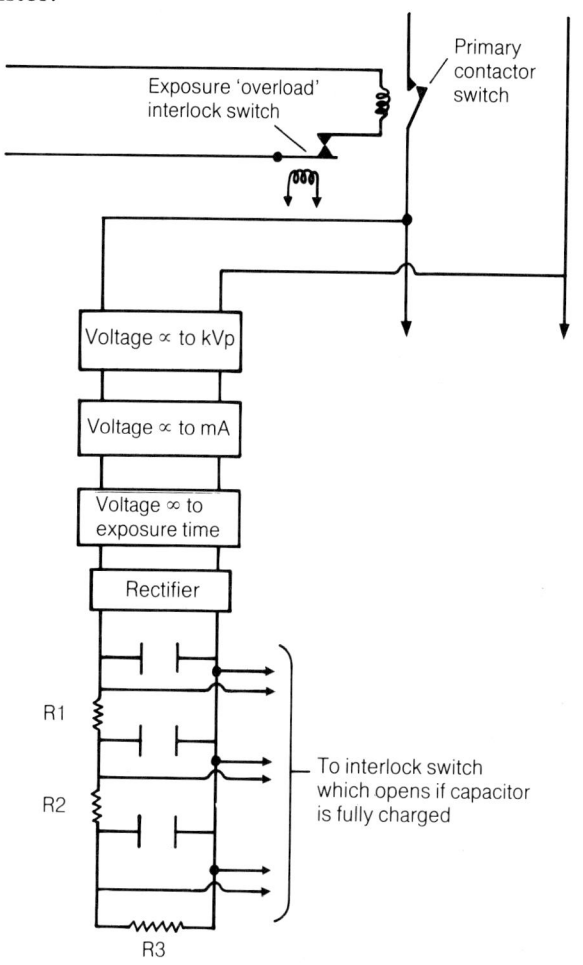

Figure 4.14 Tube overload protection against a series of exposures

We then have conditions prevailing in the three capacitors which are comparable to the conditions applying within the tube, the charge of each capacitor being proportional to the amount of heat present at each of the critical parts of the heat path through the tube. Each capacitor when fully charged represents a particular part of the X-ray tube at maximum temperature and in these circumstances a relay is opened which terminates the exposure. This system provides protection against a series of exposures.

'Loadix'

Siemens Ltd. use a method of anode thermal load indication which is very useful when the tube is used for examinations requiring heavy loading of the anode. The system is called 'Loadix' and it uses a heat sensor to measure the amount of heat radiated from the anode (Figure 4.15). The sensor provides a signal proportional to the radiated heat energy, which is then amplified and used to provide visual indication on the control panel of the extent of tube thermal loading. This usually takes the form of green, yellow and red warning lights. The green light means that the tube can be used without restriction. The yellow light means that the anode already has a high heat content and is reaching maximum safe working temperature and that an exposure may be completed but a new exposure should not be attempted until the anode has had time to cool. The red light indicates that the anode has reached maximum safe working temperature and that an exposure must not be attempted.

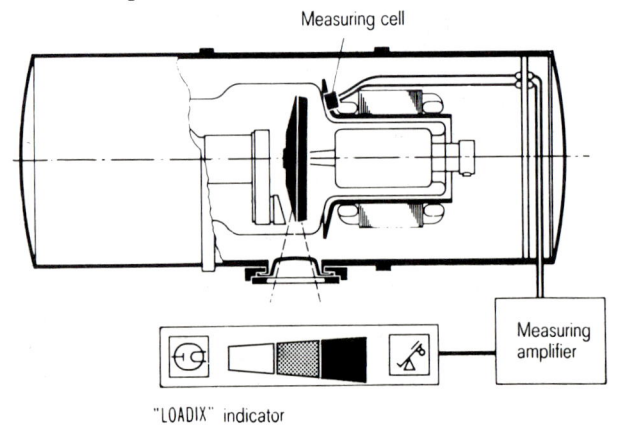

Figure 4.15 Overload protection for anode disk. A photoelectric cell checks the temperature radiation of the anode. A three colours indicator device signals level of loading of X-ray tube

This system is very useful in that it indicates the heat content of the anode due to exposures which have been or are being made. It is not, however, a substitute for overload *protection* circuits which *prevent* an exposure being made if the exposure factors would overload the tube.

THE FALLING LOAD GENERATOR

As mentioned previously, the mA meter records the *rate* of current flow and it measures this as an *average* value. As we have seen, the necessary mAs for an exposure can be obtained by using a low rate (mA) for a long time or a high rate (mA) for a short time.

We will see when we come to study rating charts that we can use a very high mA for a short time only and that if we were to continue beyond the permitted time, that the tube would be liable to damage.

The *falling load generator* reduces the mA progressively during the exposure so that the various parts of the heat path are maintained at maximum safe temperature. Because the mA starts at a very high value and progressively reduces, it follows that a given mAs can be obtained in a shorter time than would be possible using a fixed mA (Figure 4.16).

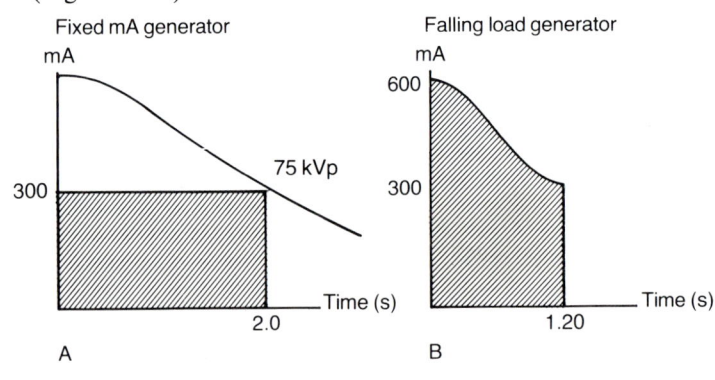

Figure 4.16 Shaded area represents 600 mAs in each case

From graph A it can be seen that to obtain 600 mAs the maximum mA we can use at 75 kVp for an exposure of 2.0 s is 300 mA.

If, however, the exposure starts not at 300 mA but 600 mA as in graph B then the 600 mAs can be obtained in say 1.20 s. The 600 mA at the start of the exposure must, of course, be reduced as the exposure progresses in line with the rating chart.

It should be borne in mind that the falling load generator does *not* give very short exposure times. It does, however, give the appropriate mAs in a *shorter* time than would be the case if a fixed mA were used. The mA may be reduced continuously during the exposure in which case it is called a continuously falling load generator, *or*, it may be reduced in a series of discrete steps in which case it is called a stepped falling load generator. The load is reduced by reducing mA and keeping the kV constant. Compensation has to be made, however, to ensure thet kV does not rise as the mA is reduced. Such compensation is, of course, automatic.

EXPOSURE TIMERS AND SPECIALIZED X-RAY GENERATORS

As it obviously reduces the tube life to maintain the target, anode, etc. and other parts of the heat path at their maximum safe temperature most modern units allow 100% or 75% of maximum tube loading to be selected. Provision is also made to allow long exposures to be made at very low tube loading when such techniques as autotomography etc. are used.

The falling load generator is ideal for use with automatic exposure control as the tube is always used within its maximum rating and there is, therefore, no longer any need to set the timer for a longer exposure than necessary to ensure that the automatic exposure device terminates the exposure and not the timer. Indeed, it should be noted that a particular mA and time cannot be selected with the falling load generator, only an mAs value.

HIGH TENSION CHANGEOVER SWITCH

When more than one X-ray tube is to be energized by a high tension transformer, i.e. over couch tube, under couch tube, skull unit, chest stand, etc., provision is made to connect the high tension supply to the particular X-ray tube we wish to energize. It is obviously important that only one tube should be energized at any one time and the circuit is arranged in such a fashion that under normal circumstances more than one tube *cannot* be energized at any one time.

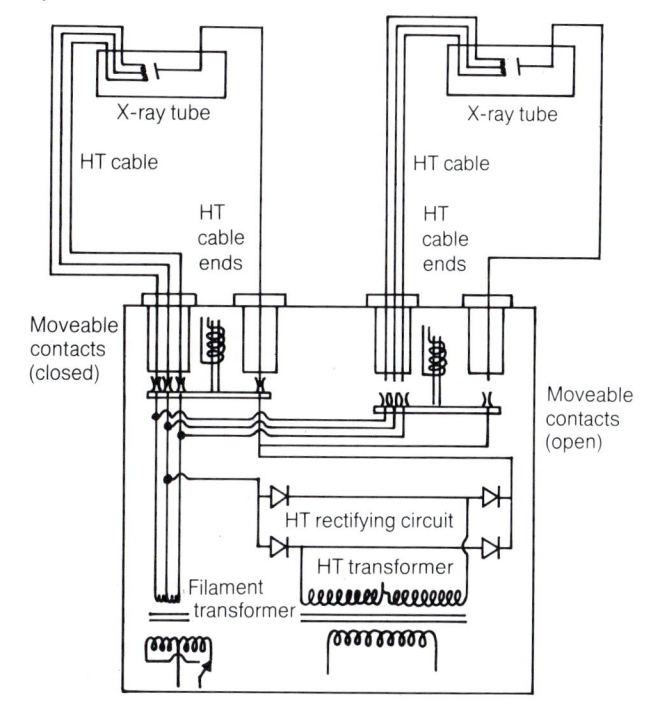

Figure 4.17 High tension changeover circuit

SHARED GENERATORS

The oil-filled casing or tank enclosing the high tension transformer etc. has a number of outlets into which high tension cables can be fitted, each pair of cables serving one X-ray tube. There may be as many as 12 such outlets supplying up to six tubes. There are a number of ways in which this situation can be exploited, for example one generator may supply a ceiling-suspended tube used with a bucky table and also the tube used with a skull unit or tomographic unit. The bucky table and the skull or tomographic unit should, of course, be in separate rooms to minimize the radiation hazard to the patient and to allow the operator to position the patient in one room whilst an exposure is being made in the other. The Code of Practice tells us that there must be a warning light, clearly visible, and close to each tube to indicate that the filament of that particular tube has been switched on so that the operator is aware that an exposure is likely to be made from it. The two rooms may share the control console as well as the generator as shown in Figure 4.18.

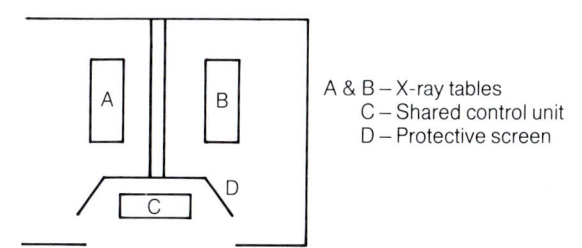

Figure 4.18 Shared generator: shared control unit

Such an arrangement saves the cost of one generator but there are also some disadvantages.

(1) Because only one console is available the operator in one room must wait until the other has made an exposure before setting up their own factors on the control console.

(2) Unless great care is taken this can lead to a situation whereby the operator uses the wrong exposure factors resulting in an increased radiation dose to the patient and staff, a waste of expensive film and a slowing down of the work rate.

(3) Any breakdown results in the loss of two rooms.

(4) There are delays in the work of one room if the other uses the generator for long periods. For this reason a generator used for fluoroscopy or angiography should never be shared.

The first two disadvantages can be overcome by using two control consoles as the exposure factors for one room can be set up independently of the other. Exposures cannot be made simultaneously as one control panel is automatically blocked off when the other one is in use. A possible layout is shown in Figure 4.19.

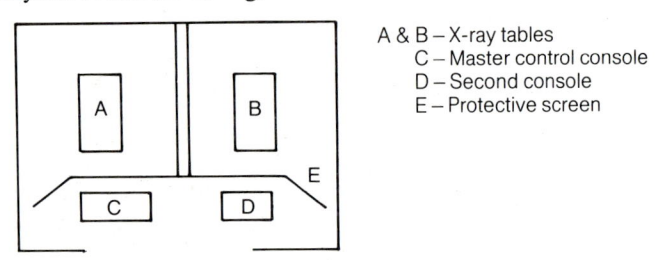

A & B – X-ray tables
C – Master control console
D – Second console
E – Protective screen

Figure 4.19 Shared generator with master control and second console

HIGH FREQUENCY GENERATORS

Until now we have considered those high tension generators which operate from a 50 (or 60) hertz electrical supply. Siemens Ltd. have recently introduced a generator which, although operating from a 50 Hz mains supply, provides high tension of approximately 10 000 Hz.

This is done by converting a 50 Hz a.c. supply to a pulsating unidirectional current by means of solid state rectifiers. Unidirectional current is smoothed by means of a capacitor so as to give a near d.c. voltage. Current is switched on and off by means of thyristors, the gates of which are supplied from a microprocessor controlled circuit, an invertor causing gate current to be switched on and off some 5000 times per second. This high frequency supply is passed to the primary of the high tension transformer and the secondary output which is, of course, twice the frequency of the primary, is then rectified before being applied to the X-ray tube. The principles of operation are indicated in Figure 4.20.

Line-voltage one or three phase

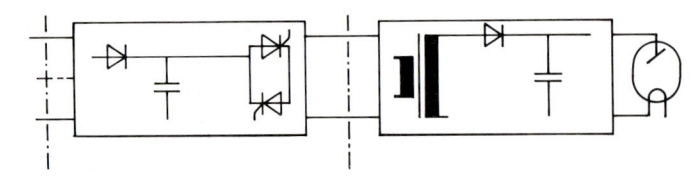

Figure 4.20 Block diagram of the high frequency generator (see also Figure 9.8, Chapter 9)

What are the advantages of this high frequency supply to and from the high tension transformer? Firstly, the secondary voltage produces, after rectification, a virtual d.c., so the unit has all the advantages associated with a constant potential circuit.

Secondly, the high frequency *primary* current means that the high tension transformer is operating in almost ideal conditions and transformer losses are very small. The greater efficiency means that the transformer can be much smaller and indeed some units are provided with the high tension transformer and the X-ray tube in one casing. These units with a microprocessor control, which is also very small, means that a relatively high powered unit can be installed in quite a small X-ray room (Figure 4.21).

Finally, because the primary current is of high frequency, the exposure time which is controlled by the thyristors can be very short. Millisecond exposures are achieved with primary switching, so this unit gives the facility of short exposure times without the need for high tension triode valves or a grid-controlled tube.

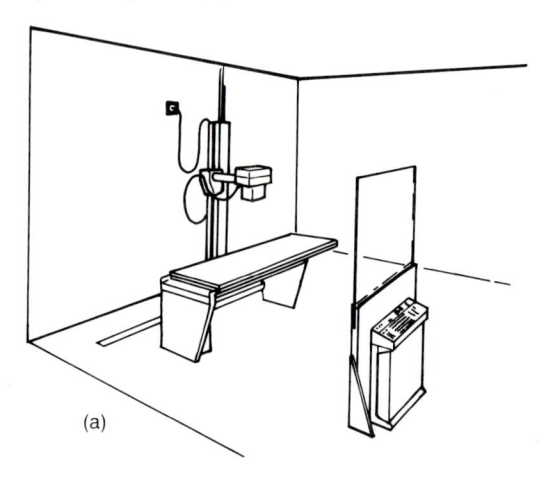

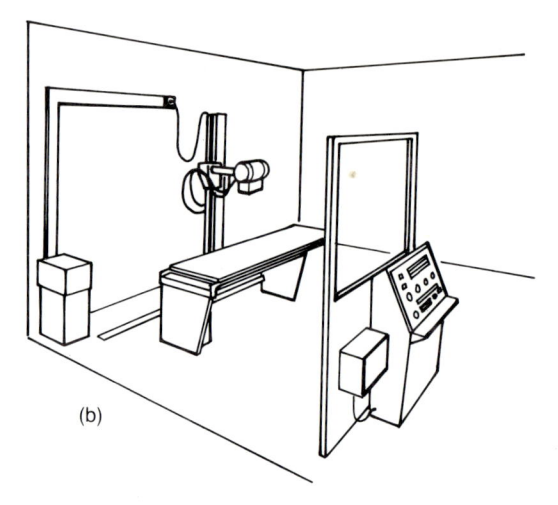

Figure 4.21 (a) medium frequency generator; (b) conventional generator. *Note* the increased space made available due to the absence of high tension cables, etc.

EXPOSURE TIMERS AND SPECIALIZED X-RAY GENERATORS

THE CONTROL PANEL OR CONSOLE

The control panel or console enables the operator to select the appropriate factors for a radiographic exposure. It may have a very simple layout as in the case of a mobile unit or be quite complex as in the case of, for example, a three-phase six-pulse unit. Whether the control panel be simple or complex however, it should be easy for the operator to read and if any difficulty is experienced by staff in interpreting the symbols used, extra labelling should be provided to clarify its use. A simple control panel is shown in Figure 4.22.

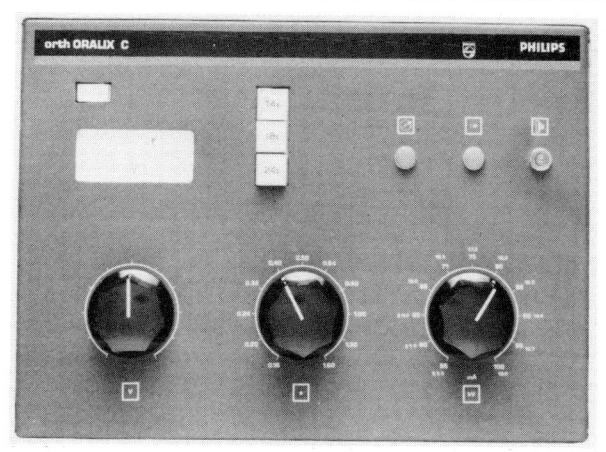

Figure 4.22 Example of simple control panel used with a low powered unit

5
Diagnostic X-ray tubes

THE STATIONARY ANODE X-RAY TUBE	56
THE ROTATING ANODE X-RAY TUBE AND SHIELD	56
The insert	56
The filament	56
Line focus principle	57
Anode rotation	58
The anode	59
Crazing of the anode surface	59
The rotor assembly	59
The stator windings	60
Stator supply circuit	62
Anode speed	62
The diagnostic X-ray tube shield	62
X-ray tube inherent and added filtration	62
Inherent filtration	62
Added filtration	62
Total filtration	62
HEAVY DUTY X-RAY TUBE	63
THE GRID-CONTROLLED X-RAY TUBE	64
THE SUPER ROTALIX METAL X-RAY TUBE (PHILIPS LTD)	65
X-RAY TUBE INSERT FOR MAMMOGRAPHY (SIEMENS LTD)	66
CODE OF PRACTICE	66
MICROFOCUS (0.1 mm AND 0.2 mm) X-RAY TUBE (SIEMENS)	66
SUPER ROTALIX CERAMIC 120 X-RAY TUBE (PHILIPS LTD)	67

Whilst the primary function of the X-ray tube is to convert electrical energy into X-rays, it may, in the case of some low powered equipment, also act as a rectifier.

Every X-ray tube consists essentially of a glass insert (containing a cathode and anode) and an oil-filled casing into which the insert is fitted.

THE STATIONARY ANODE X-RAY TUBE

The stationary anode X-ray tube (Chapter 2, Figure 2.16) is the simplest type and is used in some (but by no means all) mobile units, most dental units and all portable equipment. Its great simplicity particularly suits it to low powered simple circuits. It may be connected electrically to the high tension transformer by means of high tension cables or, alternatively and probably more likely, the stationary anode tube will be placed in the same casing as the high tension transformer – an arrangement previously described on p. 14.

THE ROTATING ANODE X-RAY TUBE AND SHIELD

Whilst the rotating anode tube is similar in many respects to the stationary anode X-ray tube it nevertheless has a number of additional features as shown in Figure 5.1.

The insert

The insert is made of borosilicate glass (a hard, heat-resistant glass, similar to Pyrex) and encloses the anode, rotor, rotor support and cathode block (into which the filament is set). During manufacture the cathode block, anode assembly and the glass of which the insert is made are all freed of remnant gas atoms. The space within the insert is then pumped out leaving it as near as possible a complete vacuum. It is important that as high a degree of vacuum as possible is preserved within the insert so that the chances of ionization occurring during an exposure are reduced as far as possible. Such ionization would lead to increased and erratic mA values, and to bombardment of the filament by positive ions.

The filament

The filament is a spiral of tungsten wire set into a nickel block. In addition to supporting the filament the cathode block focuses the electron beam on to the target area. This is achieved electrostatically, one end of the filament being in electrical contact with the cathode block which in its turn is in connection with the negative end of the high tension supply. This produces an electrostatic field of force which focuses the electrons on to the target area (Figure 5.2). Exact focusing of the electrons to the desired target area is achieved, during manufacture, by setting the filament to the correct depth in the cathode block.

DIAGNOSTIC X-RAY TUBES

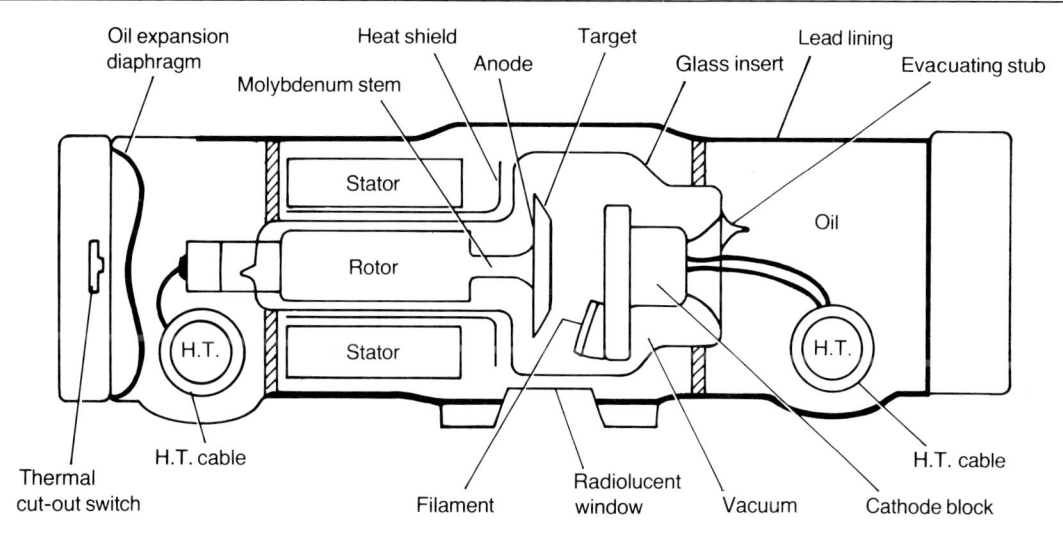

Figure 5.1 Rotating anode tube and casing

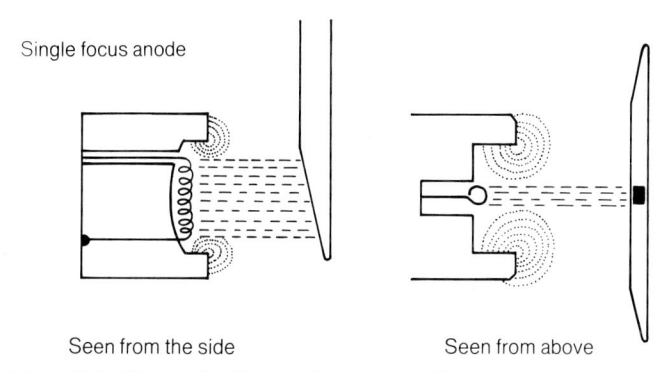

Figure 5.2 X-ray tube filament in focussing block

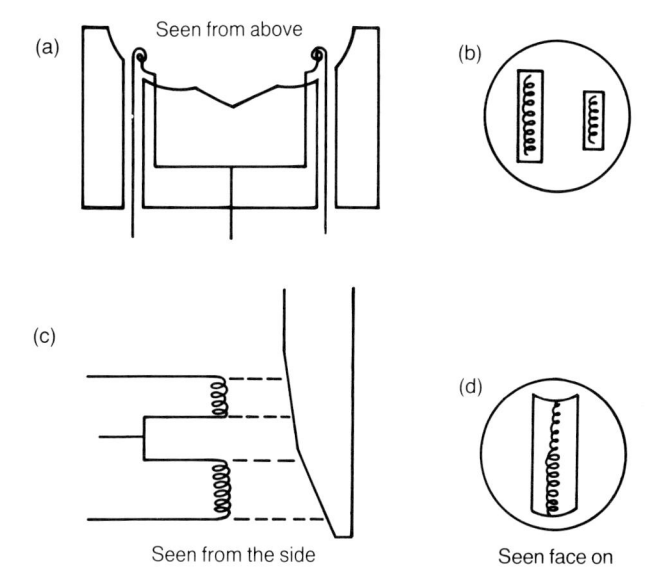

Figure 5.3 Filaments mounted side by side (a) and (b) and in line (c) (d) as in the biangular tube

Reasons for choosing tungsten as a filament material include:

(1) It is capable of stable electron emission at high temperatures.
(2) It has a high melting point (3400 °C).
(3) It has mechanical strength, long life, and can be drawn out into a fine filament.
(4) The remnant gas atoms can be removed with relative ease.

Most modern tubes have twin focii, e.g. 1.2 mm and 2.0 mm, 0.6 mm and 1.2 mm, 0.3 mm and 2.0 mm, etc.
The filaments may be mounted side by side as in Figure 5.3*a*, *b* or in line (biangular tubes) as in Figure 5.3*c*, *d*.

Line focus principle

A line has a specific length. Consider for instance a line 2 cm long. Now it will always appear to be the same length, e.g. 2 cm, so long as it is viewed 'face on', i.e. at an angle of 90° (Figure 5.4).

If, however, the line is viewed at an angle of, say, 20°, then it appears foreshortened – it looks shorter (Figure 5.5).

Note: It is only the length which appears shorter, the width is, of course, unchanged.

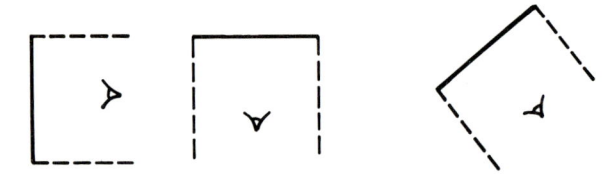

Figure 5.4 Line viewed 'face on' always appears same length

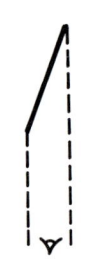

Figure 5.5 Line viewed at an angle appears foreshortened

From the foregoing it will be appreciated that the real length of a line can only be visualized by looking at it 'face on', i.e. at an angle of 90°. When viewed at any other angle it appears foreshortened.

Now it is important, from the point of view of tube loading, to have as large a focal area as possible, so that the heat produced at the target during an exposure may be spread over as large an area as possible, thus minimizing temperature rise. It is equally important, however, that the focal area be as *small* as possible to minimize geometric unsharpness of the image.

These conflicting requirements are met, to some extent, by using the line focus principle in the design of the X-ray tube, as demonstrated in Figure 5.6.

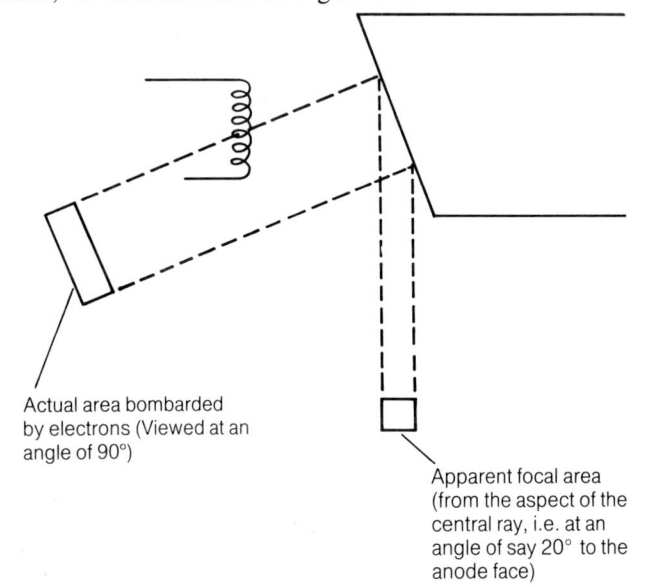

Figure 5.6 Actual and apparent focal areas

The area bombarded by electrons, the focal area, is large compared to the apparent focal area. Heat energy is therefore spread over a large area which reduces temperature rise, whilst X-rays are produced from an area which appears to be much smaller, from the aspect of the central ray. The central ray is the ray emitted from the centre of the focal area, at right angles to the long axis of the tube (Figure 5.7).

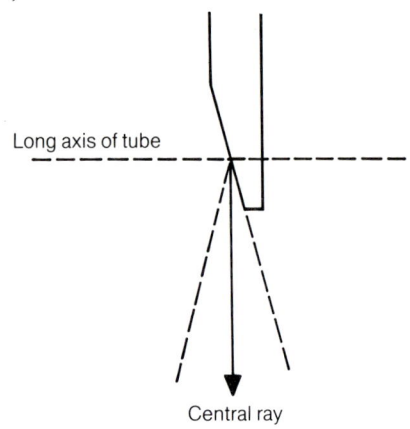

Figure 5.7 Central ray

Extra focal radiation is radiation produced outside the focal area. This extra focal radiation may be produced by electrons which have either strayed from the electron beam or by electrons which have been 'scattered' from the focal area. Extra focal radiation is produced from all parts of the anode and its support. It is, of course, much less intense than that produced from the focal area (Figure 5.8).

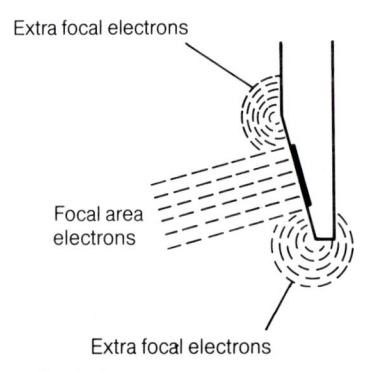

Figure 5.8 Extra focal electrons

Anode rotation

By causing the anode to rotate during the exposure the area bombarded by the electrons can be increased still further for a given apparent focal area (Figure 5.9).

DIAGNOSTIC X-RAY TUBES

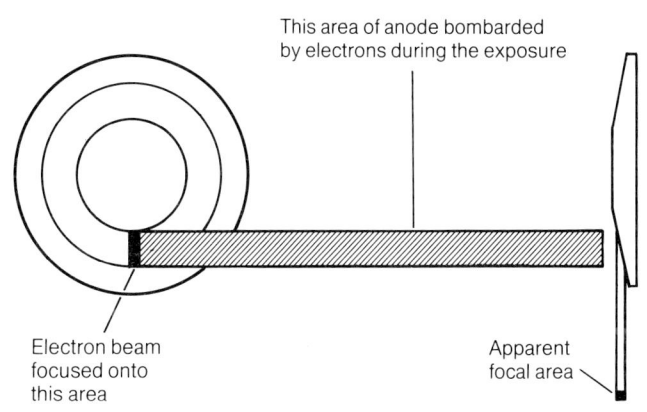

Figure 5.9 Increased area of bombardment due to anode rotation

The anode

The anode in a simple rotating anode tube is a solid disc of tungsten (or rhenium tungsten alloy) about 80 mm in diameter. Speed of anode rotation is approximately 3000 rev/min. Such a tube is used for general radiography.

Tungsten is used as a target material, for the following reasons:

(1) It has a high atomic number (74) and efficiency of X-ray production increases with the atomic number of the target.

(2) It has a high melting point (3400 °C) and is thus able to withstand the high temperatures reached by the target during an exposure.

(3) The characteristic radiation of tungsten makes a useful contribution to the beam of X-rays.

(4) It has reasonably good thermal conductivity. This is important as heat must be transferred from the focal areas to the mass of the anode.

(5) It has reasonable thermal capacity.

(6) It has low vapour pressure at high temperature which helps to preserve the vacuum within the insert.

Heavy duty, mammography and special types of X-ray tube will be described in greater detail later.

The anode angle determines not only the apparent focal spot size but also the area covered by the beam at a given focal film distance. Anode angle for general purpose tubes is usually about 17° and for skull units, image intensifiers, etc. where the required field is smaller, a narrower anode angle of about 9° may be used (Figure 5.10a). When two field sizes are required a biangular tube may be used (Figure 5.10b). The complete assembly of a biangular tube insert is shown in Figure 5.10.

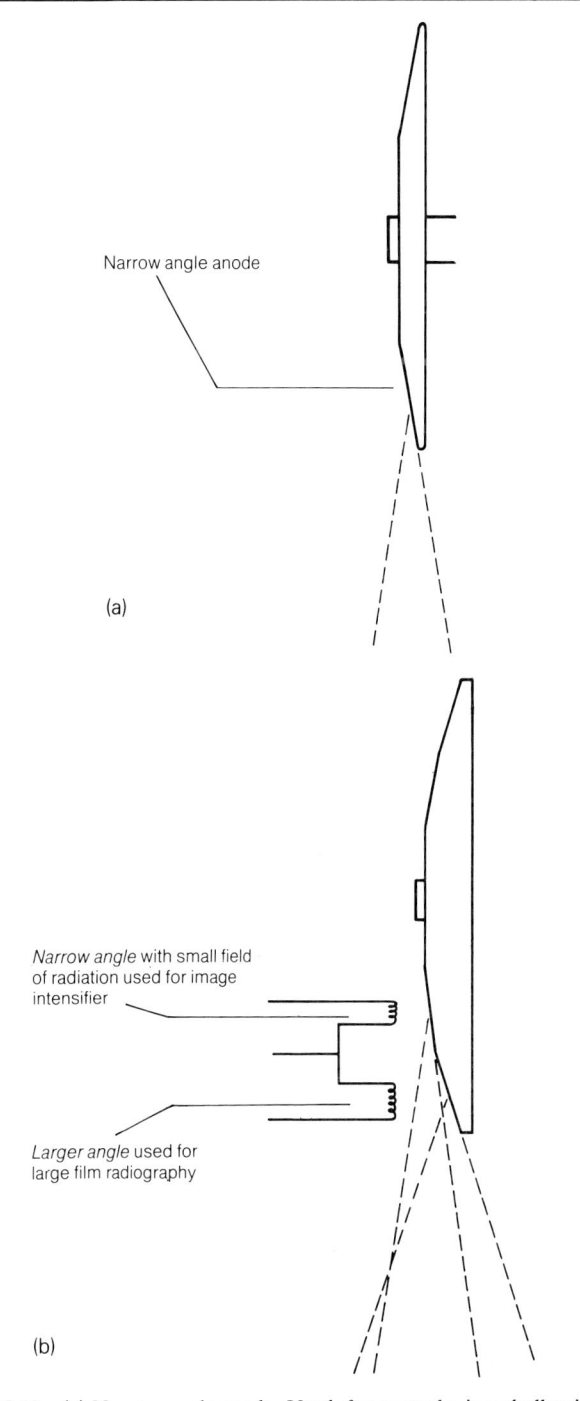

Figure 5.10 (a) Narrow angle anode. Used, for example, in a skull unit tube. The field of radiation though small covers the largest sized film used with the skull unit, i.e. 30 cm × 24 cm and provides a small apparent focus with large loading. (b) Biangular anode. Frequently used in the undercouch tube of a fluoroscopy table. *Narrow angle* with small field of radiation used for image intensifier. *Larger angle* used for large film radiography.

Crazing of the anode surface

During an exposure the surface of the target area is raised to a very high temperature. The atoms of tungsten immediately below the surface are, however, at a much lower temperature and in consequence tremendous stresses are set up in the metal. These stresses cause crazing or roughening of the target surface. Such crazing results in a loss of radiation output from the tube (photons of radiation being absorbed to a greater extent as they must now penetrate a greater thickness of metal) (Figure 5.11).

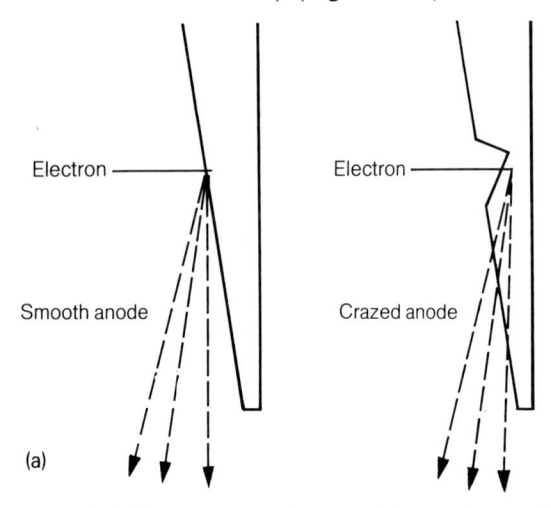

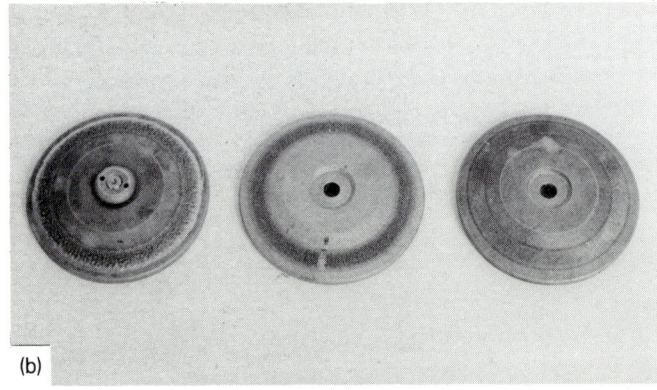

Figure 5.11 (a) Effect of anode crazing. (b) Photographs of crazed anodes

Crazing is reduced by using a rhenium tungsten alloy (10% rhenium, 90% tungsten) as the target material. Radiation output is therefore maintained at a higher level giving the X-ray tube a longer useful life.

The use of rhenium tungsten alloy as a target material helps to minimize crazing of the focal area and the use of high speed, large diameter, compound anodes permits increased loading of the focal area. The high temperatures reached by the anodes of such tubes result in thermal stresses within the anode which may cause distortion of the target angle with a consequent reduction in radiation output, a restriction in field size and in extreme cases cracking of the anode. To accommodate these stresses and to reduce the possibility of anode distortion or fracture, deliberate cracks, in the form of angled slits may be made in the periphery of the anode as shown in Figure 5.12. Alternatively, the anode may have grooves provided on each side of the focal track to allow for expansion and contraction and thus reduce the tensions within the anode. The edge of the anode is bevelled to take advantage of the line focus principle.

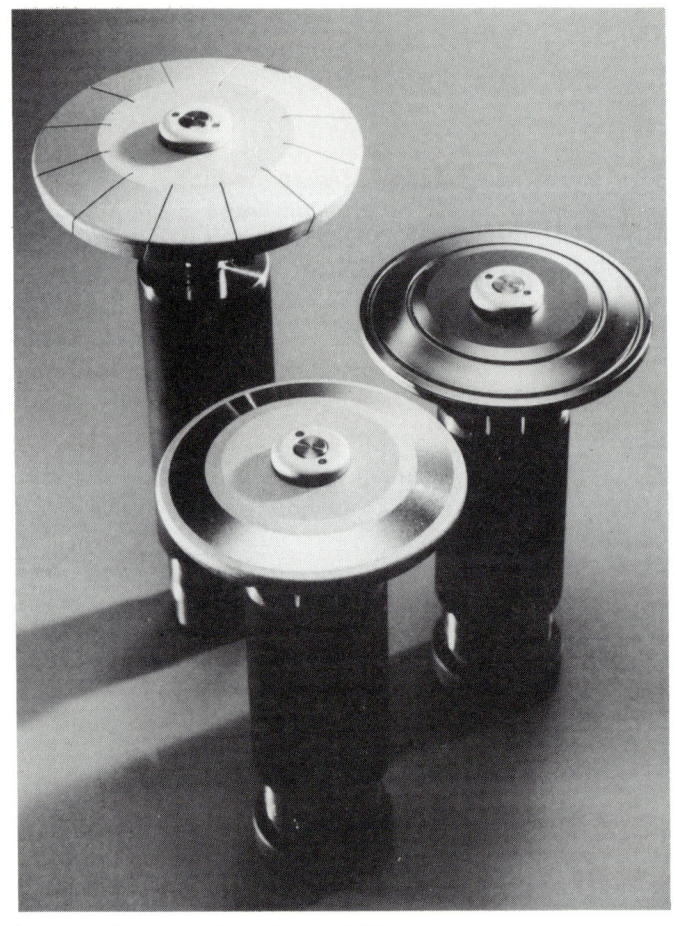

Figure 5.12 Anode discs (Philips Ltd.)

The rotor assembly

The anode disc is mounted centrally on a slender molybdenum stem which is, in its turn, secured to a copper rotor. The rotor is mounted on a steel spindle, rotation being achieved by a rotational magnetic field set up by a stator winding which, although fitted round the rotor, is situated outside the glass insert.

DIAGNOSTIC X-RAY TUBES

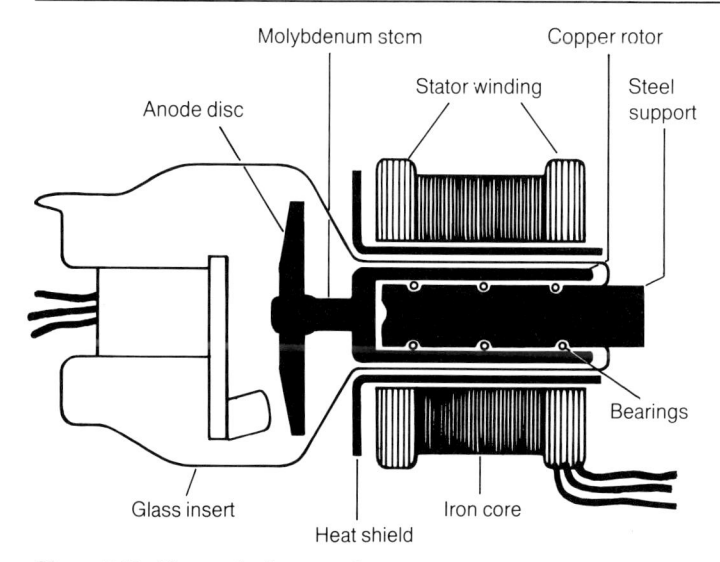

Figure 5.13 X-ray tube insert and stator

The diagrammatic representation of the anode and rotor assembly in Figure 5.13 illustrates the arrangement.

Heat produced at the target during an exposure is rapidly conducted to the mass of the anode, which experiences a rise in temperature. Subsequent conduction of heat through the molybdenum stem to the copper rotor is minimal due to the fact that:

(1) The stem is made of molybdenum, which is a metal of relatively low conductivity.

(2) The stem is of small cross-sectional area.

This thermal insulation of the rotor from the anode is of prime importance as the rotor bearings are heat sensitive, i.e. if the bearings become overheated they seize up.

As heat cannot readily pass through the molybdenum stem, it builds up within the anode causing a rapid rise in its temperature. It is for this reason, i.e. its high temperature, that heat is transferred from the anode to the oil mainly by the process of radiation, rather than being conducted through the stem.

The stator windings

The stator is composed of two windings set into a circular iron core as shown in Figure 5.14.

The rotational magnetic field is obtained by energizing two of the coils, e.g. A and B at different instants in time to the other pair, C and D; i.e. coils A and B are energized and the magnetic field associated with the alternating current flowing in the coils expands and contracts also. As the magnetic fields associated with coils A and B die away the magnetic fields associated with coils C and D expand and collapse. The magnetic fields rotate at the frequency

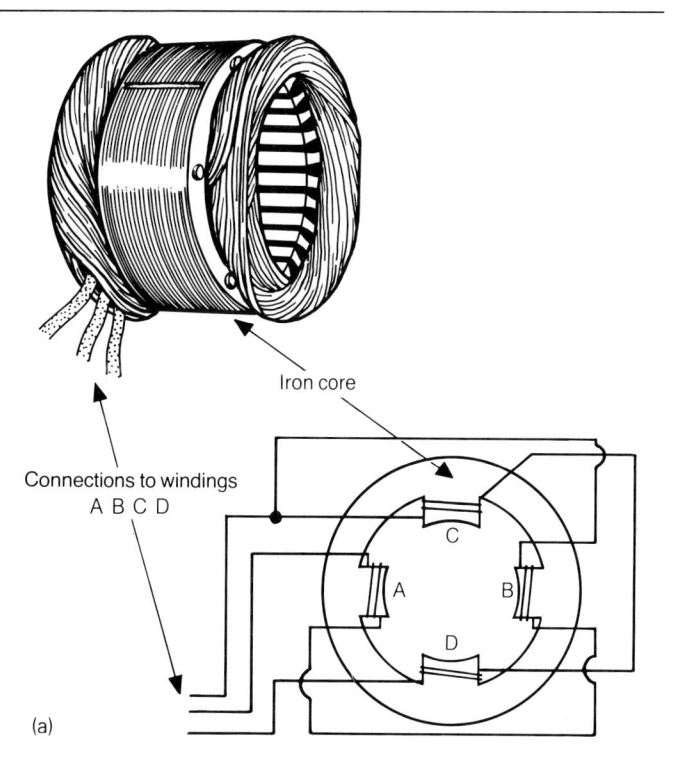

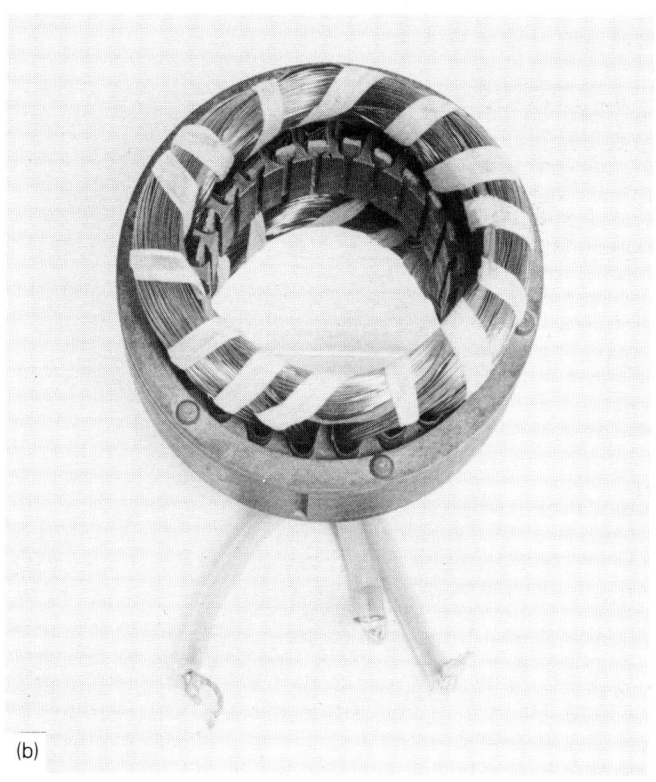

Figure 5.14 (a) Stator core and windings. (b) Photograph of stator core

of the mains supply, i.e. 50 Hz. As the magnetic fields sweep through the copper rotor a voltage is induced and current flows in the copper. The magnetic field associated with the current flowing in the copper rotor is in opposition to the force to which it was due (Lenz's Law) and in consequence the rotor begins to rotate, the speed of rotation being determined by the speed of rotation of the stator's magnetic fields which are in turn determined by the frequency of the mains supply, e.g. 50 Hz. The rotor (and anode) therefore rotate (assuming no friction) at 50 revolutions per second or 3000 rev/min.

Stator supply circuit

Current flows at peak value through coils A and B at a different instant in time to the peak current flowing through coils C and D because the currents in the two sets of windings are 90° out of phase with one another. This is achieved by placing a capacitor in series with one pair of windings (Figure 5.15).

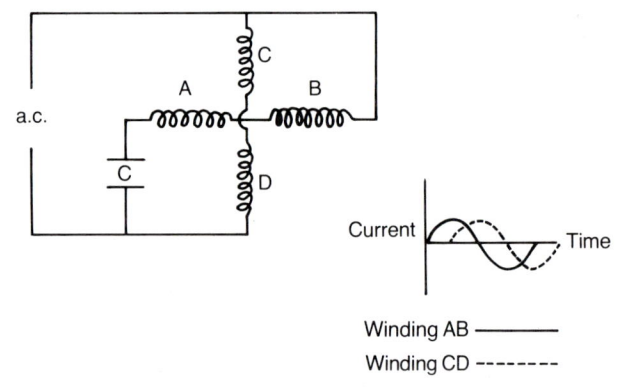

Figure 5.15 Stator supply circuit

Note: When current AB is at maximum, current CD is at zero value, i.e. they reach maximum value at different instants in time.

Anode speed

Conventional speed of anode rotation is 3000 rev/min (or slightly less). High speed anode rotation relates to speeds in excess of this, e.g. 9000 or 12 000 rev/min. The effect of this on tube rating will be discussed later.

The diagnostic X-ray tube shield

The tube shield encloses the tube insert, the latter being surrounded by oil. The shield is lead lined so that the radiation emitted by the anode is attenuated to safe levels (excepting that which passes through the tube window). Any radiation which does pass through the lead lining, called leakage radiation, must not exceed 100 mR in 1 h at a distance of 1 m from the tube focus whatever rating is used (Code of Practice).

The shield also gives access to the high tension cables. It provides attachment for the tube support, so that the tube may be mounted on the cross-arm of a floor-to-ceiling tube stand or to a ceiling-mounted gantry. The tube shield also has a flange to which can be attached filters, cones, light beam diaphragm, etc. The shield is made of steel, cast aluminium or aluminium alloy. In figure 5.16 thick lines indicate where extra lead is fitted to the inside of the shield to attenuate to safe levels all but the useful beam. The insert is held in position by the stator windings and by a collar of insulating material which fits around the filament end of the insert.

X-ray tube inherent and added filtration

Inherent filtration

This refers to the filtering effect of the X-ray tube insert, oil and radiolucent window. It is called inherent filtration because it is the filtration inherently present in the structure of the tube itself (about 0.7 mm aluminium equivalent).

Added filtration

This is filtration which is put in the path of the beam, usually at the X-ray tube window, special provision being made for such filtration at the top of the light beam diaphragm and at the top of most cones etc.

Total filtration

As the name implies, is the inherent filtration plus added filtration.

Code of Practice states that total tube filtration for a diagnostic X-ray tube must be not less than:

1.5 mm aluminium for voltages up to and including 70 kV
2.0 mm aluminium for voltages above 70 kV
2.0 mm plus 0.01 mm per kV above 100 kV

The high tension cable ends fit into two insulated sockets and the earthed metallic braid which envelopes the cables is made continuous with the tube shield by means of a collar and screw caps (Figure 5.16). Leads pass through the oil from the base of the cable sockets to complete the high tension and filament circuits. The shield is filled with oil; as the oil is heated, due to the effects of repeated exposures, it expands, the expansion being taken up by a metal bellows or diaphragm. When the bellows are fully

DIAGNOSTIC X-RAY TUBES

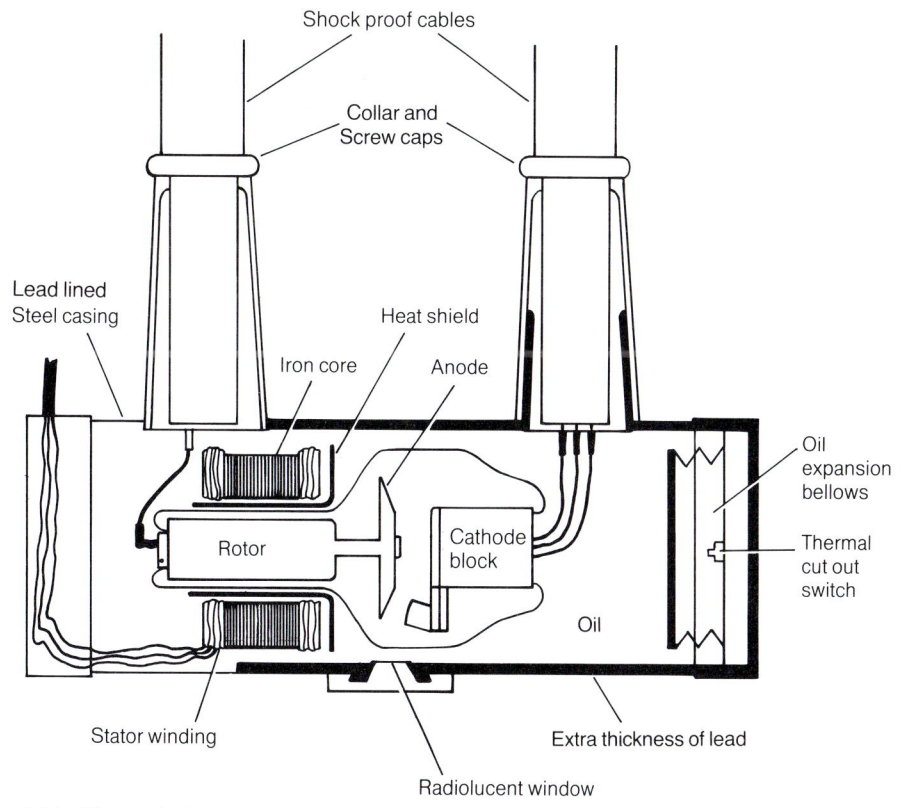

Figure 5.16 X-ray tube insert and casing. Thick lines indicate where an extra thickness of lead is needed

contracted, a microswitch is operated which prevents further exposures being made until the oil has cooled sufficiently to allow the bellows to expand and release the pressure on the microswitch. The temperature of the oil is, of course, related to the amount of heat produced at the target of the tube over a period of time, the oil gradually getting hotter as more exposures are made.

HEAVY DUTY X-RAY TUBE

The heavy duty X-ray tube, whilst basically similar to the general duty type of tube, has certain special and/or additional features. These features enable (a) *shorter exposure times* to be made, and, (b) allow *high loading* for longer periods of time.

The shorter exposure time is achieved by increasing the actual target area, i.e. by using a *larger diameter anode*, e.g. up to 120 mm, and by having *high speed anode rotation* for short exposure times. The tube will have a *compound anode*, i.e. a target area of rhenium tungsten alloy backed by molybdenum and/or graphite (Figure 5.17). Such an anode has improved thermal capacity as it can store more heat for a given temperature rise than the anode of the general duty tube previously described.

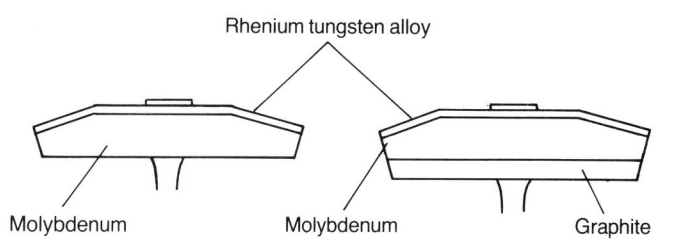

Figure 5.17 Compound anode

The greater the volume of metal, the more heat it can store for a given temperature rise.
Molybdenum has half the weight of tungsten.
Graphite has one-tenth the weight of tungsten.

The *anode angle* is usually reduced from the conventional 17–21°, to 9–14°, which improves loading for a given focal spot size.

The anode may have slits ('cracked' anode) which allow for expansion and contraction of the metal without distortion. Such a tube would normally be fitted with a *heat exchange unit*, consisting of pipes in the oil-filled casing through which water or oil is pumped before being returned via flexible pipes to a heat exchange unit, where the water or oil is cooled before being piped back to the oil-filled casing.

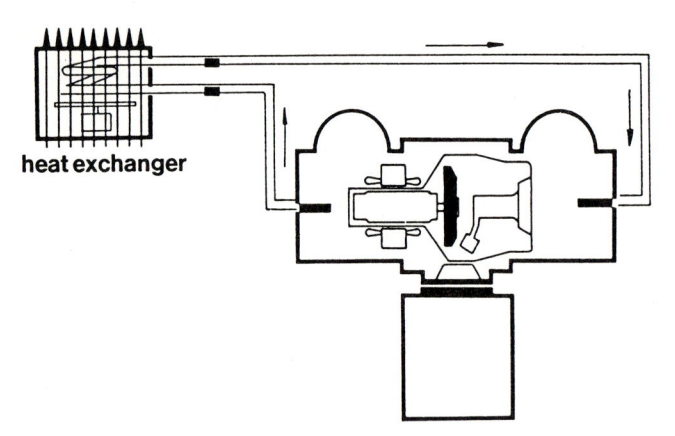

Figure 5.18 Heat exchange unit

The temperature of the anode may be monitored by a *heat sensor* which is placed inside the oil-filled tube casing, behind the anode disc (Siemens Loadix system) (Chapter 4, Figure 4.15). Information regarding the temperature of the anode is presented to the radiographer in the form of green, yellow and red indicator lights on the control panel. Green means that the tube can be operated without restriction, yellow that the exposure can be completed but a new loading must not be started (accompanied by a warning signal) and red that the tube has reached its maximum load limit and, of course, must not be used until the temperature has dropped sufficiently to ensure safe operating conditions.

Heavy duty tubes of this nature would be used whenever short exposure times and sustained high loading are needed, e.g. cine, serial radiography, etc.

THE GRID-CONTROLLED X-RAY TUBE

The grid-controlled X-ray tube acts as a secondary switch as well as a producer of X-rays. It may be drawn diagrammatically as in Figure 5.19.

The grid-controlled X-ray tube uses a negative field of force to repel filament electrons, preventing them moving from filament to target. If the negative bias is removed from the grid (by the application of a positive pulse) electrons are able to move to the target and produce X-rays.

In use the secondary circuit is energized by pressing the 'prepare' button. No X-rays are produced at the target of the tube, however, as the grid has a negative bias. At the

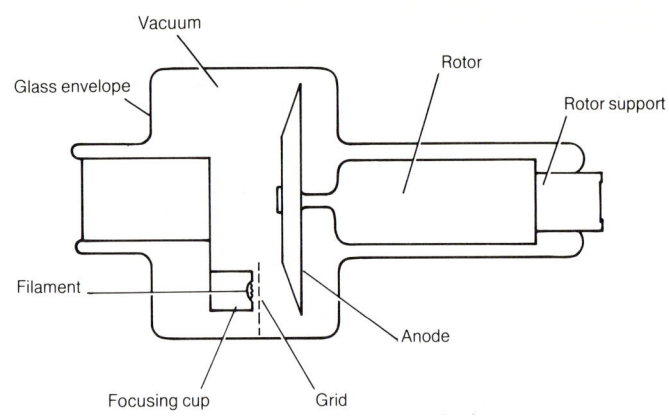

Figure 5.19 Grid controlled X-ray tube insert

start of an exposure the negative bias is removed from the grid and electrons move across the tube at high speed producing X-rays (and heat) at the target of the tube. The exposure is terminated when the negative grid bias is re-imposed. The removal and re-imposition of the negative grid voltage is performed by the timing circuit, the length of the exposure being determined by the length of time the negative voltage is removed from the grid.

As the exposure is initiated and terminated by starting and stopping electrons, which have virtually no mass and therefore practically no inertia, very rapid exposure sequences can be achieved. The grid-controlled tube is frequently used with 6- or 12-pulse circuits. Such equipment is well suited to cine fluorography, switching of the tube in this manner produces pulses of radiation which are synchronized to the movements of the film in the cine camera (Figure 5.20).

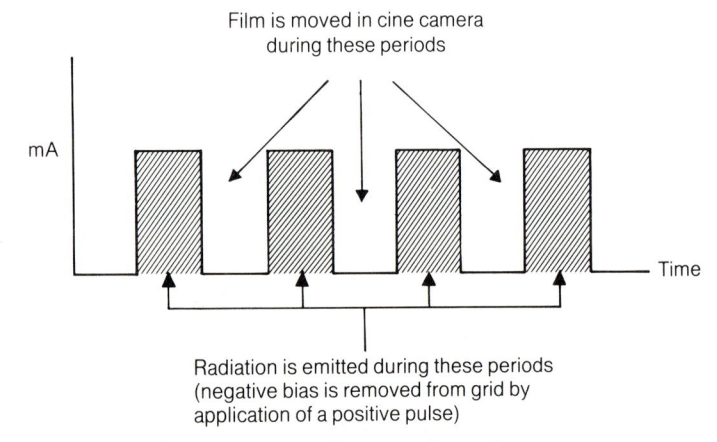

Figure 5.20 Pulsed exposures for cine radiography

Note: In appearance the grid controlled X-ray tube may appear similar to a conventional X-ray tube. This is due to the fact that there may be no actual grid in the 'grid-

DIAGNOSTIC X-RAY TUBES

controlled' tube, the electrostatic effect being achieved by making the specially shaped focusing cup highly negative with respect to the filament (Figure 5.21).

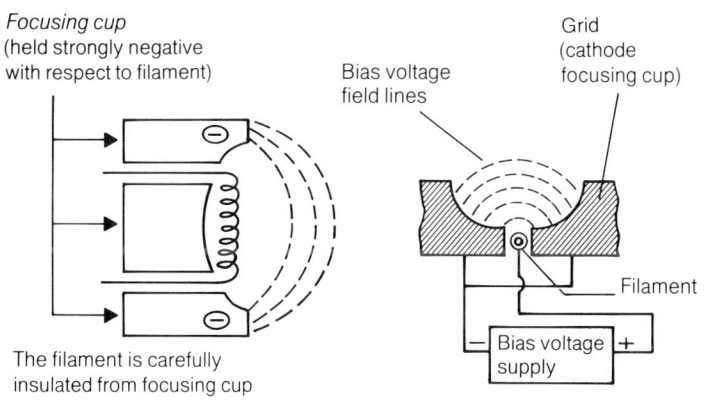

Figure 5.21 Focusing cup of grid controlled tube

THE SUPER ROTALIX METAL X-RAY TUBE (PHILIPS LTD.)

One of the limiting factors in tube loading is the maximum 'safe' temperature of the filament. This 'safe' temperature is related not only to the temperature at which it would melt (or have an unacceptably shortened life) but also to the temperature at which evaporation of the tungsten filament would become excessive. Evaporation not only makes the filament thinner but leads to the build up of a thin layer of tungsten on the inner surface of the insert.

This layer of tungsten does not constitute much of a threat in terms of filtration of the beam as the layer of tungsten is *very* thin; it does, however, form a third electrode which may lead to premature breakdown of the tube if the insert is made of glass (glass being vulnerable to electron bombardment). In this case the formation of the third electrode due to evaporation of the filament is a limiting factor in terms of tube rating.

The Rotalix 'metal' tube has an insert made of metal (steel), the central portion of which is set into glass at the anode end and ceramic at the other, as indicated diagramatically in Figure 5.22, and as a photo in Figure 5.23, the glass and ceramic acting as electrical insulators. The metal part of the tube is earthed and thus captures stray electrons. It has a window made of beryllium which absorbs less of the primary beam than glass or metal and because the metal part of the tube is earthed it is possible to bring the tube collimator much closer to the anode than in conventional tubes which results in a reduction in the effects of off-focal radiation.

As there is no danger of breakdown of the tube due to vaporization (as in the case of the glass insert), it is possible to heat the filament to higher temperatures. This leads to an improvement in rating. It also makes it possible to use higher mA values at lower kVs than was previously possible.

The metal tube is fitted with a large diameter *compound anode* (rhenium tungsten alloy target backed with molybdenum) which may contain slits to allow for expansion and contraction of the metal without distortion of the anode. The anode would normally be capable of *high*

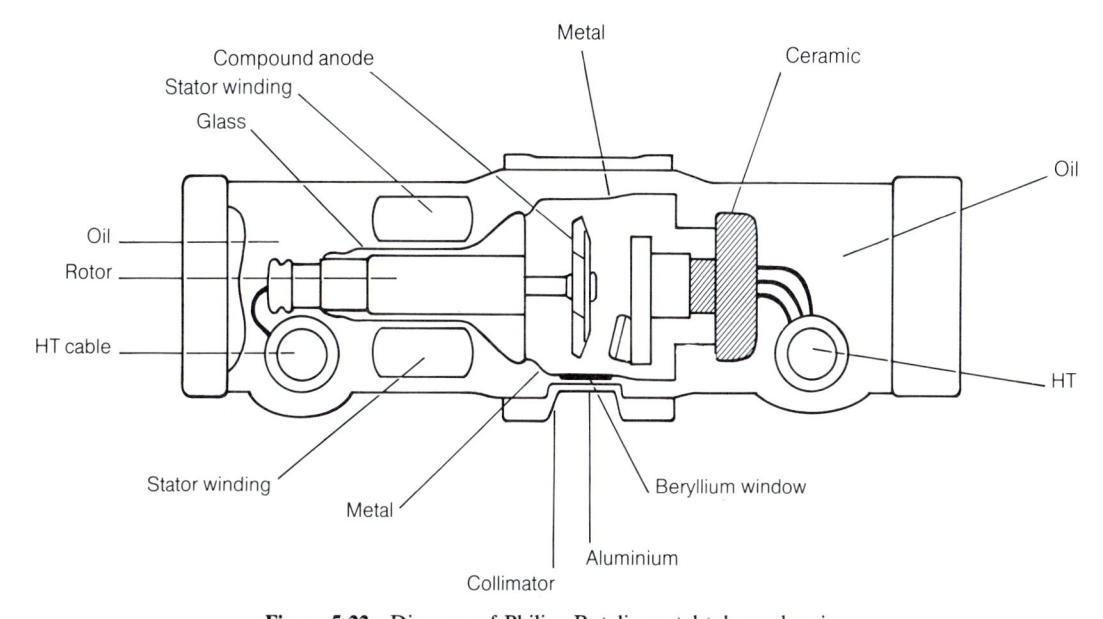

Figure 5.22 Diagram of Philips Rotalix metal tube and casing

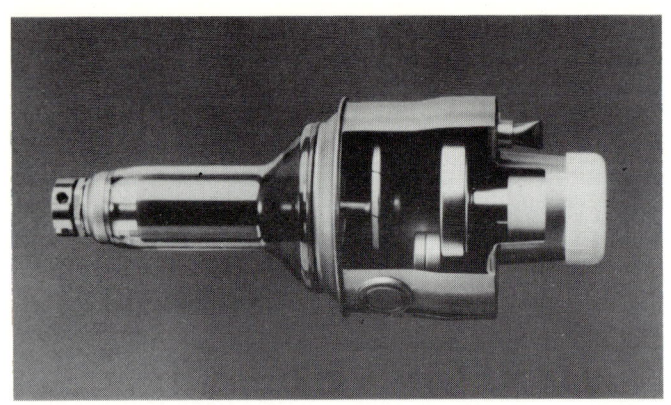

Figure 5.23 Photograph of Rotalix metal tube insert

speed rotation, the oil would be *water cooled*, and the tube used in conjunction with a *6- or 12-pulse generator* for diagnostic examinations requiring short exposure times and sustained high loading, e.g. cine radiography, tomography, serial radiography, CAT units of the later generation, etc. Focal spot sizes available are 0.3/0.7 mm, 0.6/1.2 mm, 0.6/1.8 mm. The anode angle is 11° or 12°.

Note: There is less scatter within the tube as there is no oil between the beryllium window of the insert and the window in the casing.

X-RAY TUBE INSERT FOR MAMMOGRAPHY (SIEMENS LTD.)

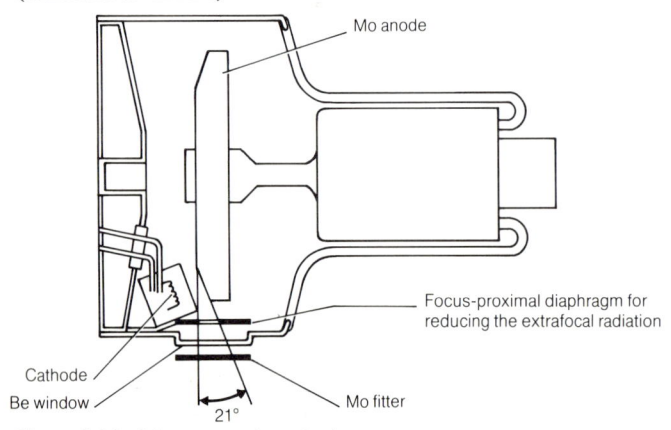

Figure 5.24 Mammography tube insert

Some mammography techniques require the use of soft radiation; such radiation is best produced by a tube operating at low kV and preferably with a molybdenum anode in place of the more commonly used tungsten (Figure 5.24). The k_α characteristic radiation of molybdenum is of much lower energy (longer wavelength than that of tungsten and therefore forms a useful part of the low energy beam needed for mammography).

The cathode end of the beam is limited by means of a diaphragm so that the radiation dose to the patient's chest wall is minimized during the exposure.

The tube has a *beryllium window* as this is less absorbent than glass, an important factor with a low energy beam, and a *molybdenum filter* rather than aluminium. Unlike aluminium, molybdenum is translucent to the characteristic radiation emitted by the molybdenum target and it therefore allows the radiation we particularly require to pass through the filter with minimal absorption. A *proximal diaphragm* reduces the effects of extra focal radiation.

The filament of the mammography tube is set much closer to the anode than that of the conventional tube which means that a given mA is obtained at a lower filament temperature. This is of importance as it results in a reduction in the amount of tungsten evaporation taking place. The deposition of such tungsten on the inner surface of the tube insert is of little importance in the conventional tube, but is a significant factor in the mammography tube which produces low energy radiation which would be much more readily absorbed than the high energy beams produced by conventional tubes. Indeed, the absorption of low energy radiation would be an advantage in the latter case.

The focal spot size of the Siemens tube is 0.6×0.6 mm, and the heat storage capacity of the tube is high enough to allow up to 60 radiographs per hour to be taken. The tube is intended for use with the Siemens Mammomat unit in conjunction with a three-phase (6-pulse) generator giving 300 mA at 25 kV. This unit is described in greater detail in Chapter 11.

CODE OF PRACTICE

In the case of tubes for general examinations which may be used for soft tissue procedures such as mammography, when the filter is removable there must be some permanent visible indication on the tube housing that the filter has been removed. Even when the main filter has been removed the total filtration must not be less than 0.5 mm equivalent of aluminium; this is particularly important in the case of beryllium window tubes, the inherent filtration of which is only equivalent to about 0.05 mm of aluminium.

MICROFOCUS (0.1 mm and 0.2 mm) X-RAY TUBE (SIEMENS)

As previously mentioned the X-ray tube may be used as a switch as well as a producer of X-rays. It will be recalled that this is achieved by making the grid of such a tube (or the focusing cup) negative with respect to the filament.

DIAGNOSTIC X-RAY TUBES

To stop all electrons from leaving the filament, i.e. to make the tube operate as an open switch, a bias voltage of some 2400 V must be applied to the grid (or focusing cup). If the voltage is of some value less than that required to *completely* stop electron flow it can be appreciated that such a bias on the focusing cup will have an effect on electron flow and indeed the negative bias tends to push the electrons together as shown in Figure 5.24. In short it acts like the 'normal' negative field of force associated with the conventional focusing cup in the conventional X-ray tube but its effect is much greater.

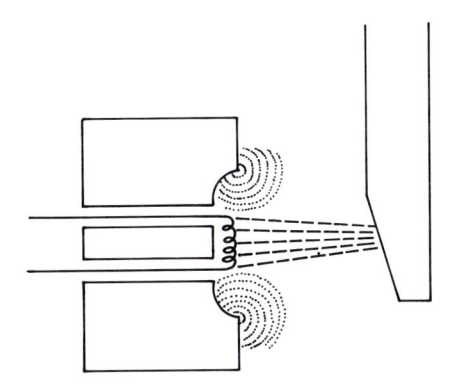

Figure 5.25 Focusing arrangement for microfocus tube

By such means and with a negative bias of 400 V a focus of 0.1 mm × 0.1 mm can be achieved and by using rather less negative bias a focus of 0.2 mm × 0.2 mm can be produced.

A microfocus tube of this nature is of course ideal for macroradiography. The 0.2 mm focus is used for macroangiography with a times two magnification factor and the 0.1 mm for macroangiography with a times three magnification factor. The 0.2 mm focus is used for angiography of the abdomen and the 0.1 mm focus for angiography of the hand or foot. Abdominal angiography with the microfocus tube is made possible by the high speed of anode rotation which is 17 000 rev/min.

SUPER ROTALIX CERAMIC 120 X-RAY TUBE (PHILIPS LTD.)

This is a heavy duty tube capable of short exposure times and sustained heavy loading. This tube differs from more conventional tubes in that the anode is rotated on an axle with bearings at each end (Figures 5.26 and 5.27). It has a large diameter compound anode disc of 120 mm diameter which is contained within an earthed metal envelope, with ceramic insulation.

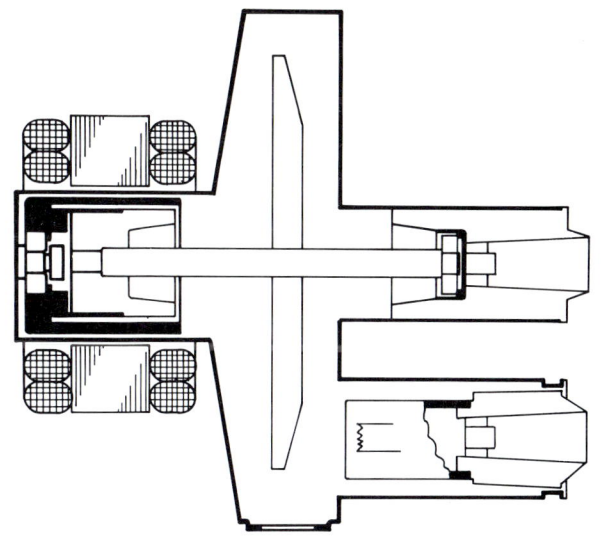

Figure 5.26 Diagrammatic representation of insert

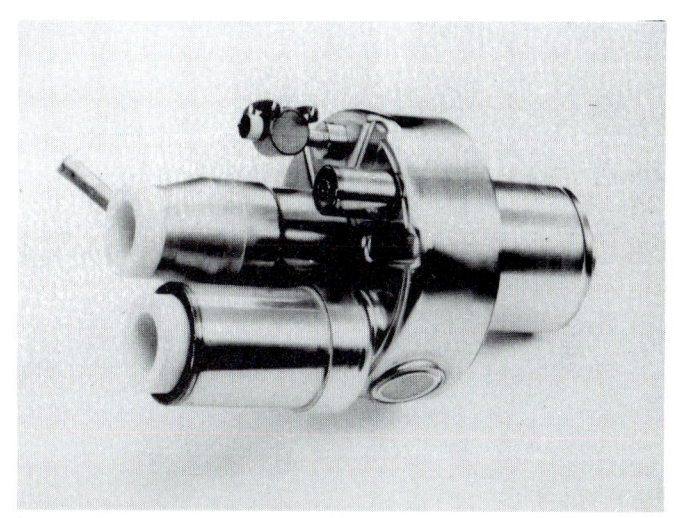

Figure 5.27 Photograph of actual insert

The target is of rhenium alloyed tungsten on a molybdenum anode disc. Focal spot sizes of 0.6 mm and 1.3 mm or 0.5 mm and 0.8 mm are available. The target angle is 13° for the former and 9° for the latter. The anode rotates at 8000 rev/min. The starting time is 1.0 s for the 0.6 mm and 1.3 mm tube and 1.4 s for the 0.5 mm and 0.8 mm tube.

The insert is contained within a steel casing which is no larger than that required for a conventional tube (Figure 5.28). An external heat exchange unit is used with this tube.

The main applications for this type of tube are serial radiography, tomographic series, cine, etc.

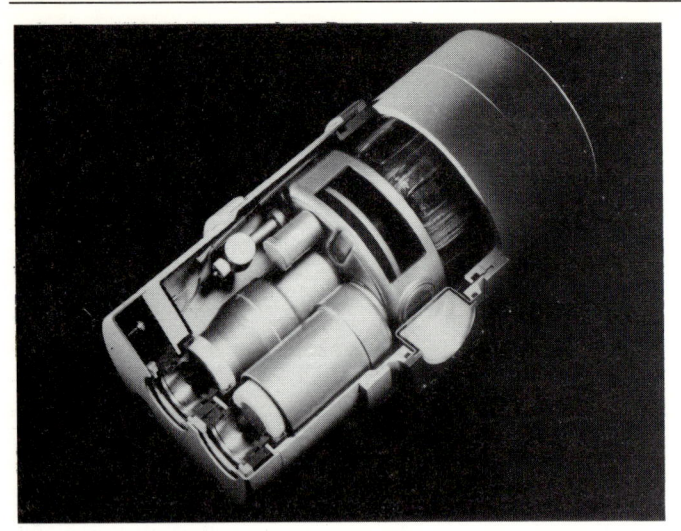

Figure 5.28 Super Rotalix Ceramic tube in housing, cut away to show internal arrangement

6
Tube rating and tube supports

HEAT AND TEMPERATURE	69
THE RATING OF X-RAY TUBES	71
Maximum power	72
TYPE OF RECTIFICATION	72
The three-phase rectified circuit	75
Focal area (focal spot size)	76
Relationship of temperature rise to area and linear dimensions of focal area	76
Speed of anode rotation	76
50 cycle stator operation	77
High speed 150 or 180 cycle stator operation	77
Continuous operation (fluoroscopy)	77
Heat transfer through the X-ray tube	77
Heat path (stationary anode)	78
Heat path (rotating anode)	78
Anode cooling chart	78
Tube housing cooling chart	79
Angiographic rating chart	80
Cine radiographic rating chart	81
X-RAY TUBE SUPPORTS	82
Floor stands	82
Floor to ceiling stands	82
The ceiling-suspended tube support	82
Motorized movements	84
Advantages of ceiling-suspended tubes	84
Disadvantages	84
'C' arm supports	84

HEAT AND TEMPERATURE

Before moving on to study tube rating let us see what is meant by heat and temperature and the various heat transfer processes.

Heat is a form of *energy*. The SI unit of energy is the *joule* and 1 J/s equals 1 W. (This unit should not be confused with the heat unit (HU) used by radiographers only). The application of heat energy to a body or the transfer of heat energy from a body causes either a change in its state (i.e. it will melt, boil, freeze or condense), or a change in its temperature. It is interesting to note that whilst a body is actually changing state its temperature remains constant. For example, the application of heat energy to a pan of water causes the temperature of the water to rise until it reaches a temperature of 100° Celsius (373 K). It then begins to change into steam. The application of greater amounts of heat energy (turning up the gas flame) does not cause an increase in the temperature of the water, it remains at 100°C; it does, however, cause it to change state (turn into steam) more rapidly. It requires a small amount of energy to make all the water boil compared to the large amount of energy needed to change all the water into steam.

Temperature is the relative hotness or coldness of a body compared to some fixed value such as the boiling point of water or the melting point of ice. Temperature may be measured in degrees Celsius, °C (centigrade), degrees Fahrenheit, °F, or degrees kelvin, °K.

The Celsius scale is divided into 100 divisions ranging from the lower fixed point (the melting point of ice) to the upper fixed point (the boiling point of water) (Figure 6.1).

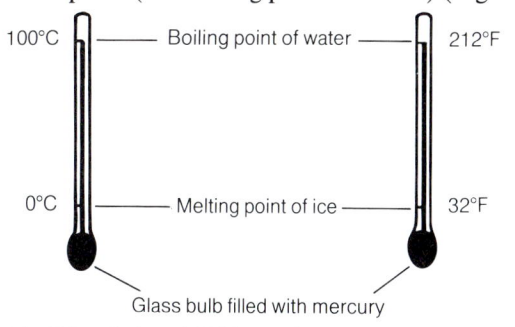

Figure 6.1 Fahrenheit and Celsius scales

It is important that you understand clearly the difference between the terms *heat* and *temperature*. For example, a cupful of boiling water and a bathful of boiling water are each at the same temperature (100°C) but the heat content is different in each case. The heat capacity of a body is defined as the amount of heat needed to raise its temperature through one degree kelvin. It is expressed in joules per degree kelvin J K^{-1}.

Heat capacity $C = mass \times specific\ heat\ capacity$

Specific heat capacity is the heat energy needed to raise unit mass of the substance through one degree kelvin. It is expressed in joules per kilogramme per degree kelvin ($J\,kg^{-1}\,K^{-1}$). (The specific heat of copper is about $400\,J\,kg^{-1}\,K^{-1}$.)

To raise the *temperature* of a body, heat energy must be given to it. Assuming that no heat is lost to the surrounding air the temperature rise experienced by the body is determined by the amount of heat energy it has been given, the mass of the body and the material of which it is composed. The applied energy may be electrical, chemical, mechanical or electromagnetic. Thus a gas flame or an electric current may be used to raise the temperature of, say, a piece of copper. Now the smaller the piece of copper the greater will be the temperature rise for a given amount of heat energy. Let us now consider the difference between the copper when it is cold and when it is heated. The cold copper, like all matter, is composed of atoms, which are bonded together to form molcules. At room temperature the molecules are vibrating and, as the copper is heated, the rate of vibration also increases. If one end of a copper bar is heated as shown in Figure 6.2, the molecules of copper in the region of the flame vibrate at an increased rate. If we touch the other end of the bar we find that it gradually gets hotter and hotter, in fact, the heat is transferred from one end of the bar to the other. The transfer of heat through the bar is achieved by the gradual increase of molecular vibration throughout the bar, vibration of one molecule causing vibration of the next until all the molecules are vibrating at the same rate (assuming no loss of heat energy to the surrounding air). At this point the temperature of the bar would be constant throughout. Transfer of heat through a solid in this way is called *conduction*. If the copper is heated to a temperature of 1080°C, it begins to melt (change its state). If the source of energy is removed the thermal activity (molecular vibration) of the copper decreases and its temperature falls until it reaches the same temperature as its surroundings (room temperature). When the copper bar is at the same temperature as its surroundings there is, of course, no further transfer of heat. From this it can be appreciated that a hot body transfers heat to a colder body and that heat transfer is at a maximum when the temperature difference between the bodies is greatest. As the temperature of a body rises, the body physically expands and occupies more space; it becomes less dense. The forces of expansion and contraction are considerable, and due allowance must be made for these effects in the design of X-ray equipment, e.g. expansion bellows or diaphragm in the X-ray tube to allow for the expansion and contraction of oil.

We have noted some of the effects of heat on a solid body. What happens when a liquid or a gas is heated? To answer this question we must compare the molecular structure of a liquid or gas to that of a solid. In a solid, the molecules of which the material is made are bonded tightly together, whereas in a liquid they are less tight and in a gas less tight again.

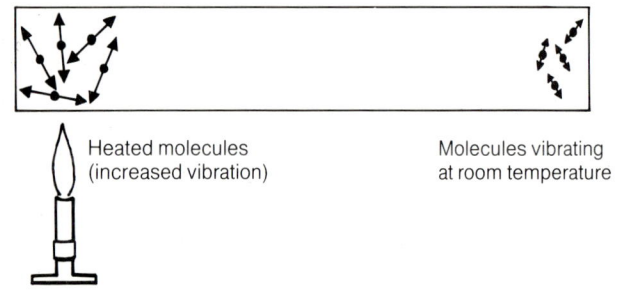

Figure 6.2 Heat transferred through the medium by the process of conduction

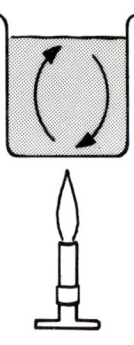

Figure 6.3 Convection

When a liquid is heated (see Figure 6.3) the molecules nearest the heat source (Bunsen flame) vibrate at an increased rate. Because the molecules in a liquid are not tightly bound to one another the molecule has space in which to increase its vibration without unduly affecting its neighbouring molecules. Because the molecule is occupying more space it becomes less dense and rises through the liquid towards the surface. Colder molecules from the surface of the liquid fall and take the place of the heated ones. These in turn are heated and rise to the surface. This movement of heated molecules in an upward direction and colder molecules in a downward direction is called a convection current. Heat is thus transferred throughout the liquid and the process is called convection. The same effect is observed in gases, e.g. hot air (heated molecules) rising from the surface of a heated body.

The third process of heat transfer is called *radiation*. A heated body emits photons or radiation, the number of emitted photons depending upon the temperature of the body, the hotter the body the greater the number of photons emitted. The emitted photons have properties similar to those of all other electromagnetic radiations, e.g. they travel in straight lines, travel at the speed of light in a vacuum, obey the inverse square law etc. (Figure 6.4). Now heat is *conducted* through a body by the transfer of molecular vibrations throughout the body and heat is

TUBE RATING AND TUBE SUPPORTS

convected through a liquid or a gas by the movement of molecules throughout the medium. In each case molecules are essential for the transfer of the heat energy. Heat transfer by the process of radiation is, however, unique in that molecules are not an essential prerequisite and heat can be transferred by the process of radiation through a vacuum. Photons of heat energy from the sun travel across 93 000 000 miles of empty space to reach the earth. Were we dependent on the transfer of heat from the sun by the processes of conduction or convection then life on earth would not be possible.

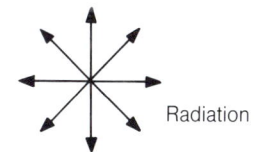

Figure 6.4 Photons are emitted in *all* directions

The rate at which heat is transferred from one body to another by the process of radiation is determined by the difference, to the fourth power, in their temperatures. (Absolute temperature = −273 °C)

Rate of heat transfer = (Temp of one body)^4 − (Temp. of other body)^4

From this it can be appreciated that radiation as a heat transfer process predominates at high temperatures.

THE RATING OF X-RAY TUBES

An X-ray tube converts electrical energy into heat and X-rays.

The *rate* of energy expenditure in heat units = $\dfrac{kVp \times mA}{time}$

Total energy expenditure in heat units = $kVp \times mA \times time$

Over 99% of the electrical energy is converted into heat.

Tube rating tells us the maximum time a specific rate of electrical energy can safely* be applied to an X-ray tube (e.g. maximum exposure time for a particular kVp and mA) or, alternatively, the maximum safe* rate of electrical energy expenditure for a given period of time (e.g. maximum kVp and mA for a particular exposure time).

The information is usually presented in the form of a graph, called a *Tube rating chart* (Figure 6.5). From such a chart the maximum kVp for a particular mA and exposure time *or* the maximum mA for a particular kVp and

* The term 'safe' in this context implies that the life of the X-ray tube will not be unduly shortened by the application of such energy.

50-CYCLE STATOR OPERATION
Radiographic Rating Chart
Ratings for Single-Phase Full-Wave Rectification

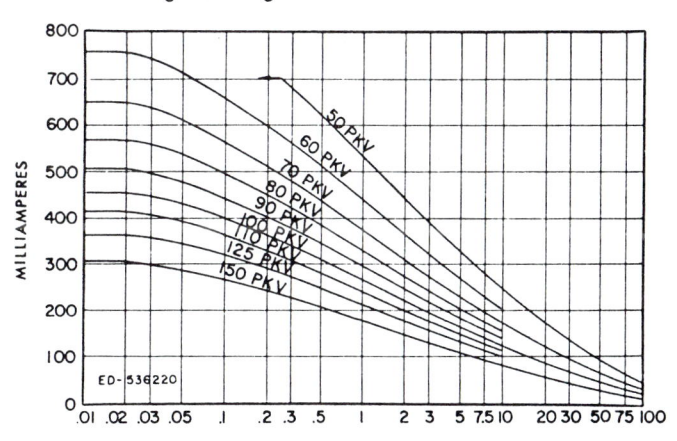

Figure 6.5 A typical rating chart

exposure time, *or* the maximum exposure time for a particular kVp and mA can be easily read off. The rating chart should specify the type of tube, size of focal area, type of rectification and speed of anode rotation to which it relates.

Although it is the product of kVp and mA which determines the rate of energy expenditure, expressed in heat units, each of these factors is subject to *individual* limitation.

Maximum kVp is governed by the physical structure and dimensions of the tube, e.g. distance between points of different electrical potential, electrical insulation, etc. Each tube is fitted with a plate on which is recorded maximum safe operating kVp, typical examples being 100 kVp, 125 kVp and 150 kVp.

Maximum mA (tube current) at low kV values is determined by the maximum temperature to which a particular filament can be raised before it burns out, or has an unacceptably shortened life.

Let us consider further the way in which maximum filament temperature limits the mA we can safely use. Although the X-ray tube may operate close to saturation condition it does not necessarily do so. From Figure 6.6 it will be noted that, although the temperature of the filament remains constant, increase in kV results in an increase in mA.

This increase in mA is compensated for by decreasing the filament heating current when the kVp is increased, and on most modern units this is done automatically.

Let us consider this in greater detail. From Figure 6.6 it can be seen that for the same filament current, say 4.8 A the tube current (mA) increases as tube voltage is increased, i.e. as the voltage rises from 25 kVp to 100 kVp

8500 r.p.m.
50 Hz – 150 Hz

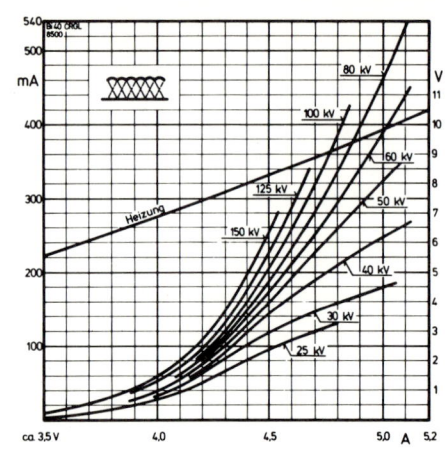

Figure 6.6 Filament heating curves

the mA also increases, and that within the space charge limited region mA decreases rapidly with reduction in kVp.

In short, the mA varies with the applied kVp even though the filament temperature remains constant. From this it will be appreciated that if, for example, the tube passes 130 mA at 25 kVp for a particular filament heating current (say 4.8 A) the mA wll rise to 390 mA at 100 kVp. It is, therefore, necessary to progressively *reduce* the filament heating current (to 4.35 A) as the tube voltage is increased from 25 kVp to 100 kVp if the mA is to remain at a steady value, e.g. 130 mA.

Conversely, when the selected tube voltage is reduced from 100 kVp it is necessary to increase the filament heating current if the tube current is to be maintained at a constant value. If, for example, we wish to maintain tube current at a value of 130 mA and reduce tube voltage from 100 kVp to 25 kVp it is necessary to increase the filament current (in this case from 4.35 A to 4.8 A).

Now, an increase in filament heating current, to maintain a particular mA at reduced kVp does *not* cause the temperature of the *target* to rise as the rate at which electrical energy (kVp × mA/time) is being converted into heat at the target of the tube is actually being decreased.

For example, in the first instance, assuming an exposure of 1.0 s,

$$\frac{100 \text{ kVp} \times 130 \text{ mA}}{1.0 \text{ s}} = 13\,000 \text{ heat units per second}$$

and in the second case,

$$\frac{25 \text{ kVp} \times 130 \text{ mA}}{1.0 \text{ s}} = 3250 \text{ heat units per second}$$

This demonstrates that the *target* is now receiving heat energy at a *reduced* rate and the limitation in rating is due to the maximum safe working temperature of the filament having been reached.

Such a limitation in the rating due to filament temperature may be indicated on the rating chart by means of an arrow as in Figure 6.7. This shows that at high kVp values it is the temperature of the *target* which limits the amount of energy we can apply whilst at low kVp values it is the temperature of the *filament* which is the limiting factor.

Maximum power

The heat produced at the target of the tube for a given exposure time is determined by the kVp applied and the current flowing (kVp × mA) and their combined effect must not cause the temperature of the focal area to rise above a certain critical value.

Note: Whilst the target would not melt until it reached a temperature of 3380°C it is the usual practice to limit the temperature to a lower value, so that the life of the tube will be extended.

It should be remembered that the production of X-rays (intensity) is directly proportional to mA and exposure time but varies to the square of the kVp. On the other hand film blackening, which is also proportional to mA and exposure time, varies to the fourth (or fifth) power of kVp.

We may consider that mA and exposure time affect the *amount* of radiation produced (i.e. number of photons) whilst kVp affects not only the amount of radiation but its average penetrating power (Figure 6.8).

TYPE OF RECTIFICATION

We will now consider how constant potential, full-wave

Change in mA
Intensity varies directly with mA
Variation of mA has no effect on penetrating power of photons.

Change in kVp
Average penetration of photons increases with kVp – average wavelength decreases

Intensity increases with increase in kVp

Number of photons varies to kVp^2

Film blackening varies to the 4th power of kVp

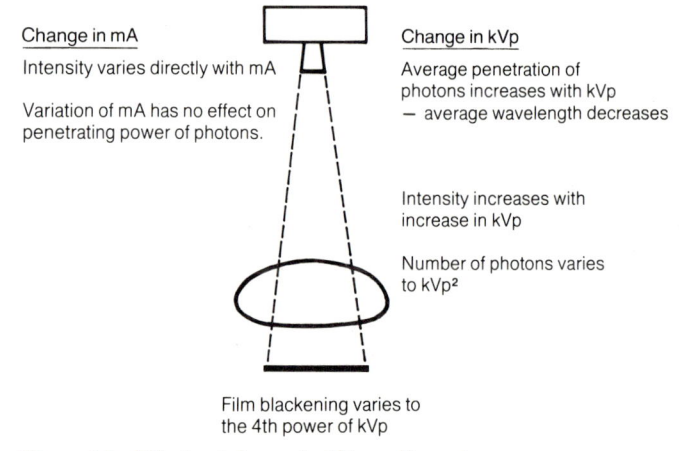

Figure 6.8 Effects of change in kVp and/or mA

TUBE RATING AND TUBE SUPPORTS

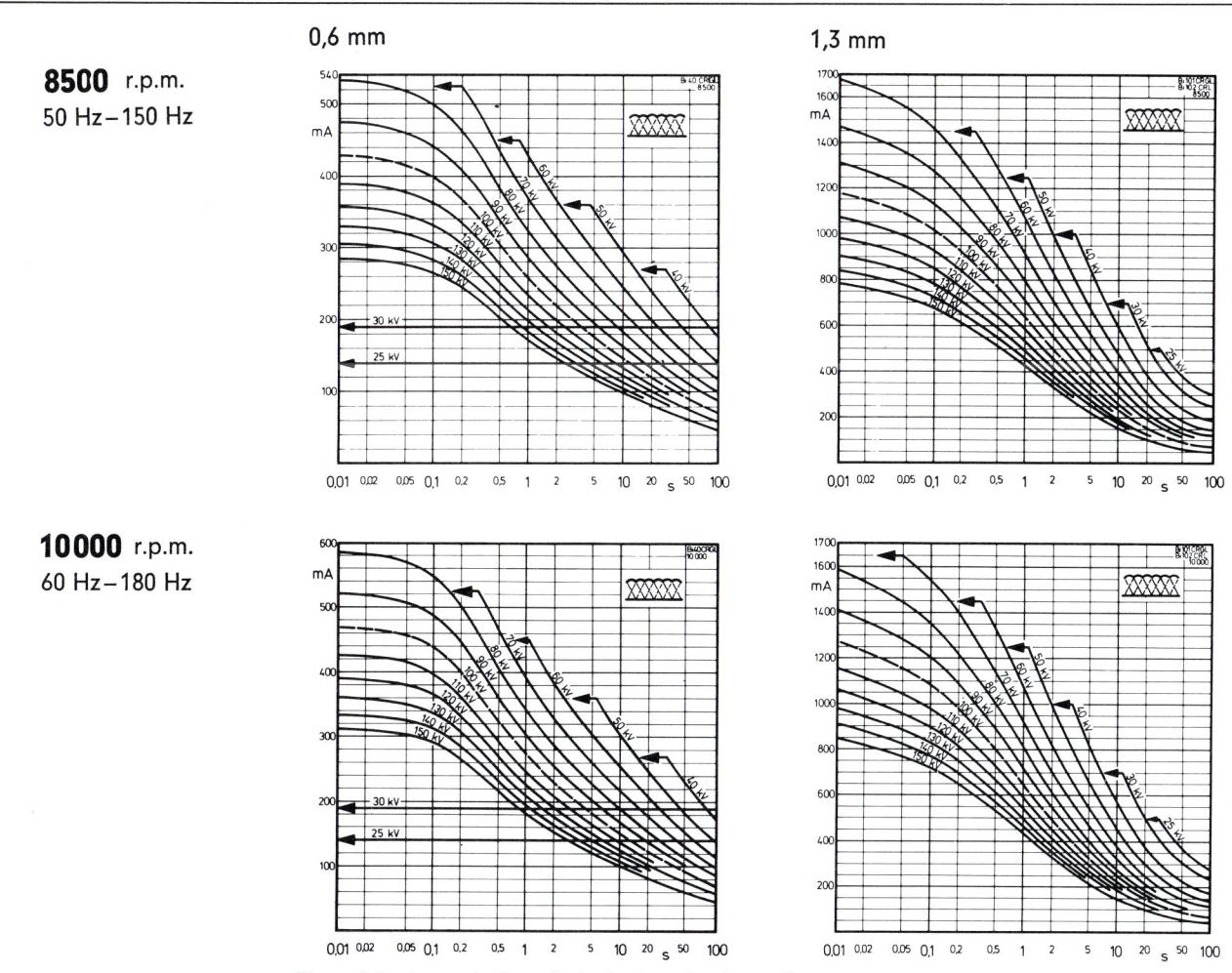

8500 r.p.m.
50 Hz – 150 Hz

0,6 mm

1,3 mm

10000 r.p.m.
60 Hz – 180 Hz

Figure 6.7 Arrows indicate limitation in rating due to filament temperature

rectified three-phase, full-wave rectified single-phase and half-wave or self-rectified voltage affects tube loading and why we need different rating charts for different types of rectification.

Assume that a series of exposures are to be made using a different type of rectification in each case and using the following factors for each exposure.

　　　0.04 s　　　50 kVp　　　100 mA

Remember that in each case the mA meter on the control panel will read an *average* value, i.e. it will measure the average current flowing over the period of the exposure.

In the case of the constant potential unit Figure 6.9 indicates the current flowing during the exposure. The current is flowing at a steady value during the exposure and consequently there are no peaks.

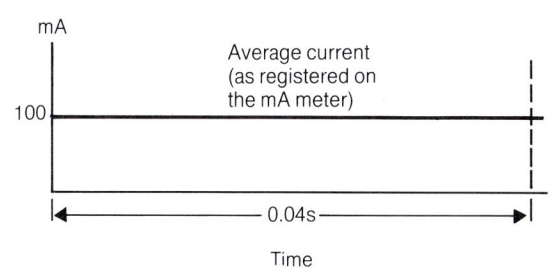

Figure 6.9 Peak and average values of current are equal with a constant potential generator

In the case of the full-wave rectified single-phase unit, however, the situation is rather different. From Figure 6.10, it will be noted that to achieve the same *average* current of 100 mA it is now necessary to have high peak values of current at instants A, B, C, D to compensate for the reduced current flow at E, F, G, H.

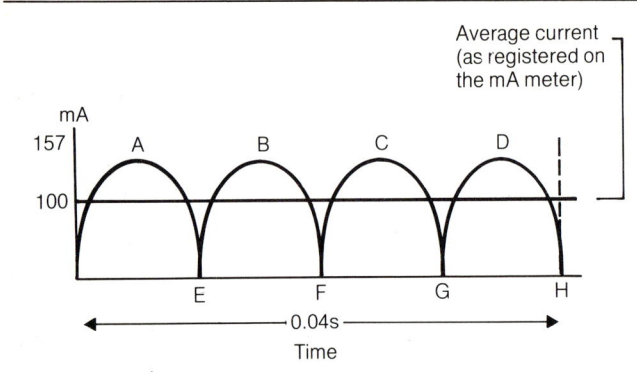

Figure 6.10 Peak and average values of current with 2-pulse generator

Now we have seen that the total heat produced at the target of the tube during an exposure time (t) is proportional to kVp × mA × t. That is to say, the same amount of heat is produced during the exposure (0.04 s) whether the average current (100 mA) is flowing at a constant rate or is produced in a series of bursts or pulses.

If, however, the current is produced in bursts, where each burst has a peak value which is 1.57 times the average value, it is easy to understand that, although the target receives the same amount of heat in *total* over the complete exposure, the surface temperature of the target is raised *at the instants of peak value* (A, B, C and D) to a much higher value than is the case when current is flowing at a constant value, i.e. at constant potential.

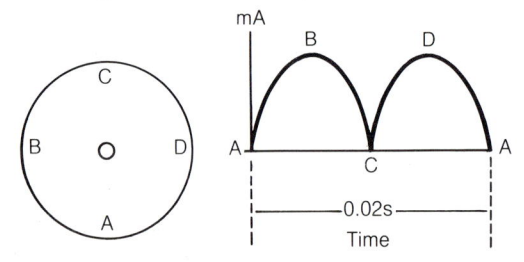

Figure 6.11 Hot spots produced during one revolution of the anode

Consider an exposure of 0.02 s. During such an exposure the anode will make one complete revolution (assuming the anode is rotating at 3000 rev/min (Figure 6.11). When the exposure starts at A the current is zero. At B the anode has made a quarter of a revolution and the current (mA) and target temperature are at maximum value. At C the current is once again at zero value and also the heating effect. At D current and heating effect are once again at peak value and at A current and heating effect are back to zero.

This results in hot spots at B and D and it is the temperature to which these parts of the target are raised which determines tube rating, but *only* for short exposure times.

To summarize,

peak value of current $I_{max} = 1.57 \times I_{average}$,

so that 100 mA average has a peak value of 157 mA.
Let us now compare this with the *self-rectified circuit*.

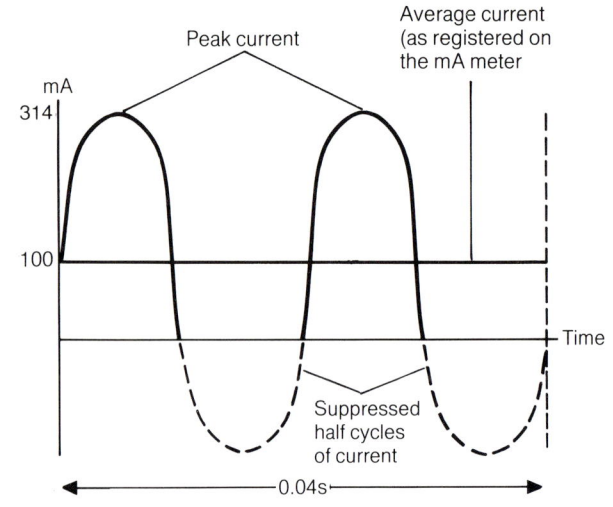

Figure 6.12 Peak and average current with a self-rectified circuit

Once again we need an average current of 100 mA but in this case the current passes in not four pulses but two as shown in Figure 6.12 (the other two pulses are, of course, suppressed). Now, if the average current is to remain at 100 mA, but, if on this occasion it is flowing for only *half* the time, the actual current flowing during each pulse must be doubled to achieve an average current of 100 mA; the actual current per pulse must be 200 mA.

Once again, peak value

$$I_{max} = 1.57 \times I_{average}$$
$$= 1.57 \times 200$$
$$= 314 \, mA$$

So that in the case of a four-valve full-wave rectified circuit a peak value of 157 mA results in an average current of 100 mA but in the case of the half-wave rectified circuit a peak value of 314 mA is needed to achieve the same 100 mA average value.

Now the intensity of the radiation produced at the target is proportional to the mA (average). Therefore the same radiographic density is achieved in each case. However, as the maximum temperature of the anode for short exposures is determined by the peak value of current, it follows that the temperature of the target will be raised to twice the value in the latter case to achieve the same mA value (and same film blackening). The energy we can safely use is therefore much reduced in the case of a half-wave rectified circuit.

TUBE RATING AND TUBE SUPPORTS

A further limitation is imposed in *self-rectified circuits*, where the temperature of the anode must not exceed approximately 1600 °C, at which temperature thermionic emission would provide sufficient electrons to constitute an inverse current as opposed to 3380 °C (temperature at which it would melt), in the case of full-wave rectified circuits.

The three-phase rectified circuit

From Figure 6.13 it can be seen that the peak value of rectified three-phase current is very close to the average value. It will also be noted that the peak value of three-phase is much less than that of rectified single-phase current.

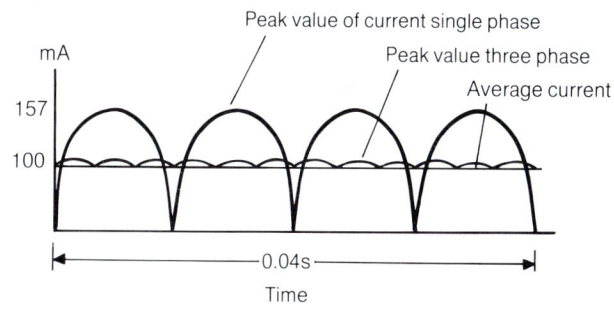

Figure 6.13 Peak and average values of current for 1-pulse, 2-pulse and 6-pulse circuits

The energy we can safely use for short exposure times, when the skin temperature of the focal area is the critical factor, is therefore much higher when using rectified three-phase current. For long exposure times, however, it is found that the energy we can use is less than that of single-phase. This is due to the fact that the voltage waveform never drops to zero and indeed remains close to peak value for the whole of the exposure. As the same average current flows in each case it follows that more energy is expended in a given period of time with three-phase than with single-phase voltage. In fact, there is an increase, in the order of about 35%, in the number of heat units produced by a three-phase circuit as compared with a single-phase circuit.

The formula for calculating heat units must now be written thus:

Heat units = $1.35 \times kVp \times mA$ (average) $\times$ time (s)

Figure 6.14 illustrates this point. The shaded area under the curves represents energy expenditure during a period of 0.01 s. The same average current flows in each case and the peak kV is the same in each case but the energy expended in 0.01 s is obviously greater in the case of the rectified three-phase voltage.

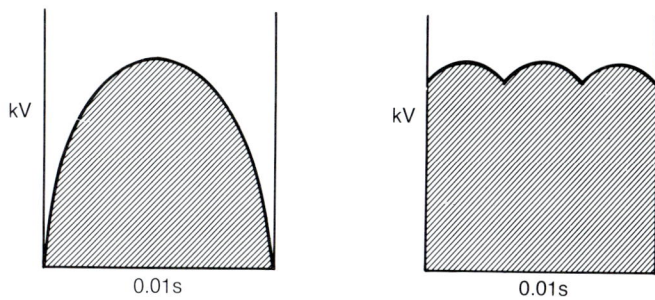

Figure 6.14 Energy expenditure during 0.01 s for 2 pulse and 6 pulse generators using the same kVp

Figure 6.15 shows the difference in tube rating between single-phase and three-phase X-ray generators.

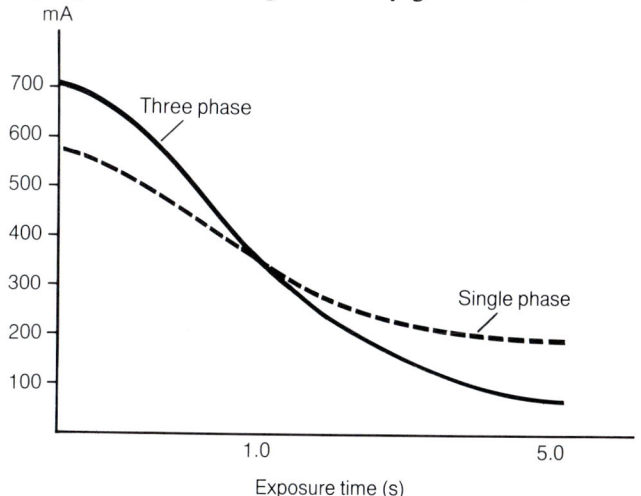

Figure 6.15 Ratings for 2-pulse and 6-pulse generators

Note: Although maximum mA at a given kVp is less at long exposure times, when using the three-phase unit, the kV is near peak value during the whole of the exposure. This results in an X-ray beam of greater intensity and shorter average wavelength than that of the single-phase unit and therefore a greater degree of film blackening for a given exposure.

Up to now we have discussed those factors which determine the rate at which electrical energy is converted into heat in the X-ray tube. The rate at which such energy can safely be used in any given tube is, of course, determined by the physical characteristics of the tube itself. These characteristics would include:
(1) Focal area,
(2) Material of which the anode is made,
(3) Diameter of the anode,
(4) Speed of anode rotation,
(5) Heat dissipation, i.e. volume of oil within the casing, forced cooling, etc.

Let us now consider some of these factors in greater detail.

Focal area (focal spot size)

The smaller the focal area, the greater is the temperature rise for a given amount of heat energy. Figures 6.16–18 may help to make this more clear.

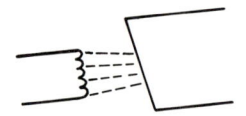

Figure 6.16 Electrical energy (kVp × mA × time) is converted into heat energy (99%) at the target of the tube

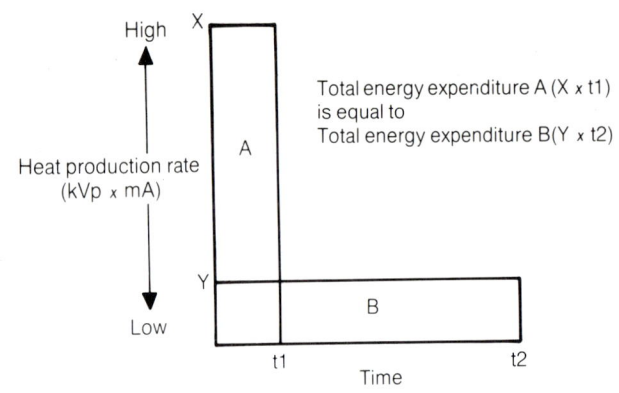

Figure 6.17 *Total* energy expenditure A ($x \times T_1$) is *equal* to *Total* energy expenditure B ($y \times T_2$) (Although time taken is different in each case)

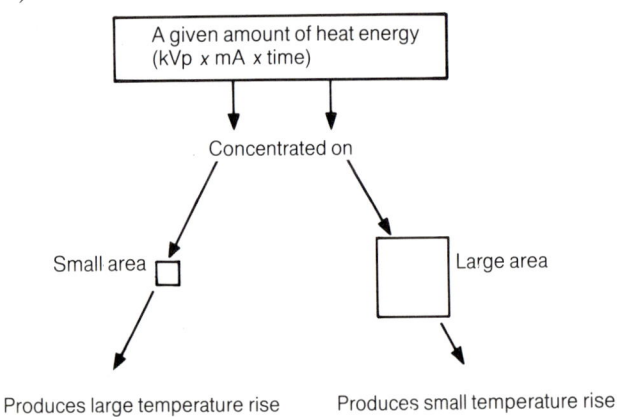

Figure 6.18 Effect of focal area on temperature rise

Relationship of temperature rise to area and linear dimensions of the focal spot

The temperature rise at the target for a given amount of heat energy is determined by its area. The rate of heat transfer from the focal area to the mass of the anode is, however, related to the peripheral dimensions of the focus as well as its actual area.

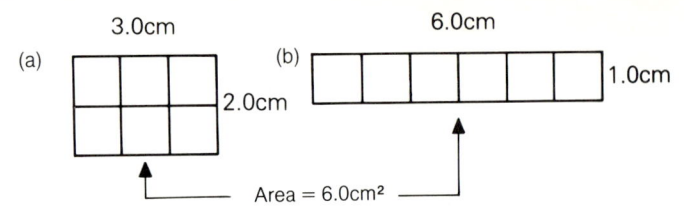

Figure 6.19 Rectangles with same area but different peripheral dimensions

Let us consider two rectangles, A and B, each having the same area but different peripheral dimensions (Figure 6.19). The peripheral dimensions of A are 10 cm whilst those of B are 14 cm and it can be readily appreciated that B conducts heat to its surroundings at a faster rate than A and in fact the rate of heat transfer varies proportionately to the peripheral dimensions rather than to the areas of the rectangles.

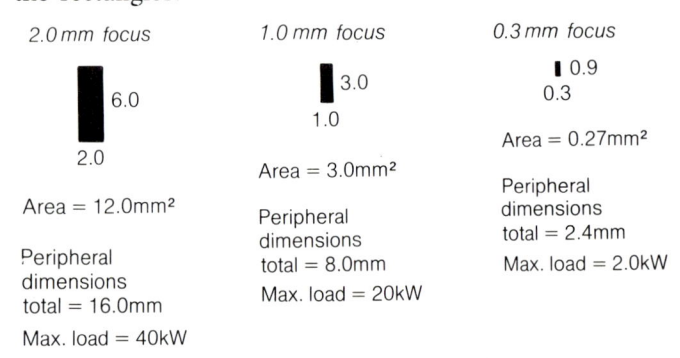

2.0 mm focus
6.0
2.0
Area = 12.0 mm²
Peripheral dimensions total = 16.0 mm
Max. load = 40 kW

1.0 mm focus
3.0
1.0
Area = 3.0 mm²
Peripheral dimensions total = 8.0 mm
Max. load = 20 kW

0.3 mm focus
0.9
0.3
Area = 0.27 mm²
Peripheral dimensions total = 2.4 mm
Max. load = 2.0 kW

Figure 6.20 Tube loading for different sized focal spots

Let us now consider the actual dimensions and areas of three focal spot sizes (Figure 6.20). (We will assume that the *actual* focus in each case is three times as long as it is broad.)

From this it can be seen that the maximum loading of the 2.0 mm sq. and 1.0 mm sq. focii varies to the ratio of their peripheral dimensions, e.g. 16 mm to 8 mm and 40 kW to 20 kW, whilst the loading of the microfocus compared with the 1.0 mm sq. focus varies more nearly to the ratio of their respective *areas*, e.g. 3.0 to 0.27 and 20 to 2.

To sum up, loading is usually related to the peripheral dimensions of the focus but for very small focal spot sizes (e.g. microfocal spots) loading is more nearly related to the focal area. This means that for a microfocus tube the rating is much less than we might at first imagine.

Speed of anode rotation

If a stator supply current with a frequency of 50 cycles per second is used to rotate the anode it will revolve 3000

TUBE RATING AND TUBE SUPPORTS

times per minute and it will take 0.02 s to make one complete revolution. If, during an exposure the anode is made to rotate at twice or even three times this speed it is possible to apply more heat to the target (Figure 6.21). In other words the rating of the tube can be increased. This is because the actual focal area is increased at short exposure times.

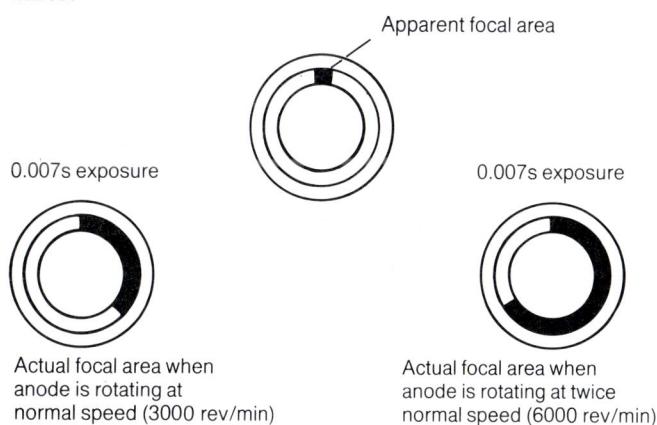

Figure 6.21 Effect of anode rotational speed on focal area

Generally speaking, if the exposure time is reduced, the mA can be increased. One of the limiting factors is the time it takes the anode to make one complete revolution. Look at the rating chart for a tube with a stator supply of 50 cycles per second (Figure 6.5) and you will see that between 0.02 s and zero the mA value for any kVp is constant, and in fact many rating charts have a time axis which starts at 0.02 s.

X-ray tube manufacturers use a range of stator supply frequencies, examples being 50, 100, 150 and 180 cycles per sec. High speed anode rotation is usually used only at high mA values and for short exposure times. For longer exposures it is recommended that a 50 cycle stator supply should be switched in so that the life of the tube may be extended, and this is done automatically in many units. A 50 cycle per second supply is also recommended when the tube is being used for fluoroscopy. The stator supply voltage is also reduced in these circumstances. The following are examples of starting and running voltages for different stator supply frequencies.

50 cycle stator operation

Intermittent operation (radiography)
Starting 115 V, 4 A, 3.6 s starting time
Running 50 V, 1.9 A, continuous
Starting time can be reduced to 1.5 s by using 230 V and 8 A.

High speed 150 or 180 cycle stator operation

Intermittent operation (radiography)
Starting and running 230 V, 3.5 A, 6.0 s starting time
Starting time can be reduced to 1.2 s by using 675 V and 10 A

Continuous operation (fluoroscopy)

Starting 230 V, 3.5 A
Running 115 V, 1.8 A
Alternatively tube stator may be switched to 50 cycle supply and 50 V operation during fluoroscopy.

Note: after *high speed* operation the anode must be slowed down rapidly. This is achieved by either applying a rectified voltage to both stator windings or by switching the stator winding to 50 cycles per second operation. Braking should slow the anode to 4000 rev/min or less in 10 s.

In some fluoroscopy units where the mA is very low the anode may actually be stationary whilst screening is in progress. Other units as indicated above use a reduced voltage and current for fluoroscopy. It should be noted that a slotted anode must always be rotating even during fluoroscopy as otherwise the electrons might pass through the slots.

We have seen that when electrical energy is converted into heat at the target of the X-ray tube, the temperature of the focal area (area bombarded by electrons) is determined by the rate at which heat energy is applied (kVp × mA), the length of time for which it is applied (exposure time in seconds), the size of the focal area, and the rate at which heat is transferred from the focal area during the exposure.

Let us now consider how heat is transferred from the target.

Heat transfer through the X-ray tube

The route followed by the heat as it is transferred from target to anode to oil to casing to outside air may be called the heat path. Heat energy is transferred through the tube from one point to another, by the process of conduction through the target and the anode; by convection through the oil surrounding the insert, by conduction through the casing and by convection and radiation from the casing to the outside air.

It should be noted that in the case of the stationary anode tube although *some* heat is radiated from the target and anode, radiation is *not* a primary form of heat transfer, most of the heat being transferred from the target to the anode and then to the oil by the process of conduction. Conversely, in the rotating anode tube, whilst heat is conducted from the target area to the mass of the anode, the amount of heat transferred by conduction from the anode to the rotor and then to the oil is relatively small, most of the heat being radiated by the anode to the oil surrounding the insert, by convection through the oil, by conduction through the casing and by convection (with some radiation) from the casing to the outside air.

It is important to clearly understand the processes by which heat is transferred from one point to another through the X-ray tube, as tube rating is closely related to the temperature reached by each of the component parts of the tube in turn, the critical points being:

(1) Tungsten target (melts at 3380 °C),
(2) Anode to rotor junction (copper rotor melts at 1080 °C),
(3) Oil surrounding the insert (maximun temperature being related to maximum safe expansion of the oil).

The part played by the various heat transfer processes in passing heat from the anode to the outside air is shown diagrammatically in Figures 6.22 and 6.23.

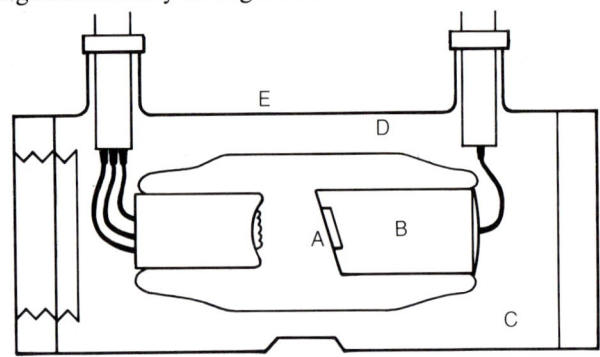

Figure 6.22 Heat path through stationary anode tube

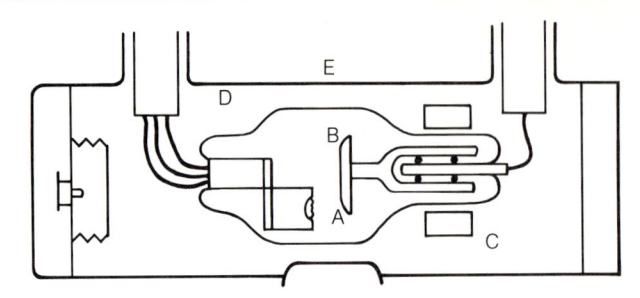

Figure 6.23 Heat path through rotating anode tube

Heat path (stationary anode) – Figure 6.22

Component through which heat is transferred	Heat transfer process
A = Target	Conduction
B = Anode	Conduction
C = Oil	Convection
D = Tube casing	Conduction
E = Outer side of the tube casing to surrounding air	Convection and radiation

Heat path (rotating anode) – Figure 6.23

Component through which heat is being transferred	Heat transfer process
A = Target and anode	Conduction
B = Vacuum	Radiation
C = Oil	Convection
D = Tube casing	Conduction
E = Outer side of tube casing to surrounding air	Convection and radiation

In addition to the rating chart previously described which relates to a *single* exposure followed by a period of rest of at least 1.0 s, there are other charts and graphs supplied by the manufacturers which are of great value to the radiographer who may be planning a series of exposures in rapid succession, for example an angiographic or cine series. There are also graphs which tell us how much heat has built up in the anode over a period of time for a given heat input as well as the amount of heat lost from the anode in a given period of time after an exposure.

Anode cooling chart

Let us look first at a typical anode cooling chart (Figure 6.24). Note the following:

(1) The chart should apply to a particular tube.

(2) The maximum number of heat units the anode can safely accept in this case is 400 000 and that it will take 11 min for the anode to cool down to ambient room temperature (assuming no further exposures are made in the meantime).

(3) In addition to providing information regarding the rate of anode cooling it also tells us how much heat will build up in the anode in a given time for different rates of heat input.

We can see from the graph that heat can be applied *continuously* at the rate of say 800 heat units/s. We know this because the curve for 800 heat units/s if extended would never reach maximum value of 400 000 heat units. This, of course, is due to the fact that after a given period of time heat is being transferred from the anode at the same rate as it is being applied and temperature of the anode therefore remains constant. If, however, we use, say, 1350 heat units/s we find that after 11 min the temperature of the anode has reached maximum safe value.

Now 80 kVp at 10 mA equals 800 heat units/s which is, of course, a very small *rate* of heat input compared with a radiographic exposure of say 80 kVp and 500 mA which equals 40 000 heat units/s. We have seen that a heat input

TUBE RATING AND TUBE SUPPORTS

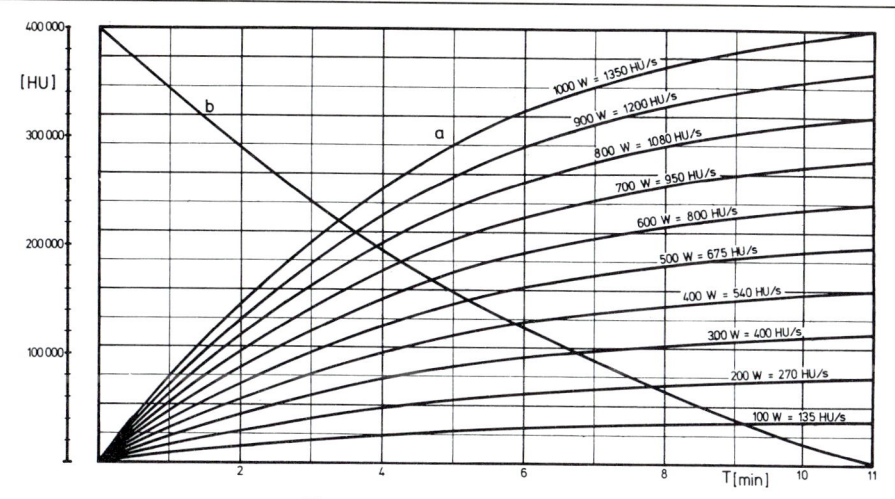

Figure 6.24 Anode cooling chart

of 800 heat units/s would *never* overheat the anode but over a period of say 10 min the heat build up would amount to 800 × 60 × 10 = 48 000 heat units and whilst the *rate* of heat input for the diagnostic exposure is much higher at 40 000 heat units/s, the *total* heat units for an exposure of say 0.25 s would be 10 000. From this it can be appreciated that there is little or no danger to the anode when very small mA values are being used but a very real danger when high mA values are selected even though the *total* heat developed over a long exposure time at a low mA is much greater than that associated with a very short exposure time at high mA.

Tube housing cooling chart

With low mA values the heat build up, which presents no difficulties so far as the anode is concerned, can and does become a problem so far as the oil in the casing is concerned. Because, as we have seen, if the temperature of the oil rises to a certain critical value its expansion will cause maximum contraction of the oil expansion diaphragm (or bellows) and a safety cut-out switch will prevent further exposures being made until the oil has sufficiently cooled. A graph supplied by the manufacturer tells us how much heat the oil in the casing can safely accommodate and the rate at which it loses heat. A typical graph is shown in Figure 6.25.

Note that once again such a chart applies to a specific tube and that in this particular case it can accommodate 1 750 000 heat units before the oil expands to such an extent that it operates the safety cut-out switch preventing further exposures being made. In the previous case we discussed we noted that whilst a heat input of 800 heat units/s would never overheat the anode it would provide a significant heat input to the oil and indeed we can calculate that it would take approximately 35 min for the

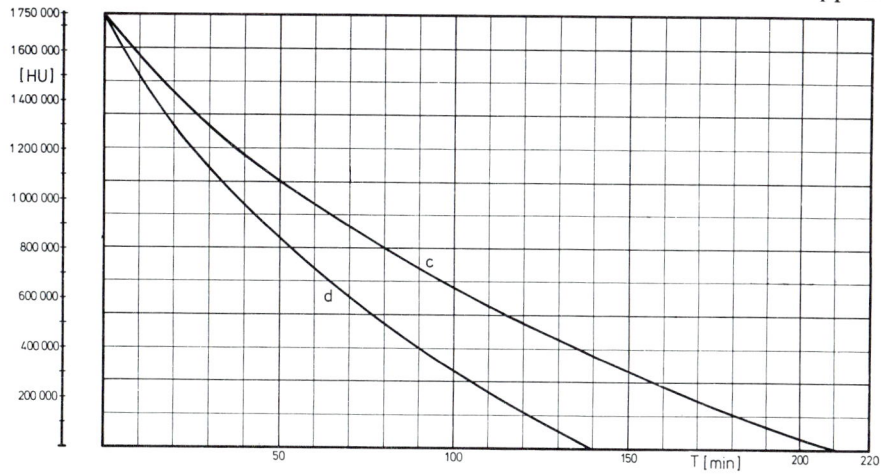

Figure 6.25 Tube housing cooling curves c – without fan d – with fan

oil in the casing to reach the critical temperature at which the cut-out switch could become operative.

Such a build up of heat in the oil may also be brought about when a series of diagnostic exposures are made over a lengthy period of time, e.g. in chest clinics, angio series, cine examinations, etc. It is worth noting that in these cases the use of an air circulator such as a fan fitted to the outer casing of the X-ray tube can improve matters dramatically and will indeed, in the case of the tube cooling graph described, allow a 50% increase in the operating time before the thermal cut-out prevents further exposures.

It is also worth noting, when comparing high speed rotating anode tubes with those operating at slower speeds, that additional heat is generated by the increased current flowing through the stator coils. The extra current is, of course, needed to provide the increased speed of anode rotation. This extra heat could be accommodated by increasing the volume of oil in the tube casing, but as this leads to an increase in tube size it is not a popular solution. Instead heat transfer is improved by circulating water through pipes which pass through the oil in the casing to a heat exchange unit which is usually fixed to the wall of the X-ray room. Remember when using such a tube that heat is transferred through the oil in the casing by the process of convection. It is advisable, therefore, when the tube is tilted through 90°, i.e. for chest examinations, to have the cathode end of the tube uppermost so that there is a greater volume of oil available for heat transfer from the anode.

Angiographic rating chart

Charts of this nature are used when planning a series of exposures which need to be made in rapid succession, as for example when using the AOT or puck film changer. It is important to note that a particular chart relates to a particular tube *and to that tube only*. It should also be noted that the tube must be rested for a specified period before the series of exposures is commenced and again before another series is started. The chart illustrated in Figure 6.26 relates to the Philips ceramic tube SRC 120 0613 and is for a tube loading of 40 kW. Charts for tube loads of 32, 100 and 120 kW are also provided for use with this tube.

Let us see how such a chart would be used. Assume that a series of exposures are to be made at a rate of 6 per second for 3 seconds and that each exposure is to be made at 75 kV 500 mA with an exposure time of 0.04 s.

We must first of all calculate the tube loading which in this case would be $75 \times 500 = 37.5$ kW. (As this tube would almost certainly be used with a 12 pulse or constant potential generator we can consider, for practical purposes, that

SRC 120 0613
LOAD DATA FOR SERIAL RADIOGRAPHY   8000/min
The table shows the number of exposures permissible per series
The intervals to be observed before and between series must not be shorter than 20 min.

TUBE LOAD kW	EXPOSURE RATE EXP /sec	3	6	10	20	25	32	40	50	63	80	100	120	160
40	12	100	100	100	82	60	42	30	22	16	-	-	-	-
	10	100	100	100	88	64	45	33	24	17	12	-	-	-
	8	100	100	100	97	71	50	36	26	19	13	10	-	-
	6	100	100	100	100	80	56	41	30	21	15	11	4	-
	4	100	100	100	100	95	67	49	35	25	18	13	10	7
	3	100	100	100	100	100	76	55	40	29	20	15	11	8
	2	100	100	100	100	100	90	66	48	34	24	18	14	9
	1	100	100	100	100	100	100	88	64	46	33	24	18	12

Figure 6.26 Angiographic rating chart

the r.m.s. factor is unity.) We would now consult the rating chart for 40 kW and looking down the exposure rate column we come to 6 and then reading across to the right we come to the column under 40 (ms) and see there the number 41. This means that we can make 41 exposures at a rate of 6/s at a tube loading of 40 kW. As we know that the tube loading we wish to use (37.5 kW) is less than

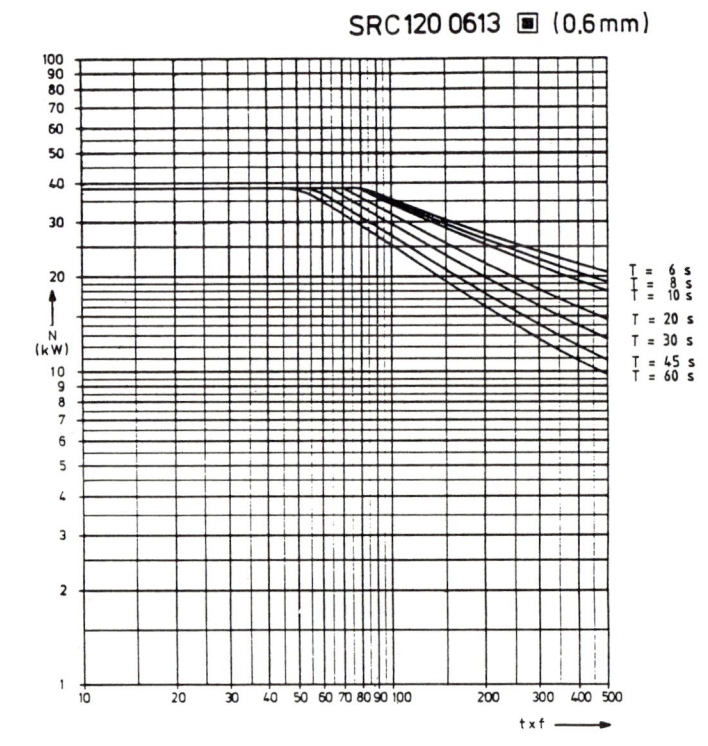

Figure 6.27 Cine radiographic rating chart

40 kW and as we need to make only 18 exposures (6/s for 3 s) we know that the series of exposures using these factors will not overload the tube and we can therefore safely proceed *providing* the tube has been rested for 20 minutes before the sequence begins.

It should be noted that some modern units using microprocessor control will make such calculations for us and will indicate on the control panel the number of exposures permissible under given circumstances and will indeed tell us how many permissible exposures remain as the examination proceeds.

Cine radiographic rating chart

This chart tells us the tube loading permissible under specified conditions. The chart illustrated in Figure 6.27 once again relates to the Philips ceramic tube SRC 1200613 and we note that it also relates to the 0.6 mm focus and an anode rotational speed of 8000 rev/min. We will once again assume that the tube is being used with a 12-pulse or constant potential generator.

The tube loading in kW is indicated on the vertical axis of the graph and the exposure time in milliseconds multiplied by the exposure rate in seconds is shown on the horizontal axis (t × f). On the right side of the graph the total time of the series is indicated in seconds (T). To use the cine rating chart we must once again calculate the tube loading in kW. Say we wished to make a cine run of 10 s duration using a 2 ms exposure at 80 kV and 250 mA and that we intend to expose the film at a rate of 75 f.p.s. The tube loading is therefore 80 × 250 = 20 kW. We must now multiply the exposure time by the f.p.s. 2 × 75 = 150. Looking at the rating chart we find 150 on the horizontal axis, then following the line upwards until it crosses the line corresponding to T = 10 s we trace the horizontal line from the intersection to the left vertical axis which indicates the permitted tube loading in kW. From this we see that we can use up to 28 kW for the cine run we have chosen and as we will be using a tube loading of 20 kW it can be appreciated that we can safely make this cine run without overloading the tube.

As we have now discussed the role of most of the major components in the typical X-ray circuit let us see how they fit into the complete circuit and how they relate to one another (Figure 6.28).

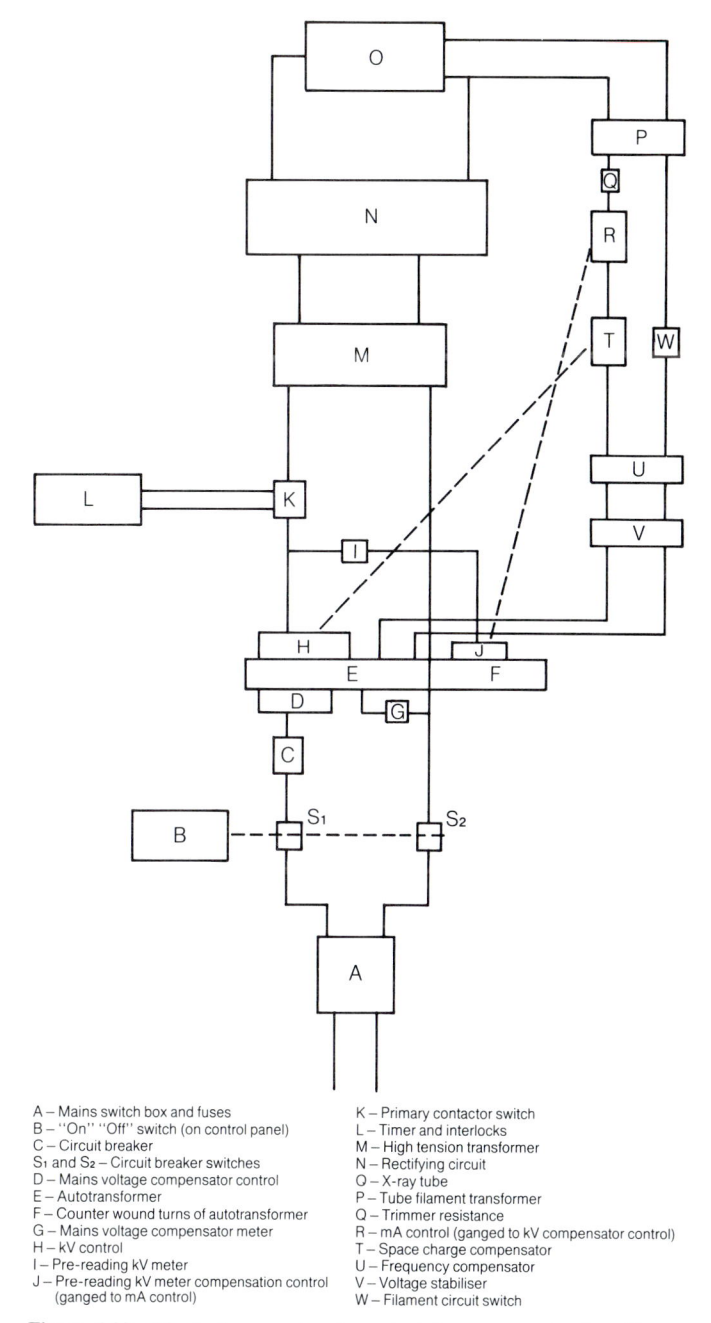

A – Mains switch box and fuses
B – "On" "Off" switch (on control panel)
C – Circuit breaker
S₁ and S₂ – Circuit breaker switches
D – Mains voltage compensator control
E – Autotransformer
F – Counter wound turns of autotransformer
G – Mains voltage compensator meter
H – kV control
I – Pre-reading kV meter
J – Pre-reading kV meter compensation control (ganged to mA control)
K – Primary contactor switch
L – Timer and interlocks
M – High tension transformer
N – Rectifying circuit
O – X-ray tube
P – Tube filament transformer
Q – Trimmer resistance
R – mA control (ganged to kV compensator control)
T – Space charge compensator
U – Frequency compensator
V – Voltage stabiliser
W – Filament circuit switch

Figure 6.28 Block diagram showing principle components of an X-ray circuit

X-RAY TUBE SUPPORTS

The X-ray tube should be mounted in such a manner as to provide the following:

(1) Movement of the tube vertically up or down.
(2) Longitudinal movement along the long axis of the X-ray table and transverse movements.
(3) Angulation of the tube.
(4) Positive locking of the tube in the desired position.
(5) Complete stability when the tube is locked in the selected position.

There are three main types of tube support:

(1) Floor or floor-to-ceiling tube stands,
(2) Ceiling-suspended tube supports,
(3) Mounting on a 'C' arm.

Floor stands

The vertical tube column is mounted on a trolley which runs along a single or double floor track. The X-ray tube is mounted on a gimbal attached to a cross-arm which moves up and down on the vertical column. The tube is usually suspended by steel cable and is counterbalanced. The range of movements is shown in Figure 6.29. The tube may be locked in any desired position or angle by means of mechanical or electromagnetic locks. It is provided with a fail-safe mechanism which ensures that the tube will not fall if the cable snaps.

Floor to ceiling stands

Extra stability may be achieved by having the vertical tube column run along a ceiling track as well as the floor track just described. The additional ceiling support tends to offset the inbalance caused by the weight of the X-ray tube.

The ceiling-suspended tube support

Compared with the tube stand just described, which is restricted in its transverse movements, the ceiling-suspended tube has no such restriction and therefore offers much greater flexibility in use. Its range of movement is shown in Figure 6.30.

A = Vertical tube support
B = Cross arm
C = X-ray tube
D = Trolley to which vertical tube support is attached
E = Floor track

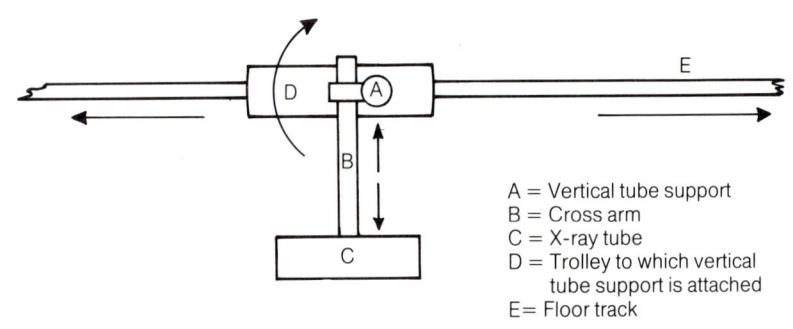

Figure 6.29 Vertical tube stand viewed from above

TUBE RATING AND TUBE SUPPORTS

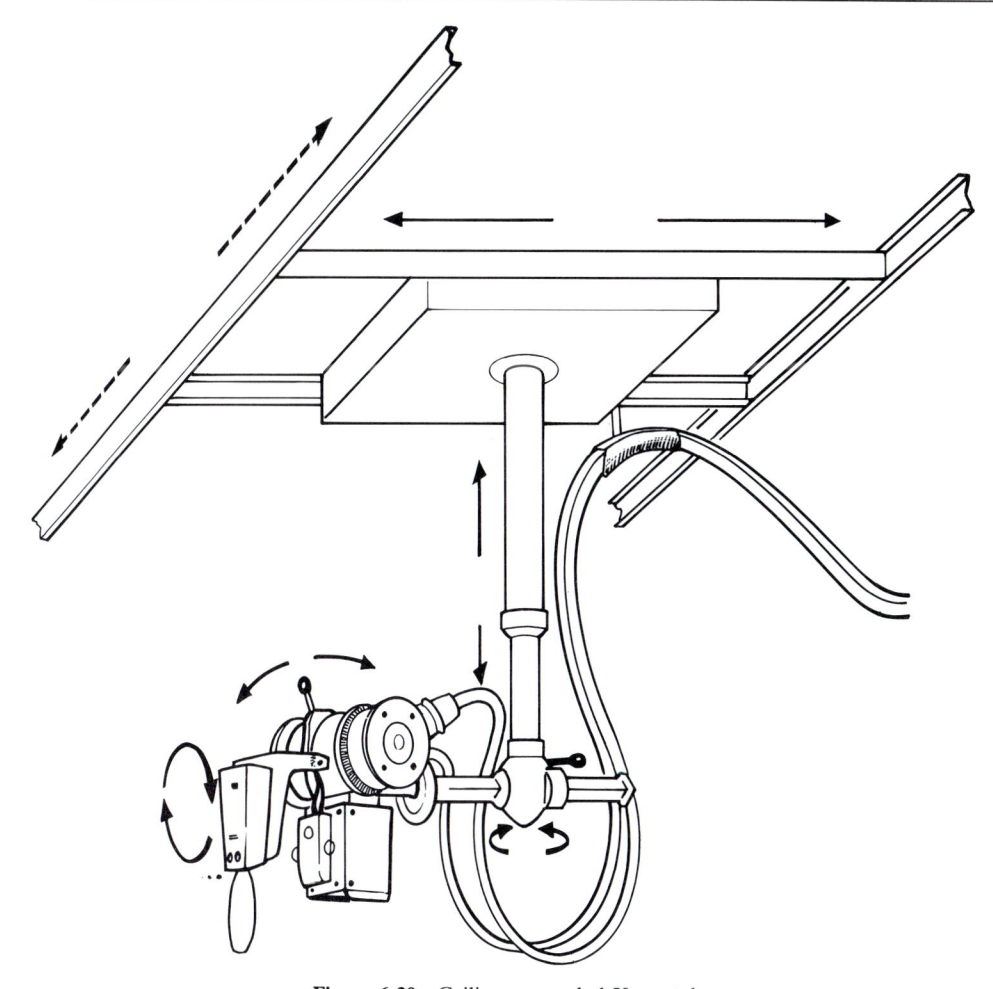

Figure 6.30 Ceiling-suspended X-ray tube

It will be noted that longitudinal movement is achieved by moving the tube and transverse carriage along the fixed track in the direction of the broken arrows. Transverse movement is achieved by moving the tube and cradle (from which it is suspended) along the transverse carriage in the direction of the black arrows. The transverse movement may be locked whilst the tube is moved in a longitudinal direction and conversely the longitudinal movement may be locked when the tube is moved in a transverse direction. If both locks are left off the tube may be moved diagonally or even in circles. The tube is usually suspended on a telescopic arm, Figure 6.31(b) by means of which it is raised or lowered, the movement usually being motorized. The switches controlling the various movements etc. of the tube may be gathered together on a control unit as shown in Figure 6.31(a).

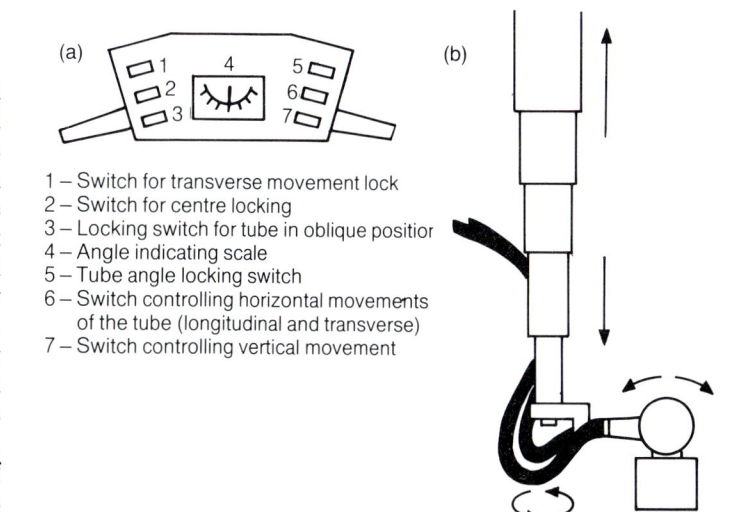

1 – Switch for transverse movement lock
2 – Switch for centre locking
3 – Locking switch for tube in oblique position
4 – Angle indicating scale
5 – Tube angle locking switch
6 – Switch controlling horizontal movements of the tube (longitudinal and transverse)
7 – Switch controlling vertical movement

Figure 6.31 (a) Handlebar control unit. (b) telescopic tube support

Motorized movements

The up and down movements of the tube are usually motorized whilst movement of the tube in a longitudinal or transverse direction is usually controlled manually. Electromagnetic locks effectively hold the tube in the desired position or angle. Automatic stops at selected focus to film distances are usually provided as well as automatic stops which limit the longitudinal and transverse movements of the tube and thus prevent it banging into walls etc.

Switches to control the motorized movements and the electromagnetic locks are usually mounted on a conveniently placed control box which is located either at the front of the tube itself or on a rod which is attached to the ceiling cradle.

An automatic cut-out switch is fitted to the base of the light beam diaphragm – this switches off the electric motor drive if the encircling metal band at the base of the light beam diaphragm is depressed. This prevents the tube being driven inadvertently into the table top or the patient!

Advantages of ceiling-suspended tubes

Advantages in the use of ceiling suspended tubes include:

(1) Uncluttered floor space due to absence of floor track.
(2) Greater area of the room made available for radiography due to increased transverse movement of the tube.
(3) Greater flexibility in the use of other equipment, e.g. chest stand, pedestal bucky, etc.
(4) Ability to radiograph patients on accident trolleys, wheelchairs, etc.
(5) Ability to take lateral views from either side of the table.

Disadvantages

(1) Possible need to reinforce the ceiling, to provide necessary strength to hold the tracks, suspension and tube.
(2) Need for minimum room height.
(3) Extra length of high tension cable needed to cover the increased area.

'C' arm supports

The 'C' arm is used with mobile image intensifier units, skull units, etc. These will be described in greater detail later. Suffice to say at the moment that the X-ray tube is positioned at one end of a metal arc whilst the counterbalance or image intensifier is mounted at the other.

7
Control of scattered radiation, X-ray tables and 'bucky' stands

SCATTERED RADIATION	85
Formation of the radiographic image	85
STATIONARY GRIDS	87
Parallel grid or non-focused grid	87
The focused grid	89
Cross-hatch grids	90
The grid cassette	90
The all metal grid	90
Metal filter	91
Assessing the efficiency of a grid	91
MOVING GRID MECHANISMS	92
Operation of the reciprocating bucky	92
Disadvantages	92
Oscillating 'vibrating' movement	92
Siemens catapult bucky	93
INTERCHANGEABLE GRIDS	93
SIEMENS 'SLOT' TECHNIQUE	93
LIMITATION OF THE PRIMARY BEAM	94
The light beam diaphragm	95
Use with automatic exposure control	96
Use in theatre with optical viewfinder	96
Undercouch tube – automatic beam collimation	96
Crossed light beam centring device	97
X-RAY TABLES	97
Floating top table	97
Variable height table	98
Other 'bucky' assemblies	98
The vertical bucky	98
The Versatilt bucky	98

SCATTERED RADIATION

Formation of the radiographic image

As radiation traverses the patient's tissues during a diagnostic exposure it is attenuated by the processes of photo-electric absorption and compton scatter. The processed radiograph is a pattern of densities forming a shadow image of the structures penetrated by the radiation. The extent to which the radiation is absorbed is determined by the atomic number of the tissues encountered. Bone, for example (atomic number 14), absorbs more radiation than soft tissue (atomic number 7.4) or fat (atomic number 6.0). The image is formed by emergent primary radiation reaching the film. Contrast is determined partly by the extent to which primary radiation penetrates the various body structures and partly by the effects of scatter.

The optimum kVp is that which will adequately penetrate the part under examination so as to outline it against surrounding tissues and demonstrate its structure. When the atomic number of the structure is the same as its surroundings it cannot be differentiated, e.g. gall bladder, alimentary tract, etc., and in these circumstances it is necessary to use a contrast agent with a different, in this case a higher, atomic number to demonstrate the part against its surroundings.

Scattered radiation is radiation deviated in direction from that of the primary beam. At low kVp values scatter tends to be sideways and backwards in direction whilst at increasing kV values the proportion of scattered radiation in a forward direction is increased. The effects of scattered radiation are always deleterious in diagnostic radiography. As forward scatter falls indiscriminately on the film it has the same effect as general fog. Scatter reaching the film thus reduces contrast. Figures 7.1–5 illustrate some of the factors which affect the amount of scatter reaching the film.

So far we have discussed a number of ways in which the amount of scatter reaching the film can be reduced. These include:

(1) Smallest possible field size, e.g. beam collimation.

(2) Lowest possible kVp consistent with adequate penetration of the part in question.

(3) Use of the displacement band to reduce the thickness of the part under investigation.

(4) In special cases, use of the air-gap technique.

Whilst these measures limit the amount of radiation

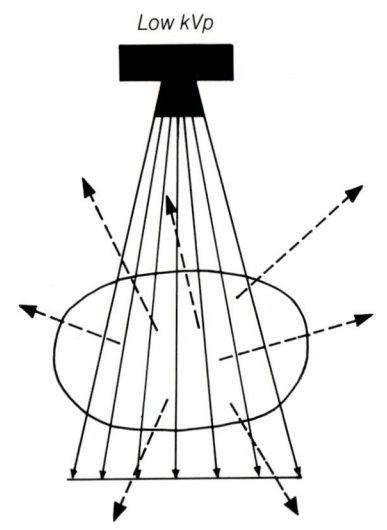

Figure 7.1 Low kVp. A greater proportion of the radiation is scattered backwards and to the sides at low kVps, thus *less* scatter reaches the film

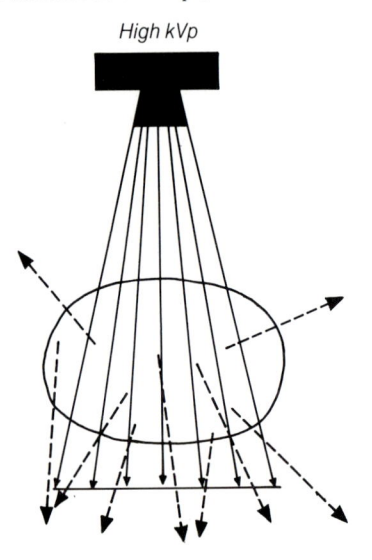

Figure 7.2 High kVp. A greater proportion of the radiation is scattered in a forward direction, thus *more* scatter reaches the film

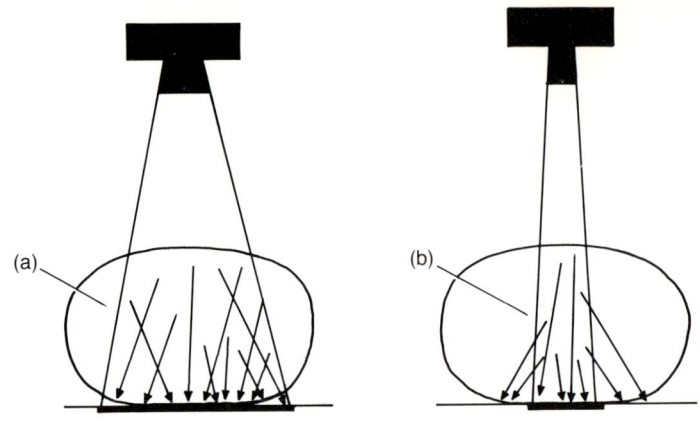

Figure 7.3 (a) Large field size, large amount of scatter produced. (b) Small field size, small amount of scatter produced. Moral – 'cone down'

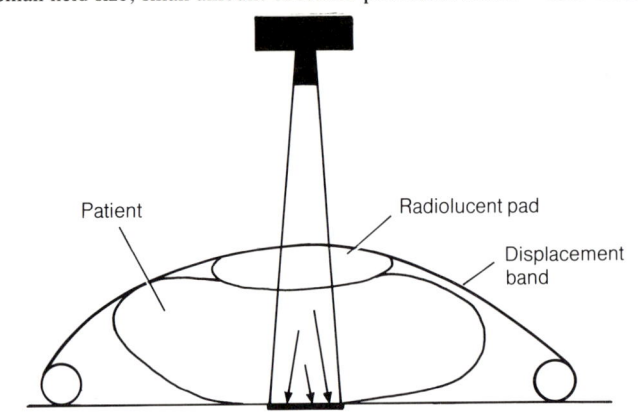

Figure 7.4 The greater the thickness of tissue the greater the amount of scatter. Moral – displace fatty tissues by means of a radiolucent pad and a displacement (compression) band

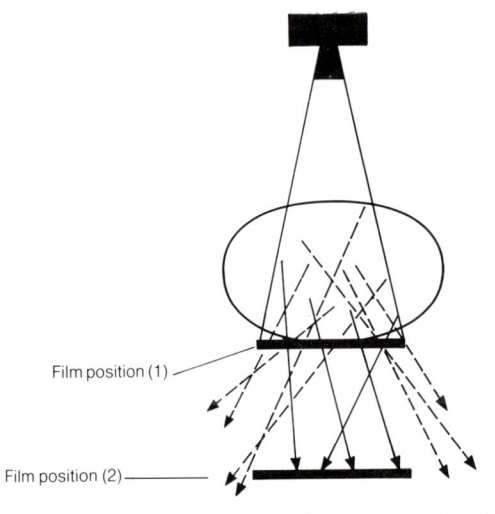

Figure 7.5 Air-gap technique. All of the scatter reaches the film in position (1) but only that shown as solid lines reaches the film in position (2)

reaching the film, they may not, in themselves, be sufficient to produce satisfactory radiographs of thicker parts such as the abdomen. The relatively high kVp needed to penetrate the part, and the thickness of the part itself results in a large amount of scatter being produced and consequently a radiograph lacking in contrast.

In these circumstances a secondary radiation grid must be used to absorb scattered radiation *before it reaches the film*. It should be borne in mind that whilst the measures described up to now reduce patient dose, the use of a grid always necessitates increased exposure dose to the patient.

The secondary radiation grid consists of alternate parallel strips of radio-opaque and radiolucent material. The radio-opaque strips or slats are usually made of lead or tungsten and the radiolucent spacing material of aluminium, paper or wood (Figure 7.6). It has a protective covering, front and back, of thin aluminium or plastic and protective strips around the edges of the grid.

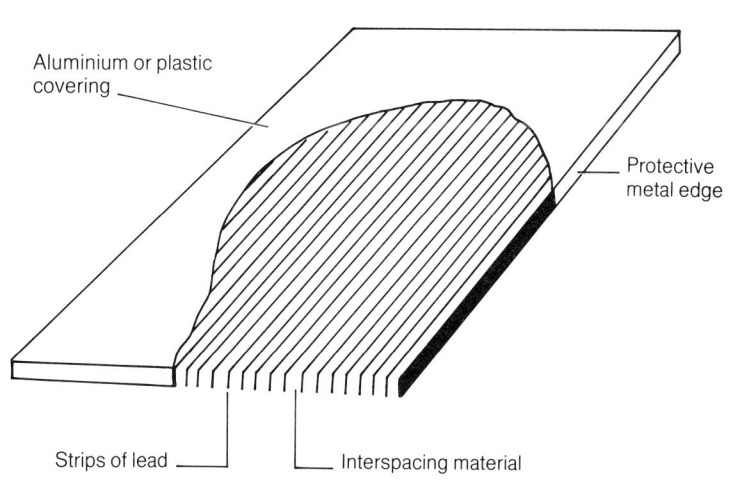

Figure 7.6 Diagrammatic representation of a parallel secondary radiation grid

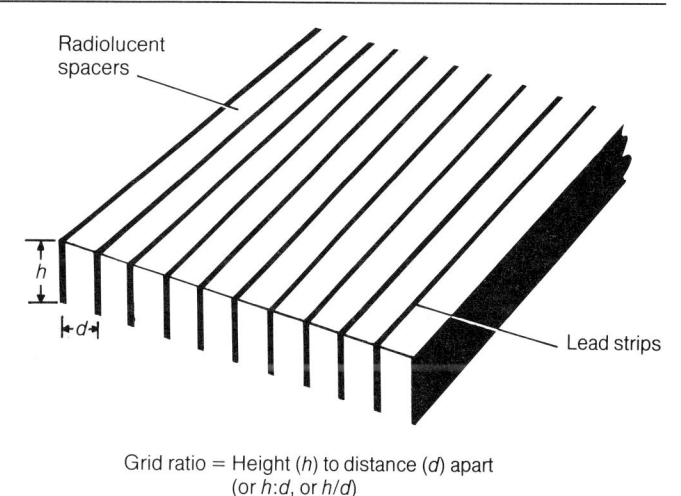

Figure 7.7 Non-focused or parallel grid

Grid ratio = Height (h) to distance (d) apart (or $h:d$, or h/d)

Grid ratio is the relationship between the height of the lead strips to their distance apart. The higher the grid ratio the more effective is the grid in the absorption of scatter (see Figure 7.7).

The grid factor, however, which is the number of times we must increase the exposure when using a particular grid as opposed to the exposure required without the grid, also increases with grid ratio.

Grid ratios from 4:1 to 16:1 are available and most units have the facility of interchangeability of grids. A low ratio grid is used for low kV work and one of high ratio for techniques involving the use of high kVp, or the production of large amounts of scatter.

Grid lattice is the number of lead (or tungsten) strips per centimetre measured across the grid (i.e. at right angles to the grid lines).

STATIONARY GRIDS

There are three main types of grid, the *parallel grid* (Figure 7.6) in which the lead strips, separated by radiolucent spacers, are positioned parallel to one another, the *focused grid* and the *cross-hatch grid*. The focused grid is similar to the parallel grid in so far as it also is made up of lead strips with radiolucent spacers but in its case the strips of lead are angled towards the edges as shown later in Figure 7.14. Note that peripheral radiation, absorbed by the outer strips of lead in the parallel grid, is able to pass through the angled strips of lead in the focused grid without hindrance. The *cross-hatch grid* is composed of lead strips placed at right angles to one another. The scatter is thus absorbed from all angles. Note that when using this grid the beam must be centred to the centre of the grid and that no off-centring or tilting of the beam is permissible.

Parallel grid or non-focused grid

The parallel grid is frequently used in conjunction with a mobile unit for radiography in the ward or theatre. The focus–grid distance is not critical (as it is with the focused grid) but it should not be too short as the peripheral cut-off increases as the focus–grid distance decreases (Figure 7.8).

Limitation of field size also reduces peripheral cut-off as shown in Figure 7.9.

Centring of the beam to the grid is not critical providing part of the grid is positioned under the area of interest (Figure 7.10).

The radiation must be kept as nearly as possible parallel to the strips of lead. This means that the tube can be angled parallel to the strips but not against them (Figure 7.11). The grid should not be tilted transversely otherwise there will be marked cut-off on one side (Figure 7.12).

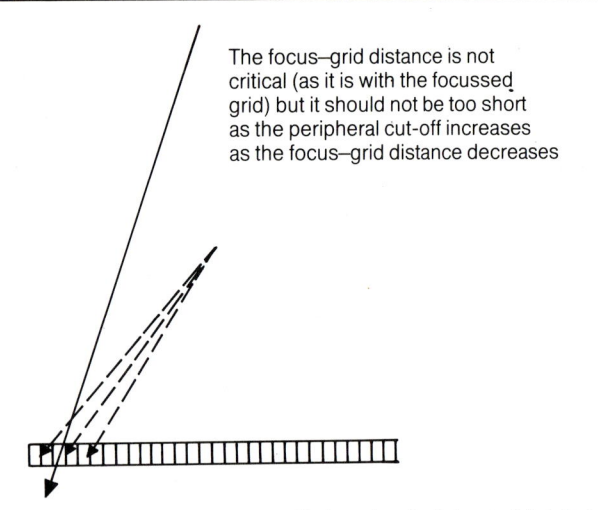

88 EQUIPMENT FOR DIAGNOSTIC RADIOGRAPHY

Figure 7.8 Dotted lines indicate radiation absorbed due to f.f.d. being too short

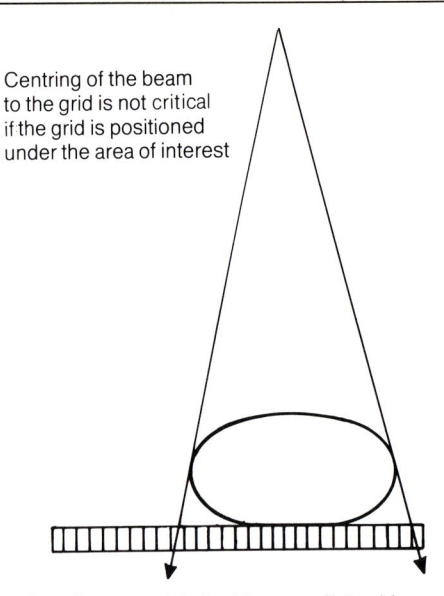

The focus–grid distance is not critical (as it is with the focussed grid) but it should not be too short as the peripheral cut-off increases as the focus–grid distance decreases

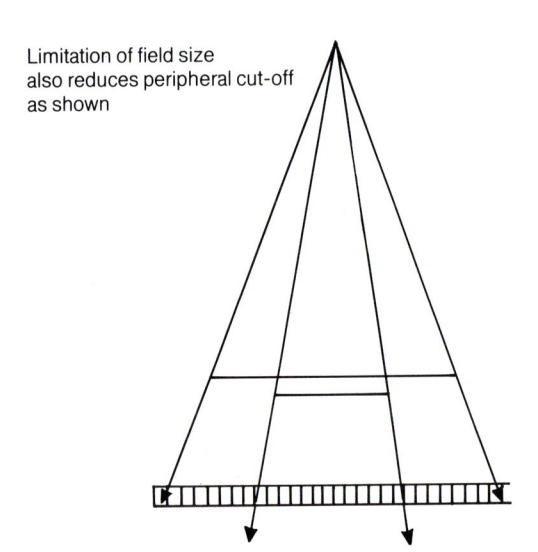

Figure 7.9 Increased cut off due to large field size

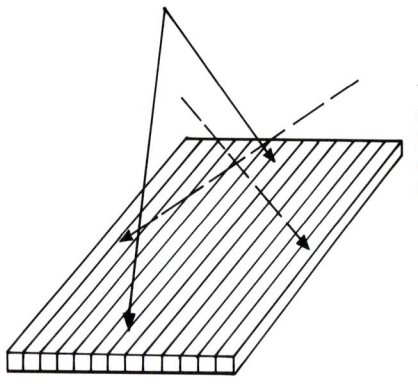

Limitation of field size also reduces peripheral cut-off as shown

Figure 7.10 Centring not critical with a parallel grid

Centring of the beam to the grid is not critical if the grid is positioned under the area of interest

Figure 7.11 Tube should not be angled across the grid

The radiation must be kept as nearly as possible parallel to the strips of lead. This means that the tube can be angled parallel to the strips but not against them

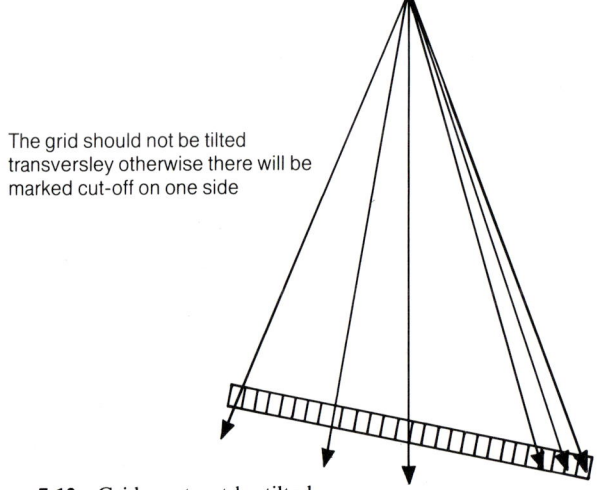

Figure 7.12 Grid must not be tilted

The grid should not be tilted transversley otherwise there will be marked cut-off on one side

Some parallel grids have shorter lead strips at the edges, to allow more peripheral radiation to pass through (Figure 7.13).

The following points should be noted when using a stationary parallel grid.

(1) use a relatively long focus–grid distance particularly when using a large field of radiation.

(2) Limit the field size as far as possible.

(3) Don't angle the beam of radiation into the lead strips by either tilting the beam transversely or angling the grid transversely.

CONTROL OF SCATTERED RADIATION, X-RAY TABLES AND 'BUCKY' STANDS 89

Some parallel grids have shorter lead strips at the edges, to allow more peripheral radiation to pass through

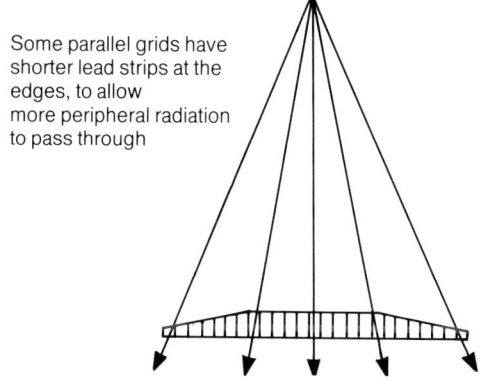

Figure 7.13 Parallel grid prismatic section

The focused grid

The *focused grid* is composed of strips of lead angled towards the edges as shown in Figure 7.14.

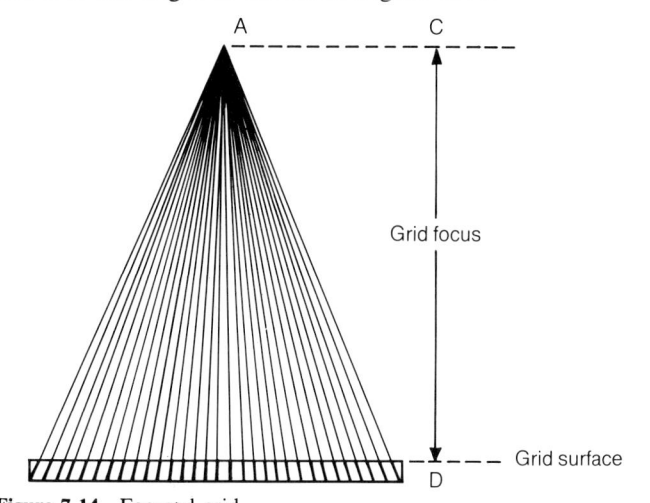

Figure 7.14 Focused grid

The lead strips are set at particular angles; if these angles are extended as shown they intersect at point A. Distance C–D is the grid focus.

If the tube focus is positioned at point A primary radiation passes through the interspaces parallel to the lead strips.

It should be noted that even when the tube is positioned at the correct focal–grid distance (grid focus) some *primary* radiation is absorbed by the lead strips. The greater the lead content of the grid, e.g. the greater the number of lines per cm or the thicker the lead the greater the absorption of primary radiation.

If the focal–grid distance is greater or less than the grid focus there is geometric cut-off. The primary radiation, instead of passing through the interspaces parallel to the

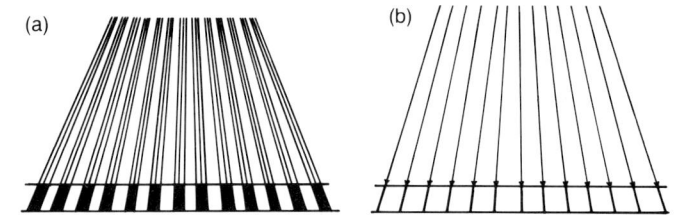

Figure 7.15 (a) Focused grid with high lead content – absorption of scattered radiation good but absorption of primary high. (b) Focused grid with low lead content – absorption of secondary poor but absorption of primary is also low

strips of lead is partially or completely absorbed by the lead (Figure 7.16).

If the focal-grid distance is greater or less than the grid focus there is geometric cut-off.
The primary radiation instead of passing through the inter-spaces parallel to the strips of lead strike the lead and are partially or completely absorbed

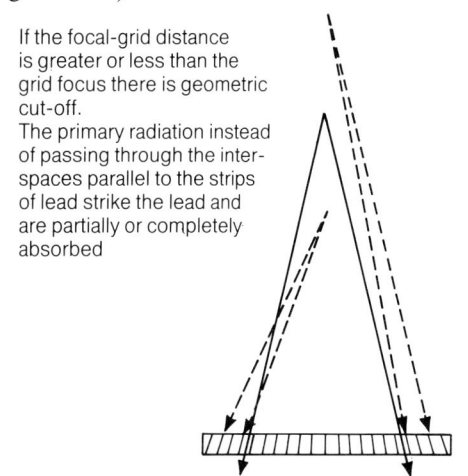

Figure 7.16 Absorption of primary due to incorrect grid focus distance

If the grid is tilted transversely to the beam of radiation there is cut-off, particularly at one side of the grid (Figure 7.17). If the beam is off-centred transversely to the length

If the grid is tilted transversley to the beam of radiation there is cut-off by the grid

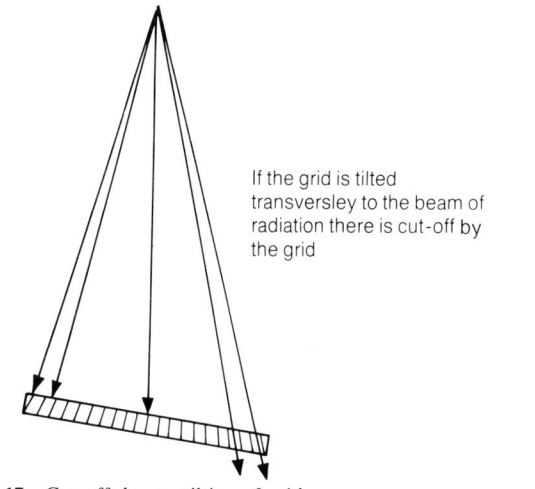

Figure 7.17 Cut-off due to tilting of grid

of the strips of lead there is marked cut-off (Figure 7.18).

If the beam is off centred transversley to the length of the strips of lead there is marked cut-off

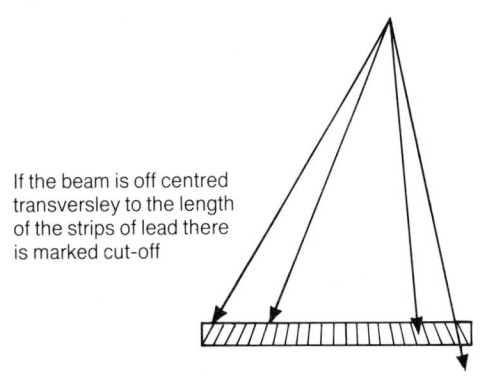

Figure 7.18 Cut-off due to incorrect centring of tube to grid

If a focused grid is used with the wrong surface towards the tube there is marked absorption of the peripheral rays (Figure 7.19). The extent to which the radiation is absorbed is dependent on the kVp used and the thickness of the lead strips. The radiograph shows normal density in the mid-line portion but fades off rapidly towards the edges. If the reason for this fault is not immediately comprehended and rectified (by turning the grid over) repeat exposures may be made resulting in increased and unnecessary dosage to the patient.

Wrong surface of grid to tube

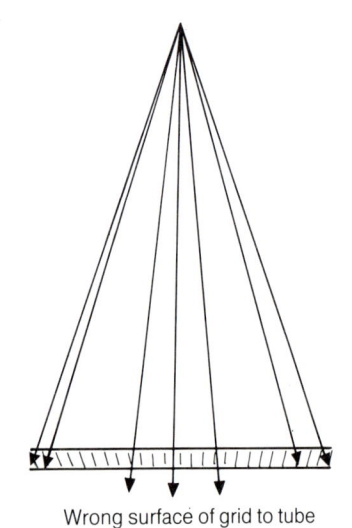

Figure 7.19 Cut-off due to grid being upside down

Ideally, a grid should absorb as little of the primary radiation as possible, e.g. the grid factor should be as close to unity as possible. *Grid loss* is a term frequently used to denote the amount of primary radiation absorbed by a grid.

Cross-hatch grids

Cross-hatched grids consist of two parallel or focused grids placed at right angles to one another (Figure 7.20). The pattern recorded on the radiograph is of tiny squares. When a high kV is used, as in examinations such as biplane angiocardiography, a lot of scatter is produced in all directions and a cross-hatch grid may be used to good effect. The X-ray beam must be centred to the grids and be at right angles to them. If it is necessary to tilt the beam a single grid must be used, otherwise the beam will be directed into one or other of the grids. The exposure must be increased when using a cross-hatch grid, and if the X-ray tubes are already being used at or near maximum loading, e.g. in biplane radiography, it may be necessary to sacrifice the improved quality achieved with a cross-hatch grid, and accept the results obtainable with a single grid.

Cross hatch grid

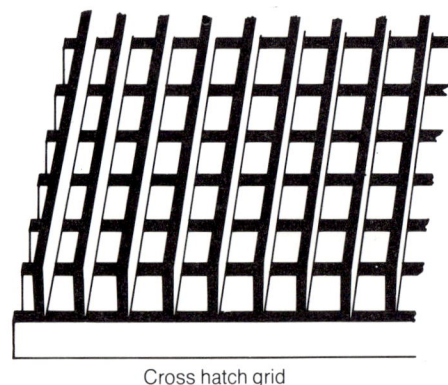

Figure 7.20 Cross-hatched grid

The grid cassette

Whilst the stationary grid may be used by simply placing it on the cassette, it is possible to obtain cassettes in which the grid is fitted as an integral part. Whilst grid cassettes are very convenient in use, if a number of exposures have to be made, e.g. in the ward or theatre, a number of grid cassettes, possibly of different sizes, will be required and the expense may be prohibitive.

The all metal grid

This uses aluminium as an interspacing material and as a protective covering. A number of different ratios are available as focused or parallel grids. The aluminium interspacing material absorbs more primary than organic material, but their sturdy construction renders them particularly useful for theatre and mobile radiography. (Examples of organic material are paper, wood, plastic, etc.)

Metal filter

A sheet of metal, e.g. lead foil (0.1 mm), may be placed on top of the cassette to absorb scattered radiation. Although some primary radiation is absorbed as well as scatter, the metal sheet does tend to absorb more scatter than primary (Figure 7.21). The reasons for this are twofold. First, because the scatter is travelling through the metal at a greater angle than the primary it must perforce travel through a greater thickness of metal and, secondly, because the scatter has less energy, i.e. longer wavelength than the primary, it is more readily absorbed. The advantage of this method of scatter absorption is that there is no critical focal-grid distance to be considered and the central ray may be directed in any direction. It may also be used in conjunction with a moving grid to further enhance contrast. The greatest disadvantage is that the exposure must be increased significantly to offset the high absorption of primary radiation.

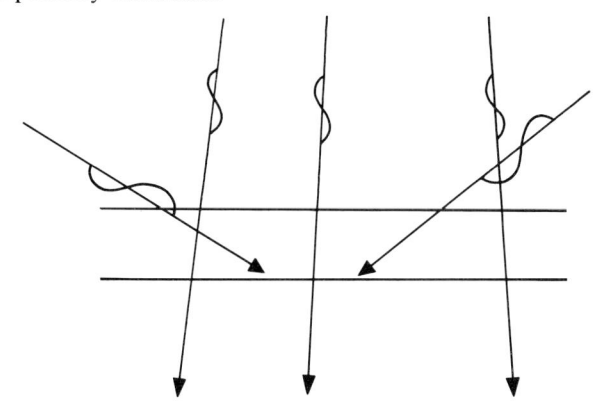

Figure 7.21 Metal filter used to absorb scatter

Assessing the efficiency of a grid

The grid is made up of alternate strips of metal and interspacing material. The function of the metal strips is to absorb scatter and that of the interspacing material to support the metal strips at the required angle and position with minimal absorption of primary.

The higher the atomic number and density of a material the greater are the chances of that material absorbing radiation. (Absorption $\propto Z^3$.) The metal of choice for the strips in a grid is usually lead (atomic number 82), but some manufacturers use tungsten (atomic number 74) as an alternative material. Siemens Superfine Grids, for instance, with 50 strips to the cm use tungsten as the absorbing metal with which the strips are formed. The ratio of this particular grid is 5:1, and its selectivity is poorer than an 8:1 grid with 40 lead strips per cm. However, it is not as critical as regards centring and focusing, and as there are so many strips to the cm they are practically invisible on the radiograph at normal viewing distance. Such a grid is particularly useful for theatre and mobile radiography.

Whilst the metal strips must be good absorbers of radiation the interspacing material must absorb as little radiation as possible.

Grid ratio indicates to some extent the radiographic efficiency of a grid, but it does not tell us the whole story. For instance, by increasing the number of lead strips in a grid we increase its efficiency so far as absorption of scatter is concerned. However, by putting more lead strips in the grid we also reduce the amount of primary radiation reaching the film. If the thickness of the lead strips remains constant and we continually increase the number of lead strips we would end up with a grid consisting of a solid sheet of lead – the absorption of the secondary radiation would be very high, possibly approaching 100%, but the absorption of the primary would also be so high that we would get virtually no image-forming radiation through the grid to the film. What is needed is a high degree of secondary absorption with minimal absorption of primary. The efficiency of a grid can best be described by considering the ratio of these two factors to one another.

The ratio of the amount of primary radiation passing through a grid to the amount of scatter passing through the grid is called the selectivity of the grid.

$$\text{Selectivity} = \frac{\text{Transmitted primary}}{\text{Transmitted scatter}}$$

A variation in selectivity of at least 20% is needed between two grids before any difference becomes apparent radiographically.

An example will help make this clear. Table 7.1 shows the selectivity, at different kV values of two grids, each having about the same grid ratio but different numbers of lead strips to the cm.

Table 7.1 Selectivity of two grids at different kV values

	75 kV	100 kV	125 kV	150 kV
Grid A 40 strips per cm (12:1)	8.5	5.8	5.2	5.1
Grid B 24 strips per cm (12.8:1)	16.0	12.0	11.0	10.1

The fine line grid (A) has a lower selectivity than grid (B) at all kV values. This means that, although grid (A) has a large number of lines per cm which will not be readily apparent on the radiograph, the elimination of scatter is not as good as that of grid (B) and the film will, therefore, have less contrast.

MOVING GRID MECHANISMS

Whilst stationary grids absorb scatter they also record a pattern of their grid lines on the radiograph. However, if the lines are close together (large number of grid lines to the cm) their presence tends to be unobtrusive and they may be quite difficult to detect when viewing the radiograph at the normal distance.

We also noted, however, that if there are a large number of grid lines per cm the increased number of strips is usually accommodated by making each of the strips of thinner metal (lead or tungsten). Consequently, the selectivity of such a grid is usually lower than that of a grid with fewer lines per cm providing the lesser number of strips are made of thicker lead and the grid ratio remains constant.

The better grid to use in practice will obviously be the grid with the greatest selectivity, e.g. the grid which allows the greatest transmission of primary with the maximum absorption of scatter but only if the coarse pattern of grid lines can be eliminated from the radiograph. Elimination of grid pattern is achieved by causing the grid to move during the exposure.

It should be noted that everything said previously about stationary grids applies equally to moving grids, e.g. there should be minimal off-centring of the beam to the grid. A focused grid should be used at the correct FFD. Care should be taken to position the grid with the correct surface to the tube and the beam should not be directed against the grid lines etc. It is obvious that if the grid is moving during the exposure it cannot remain centred to the tube. Some degree of off-centring is inevitable, but this is minimized by making the grid move as short a distance as practicable during the exposure (usual distance is about 4.5 cm).

Other disadvantages include the possible vibration of the cassette due to movement of the grid and the unavoidable increase in geometric blurring and enlargement of the image due to the increase in object film distance, needed to accommodate the moving grid and its associated mechanism.

The types of grid movement in general use are:

Reciprocating movement	Grid moves fast in one direction and slowly in the other, maintaining this sequence throughout the exposure
Oscillating (vibrating) movement	Grid moves back and forth across the film during exposure
Catapult movement	Grid makes one movement across film. Initial speed is very high, then it moves more and more slowly.

The single stroke, potter bucky movement, using a single, timed movement of the grid across the film during an exposure, was popular for many years, but is now almost obsolete.

Reciprocating movement

Pressing the exposure switch on the unit energizes an electromagnet which pulls the grid rapidly across the film and simultaneously tensions a spring. The exposure is started when contacts are closed shortly after the grid begins to move. Just before it reaches the end of its travel the grid breaks a contact which stops current flowing in the electromagnet and the grid is pulled across the film, by the spring, in the opposite direction. This time, however, movement is slowed by the oil in a hydraulic system. Just before it reaches the end of its travel the grid operates a contact which energizes the electromagnet once again. This sequence continues, fast in one direction, slow in the other, until the end of the exposure.

A short exposure takes place whilst the grid is moving fast and a longer exposure extends into the slow return movement. Still longer exposure take place whilst the grid is moving alternately fast and slow.

Disadvantages

(1) The grid is stationary for a brief fraction of time at each reversal of movement. There is the possibility of synchronism occurring. Synchronism occurs when the grid lines are in the same position for each pulse of radiation. Such a danger can be reduced by using a different type of grid movement, e.g. a vibrating grid movement whose frequency of alternation is not constant but decreases rapidly with time.

(2) The rapid and slow movements of the grid can easily cause vibrations to be set up in the X-ray table or erect bucky. Such vibration inevitably leads to loss of film quality.

Oscillating 'vibrating' movement

The grid, supported by four leaf springs, makes a backwards and forwards movement over the film.

When the exposure switch is put into 'prep' an electromagnet is energized and it pulls the grid across to the limit of its travel. The grid is held in this position with the springs tensioned ready for an exposure. When the exposure switch is pressed, a relay is operated which stops current flowing to the electromagnet and the grid is released. The grid is now free to move back and forth under the influence of the springs. Shortly after the grid begins its movement it operates a relay which starts the exposure.

CONTROL OF SCATTERED RADIATION, X-RAY TABLES AND 'BUCKY' STANDS

The grid continues to vibrate during the exposure but the frequency of vibration is not constant and the grid vibrates slower and slower until it finally comes to rest after 15–30 seconds, which is long enough for any diagnostic exposure (Figure 7.22).

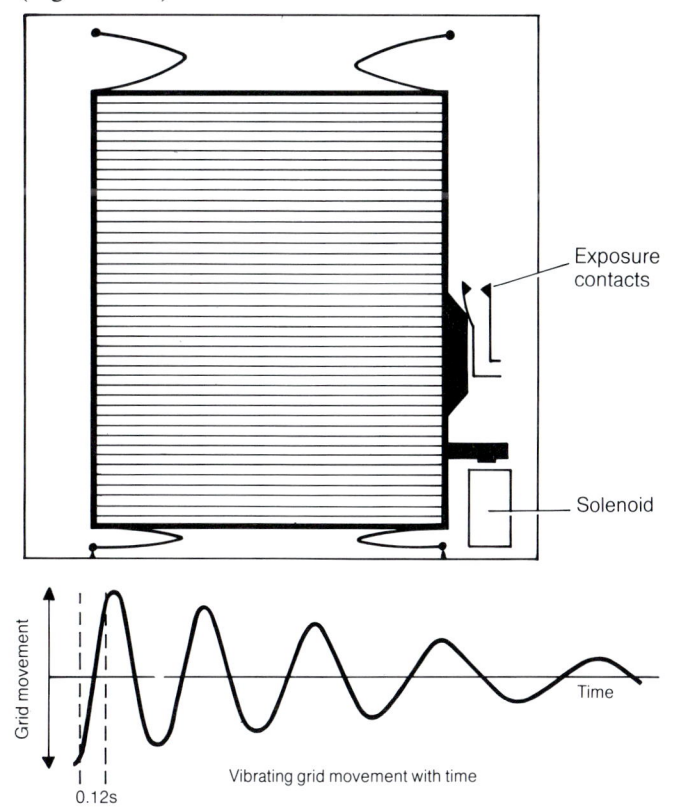

Figure 7.22 Vibrating grid mechanism and graph showing grid movement against time

Siemens catapult bucky

The grid moves initially at high speed then slows down in an exponential fashion.

The exposure is initiated shortly after the grid begins to move, i.e. when the grid is moving at its fastest. In this way short exposures occur whilst the grid is moving very fast and longer exposures extend into the time the grid is moving more and more slowly. This type of movement ensures grid movement during the exposure, whether the exposure is long or short.

The grid in this case is driven by an electric motor. There is no reversal of grid movement and the constantly changing rate of movement ensures that synchronism does not occur (Figure 7.23).

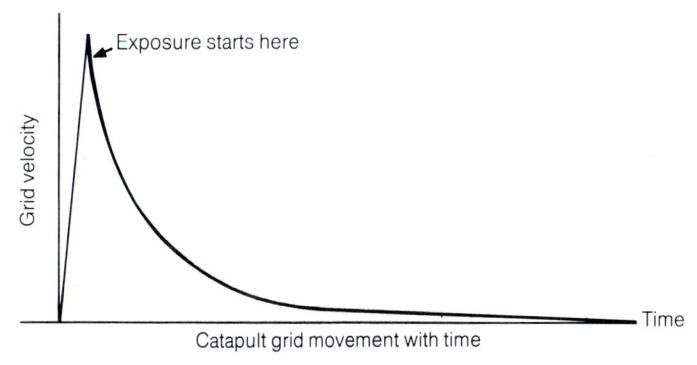

Figure 7.23 Catapult grid movement

INTERCHANGEABLE GRIDS

Most modern moving grid assemblies have grids which are supported in a metal frame and secured by catches. Releasing the catches allows the grid to be lifted from the frame and removed. A series of grids with different characteristics, e.g. different ratios, are available enabling the radiographer to choose the grid he feels most appropriate for a particular examination or kVp used.

SIEMENS 'SLOT' TECHNIQUE

Besides the conventional grid movements previously described, which are available in one form or another on all Siemens X-ray tables, some have an additional facility using the slot technique (Figure 7.24).

Using this technique the X-ray tube swivels about an axis, located at the tube focus, when an exposure is made. The X-ray beam is collimated to a narrow transverse slit approximately 1 cm in width which sweeps down the patient (and film) during the exposure. A second collimator located under the table top but above the cassette ensures that the slit of radiation does not exceed 1.0 cm when it reaches the film. Figure 7.25 illustrates the technique.

During the exposure the tube rotates and the narrow transverse beam of radiation passes down the patient. The primary and secondary slit diaphragms move down the table, as shown in Figure 7.25, exposing only a section of the film at a time. The film is thus exposed by a slit of radiation which moves continuously over the film during the exposure. There is no 'grid' as such and therefore patient dose is reduced by as much as 50%. The disadvantage of this technique lies in the fact that the film is exposed in sections and although the exposure is continuous the exposure *time* is obviously extended. For short exposure times, i.e. when there is likelihood of physical movement, the more conventional moving grid technique is used.

LIMITATION OF THE PRIMARY BEAM

We noted previously that the larger the field irradiated the greater is the amount of scatter produced. Restriction of the X-ray beam to the desired limits, with consequent reduction in scatter, may be achieved by the use of *cones*, *diaphragms* (single or multiplane) or, more usually, the *light beam* diaphragm. The *cone*, made of metal and sometimes lined with lead, restricts the beam to a specific area, the dimensions of which are determined by the length of the cone, its diameter and the focal film distance at which it is used. Cones project a circular field of radiation (Figure 7.26) but collimators can be obtained which give a rectangular field. The latter are generally more effective, excepting those cases especially suited to a circular field, e.g. radiography of the skull, sinuses, etc.

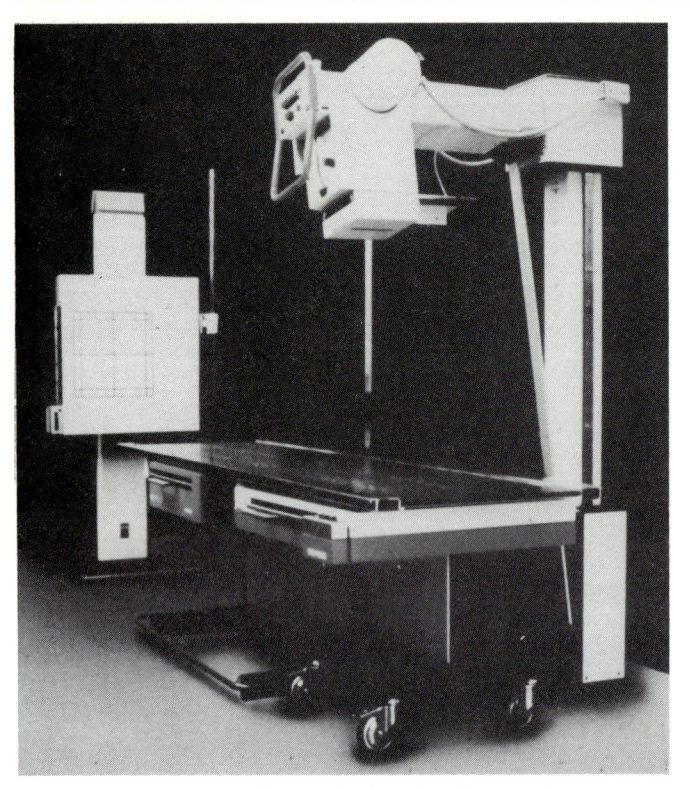

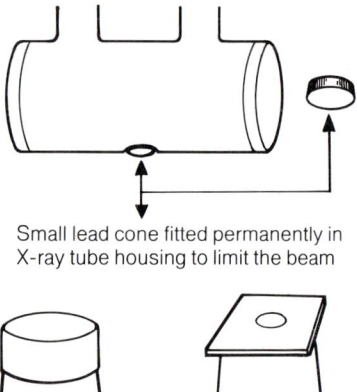

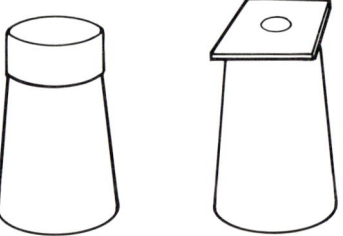

Figure 7.24 Siemens unit (Multix CPS) with choice of SLOT or conventional grid movement

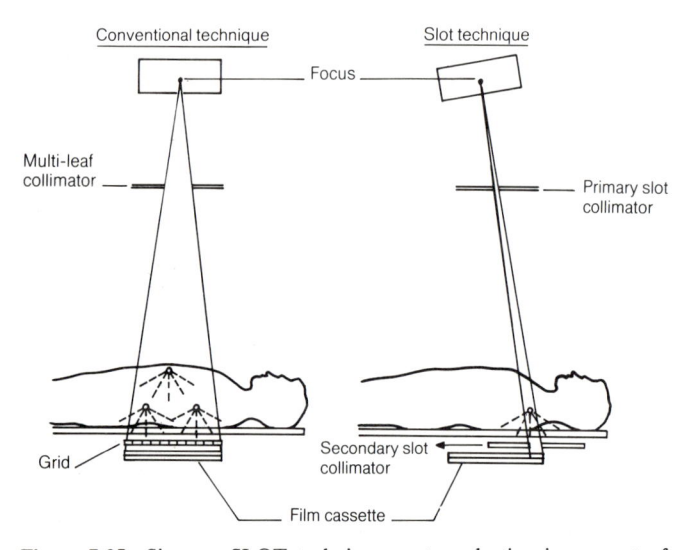

Figure 7.25 Siemens SLOT technique, note reduction in amount of scatter produced compared with conventional technique

Figure 7.26 Different types of metal cones

Another simple means of beam collimation is provided by the *plate diaphragm* which is simply a metal plate with a hole in it (Figure 7.27). The diameter of the hole determines the field covered at a particular focal film distance. A set of such diaphragms are provided as accessories for use with the skull unit. Although cheap and simple to use, single diaphragms do not give a sharply defined field because of the effects of the penumbra.

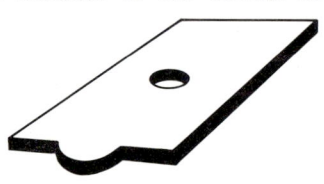

Figure 7.27 Plate diaphragm

CONTROL OF SCATTERED RADIATION, X-RAY TABLES AND 'BUCKY' STANDS

Penumbra, at the edge of the field, can be reduced by using cones or multiplane diaphragms. The longer the cone the less the penumbra.

Single plane diaphragms with a variable aperture (Figure 7.28), either circular or rectangular, whilst more flexible in use than the plate diaphragm also suffer from the problem of penumbra at the edge of the field of radiation.

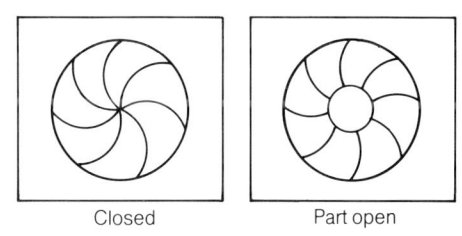

Figure 7.28 Variable Aperture Diaphragm (Iris Diaphragm) with lead leaves

The light beam diaphragm

This utilizes lead leaves, usually multiplane, to collimate the beam of radiation. The field covered is indicated by a beam of light which follows the same path as the X-ray beam. The lead leaves in each of the sets (A) and (B) can be moved in or out as indicated by the arrows (Figure 7.29). Pairs of lead leaves (1–2) and (5–6) and (3–4) with (7–8) move in and out in unison. However, each set of pairs (i.e. 1256 and 3478) can be moved independently of each other, making it possible to produce a rectangle of any dimensions, within the maximum limits of the housing.

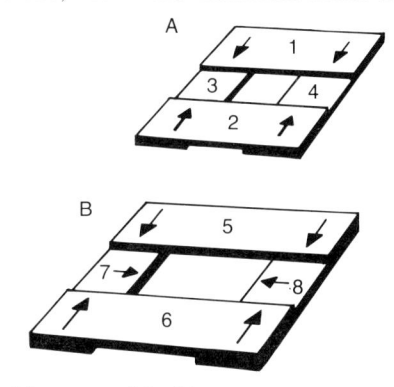

Figure 7.29 Movement of lead leaves

Movement of the leaves is controlled by levers or knobs. Linear movement of the former or rotation of the latter operates a drive which moves the diaphragm in or out. The field covered is indicated by the light from a high intensity lamp which is focused on to a radiolucent mirror, usually silvered plastic (aluminium equivalent about 0.5 mm) which is positioned at an angle of 45° to the central ray (Figure 7.30). Because such a lamp has a short life it is usual for it to be operated by a press button, self-cancelling switch which stays on for only a limited period, usually about 15 seconds. A separate spring-loaded switch is sometimes provided to allow increased light output for a limited period of time when the light beam diaphragm (LBD) is being used in a well lit room. A scale indicates the dimensions of the field covered at different focal film distances. The front of the LBD is made of clear plastic and either intersecting black lines or a black dot indicate the centre of the beam when the light shines on to the patient.

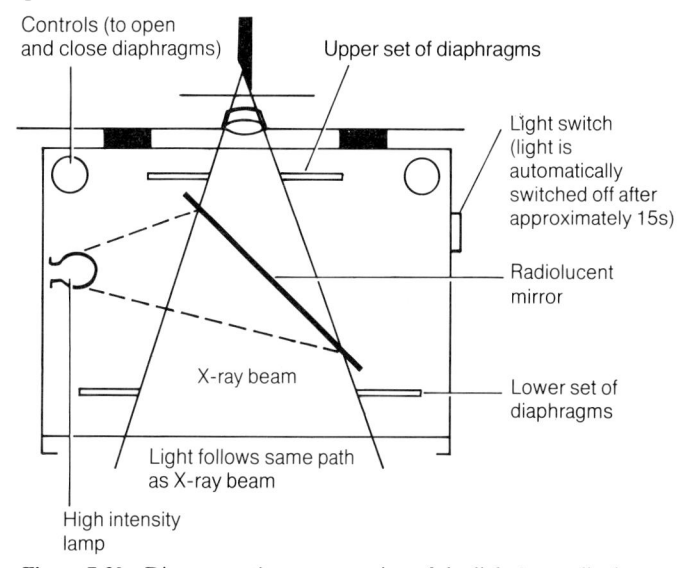

Figure 7.30 Diagrammatic representation of the light beam diaphragm

The light beam diaphragm can be rotated through 90° on its mounting, to allow the rectangular field to be lined up to the cassette when it is used on the table top. The underside of the LBD may be fitted with channels to allow the fitting of cones to provide a circular field for such examinations as the skull, sinuses etc. When the LBD is fitted to a tube with motorized movements (e.g. a ceiling-suspended tube) there may be a metal ring fitted to the face of the LBD. It is held off the face of the LBD by two coil springs. Compression of one or both of these springs operates a microswitch which breaks the circuit to the electric motor and stops the movement of the tube. This ensures that careless usage or a faulty electric switch does not cause the tube to be driven down on to the patient and cause injury, as the tube movement is stopped when the LBD touches the patient, compressing the springs and operating the cut-out switch.

It must be remembered that the beam of radiation and the beam of visible light are diverging, therefore the area indicated by the light on the patient's skin is always smaller than the area covered by radiation on the film (Figure 7.31). Care must therefore be taken not to irradiate too large an area, especially when such examinations as lumbosacral junctions etc. involving a large skin surface to film distance, are being undertaken.

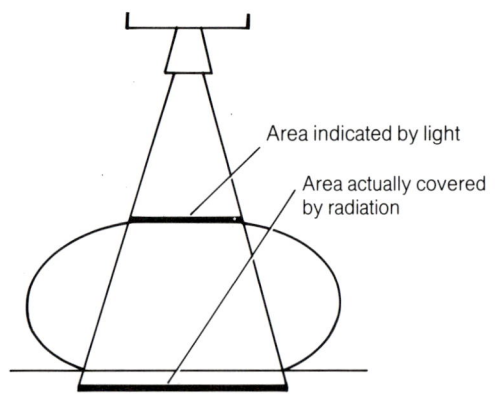

Figure 7.31 Area indicated on skin surface is always smaller than area of film exposed

Use with automatic exposure control

When a light beam diaphragm is fitted to a unit using automatic exposure control, such as the iontomat, the position of the ionization chambers (measuring fields) relative to the X-ray beam and the patient may be indicated by using a perspex sheet on which is marked the outline of the measuring fields. This is fitted to the front of the LBD and projects the outline of the measuring fields on to the patient's skin. The radiographer is thus able to ensure that the measuring field is under the patient and not exposed directly to radiation. A different plate must be used for each focal film distance.

Use in theatre with optical view finder

When the ambient lighting conditions are very bright, e.g. in the operating theatre, it may be difficult to see the light beam projected on to the patient's skin. In these circumstances an optical viewfinder is sometimes used. With this system the light source is replaced by an optical system. Light from the patient is reflected by the mirror on to a ground glass screen via an optical system (Figure 7.32). The radiation field is then viewed by the radiographer on the ground glass screen.

Undercouch tube – automatic beam collimation

When using an overcouch tube, the lead leaves of the light beam diaphragm can be adjusted manually so as to cover exactly the field required for a particular examination. The radiation field can be seen as an area of white light

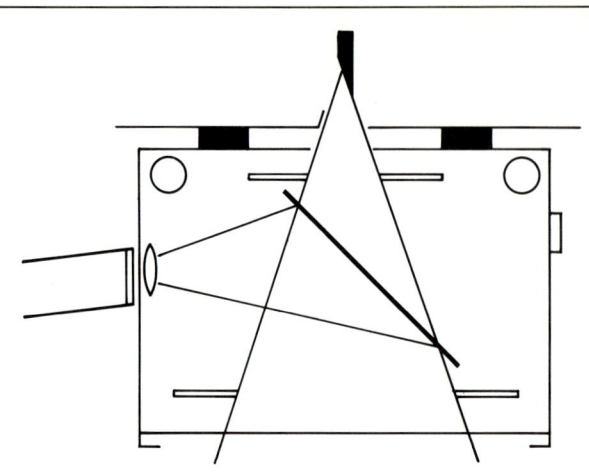

Figure 7.32 Light beam diaphragm with optical viewer

on the patient's skin and changes in field size due to variation in focal film distance can be compensated for by manipulation of the lead leaves.

As the undercouch tube is relatively inaccessible manual control of the diaphragms is obviously impracticable. The lead leaves are therefore driven in and out by small electric motors which are controlled by switches located either on the explorator panel or on a remote control trolley. If the beam of radiation from the undercouch tube is collimated, so as to just cover the fluorescent screen when it is fully compressed, the radiation will overshoot the edges of the screen when there is minimal compression (when the focal-screen distance is at a maximum) (Figure 7.33). If the radiation hazard is to be kept to a minimum it is necessary

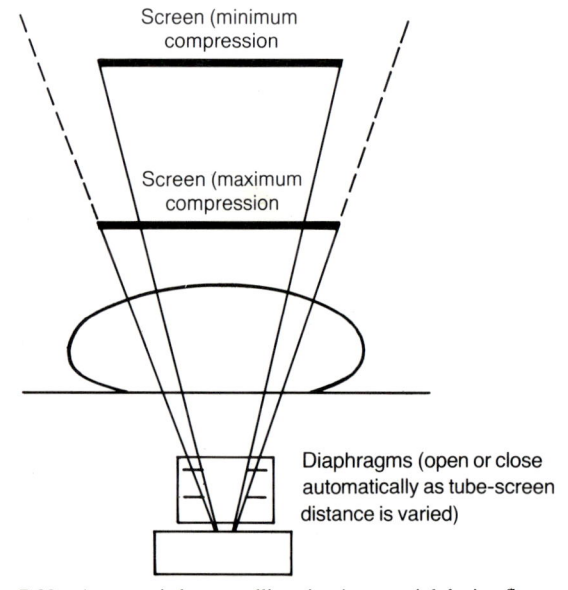

Figure 7.33 Automatic beam collimation is essential during fluoroscopy

CONTROL OF SCATTERED RADIATION, X-RAY TABLES AND 'BUCKY' STANDS

for the diaphragms to close as the focal-screen distance is increased and opened when it is decreased. It is essential that this collimation is automatically controlled if there is to be complete coverage of the fluorescent screen at all focal-screen distances with minimal danger of radiation dose to staff. It should be noted that the foregoing refers to *maximum* screen coverage, the radiologist is still quite free, of course, to reduce the field to as small an area as he wishes *within* this controlled area.

Similarly, in cassetteless radiography the beam is automatically collimated to the selected film format as described in Chapter 11.

Crossed light beam centring device

This device indicates the centre of the X-ray beam by means of two intersecting white lines which form a cross on the patient's skin.

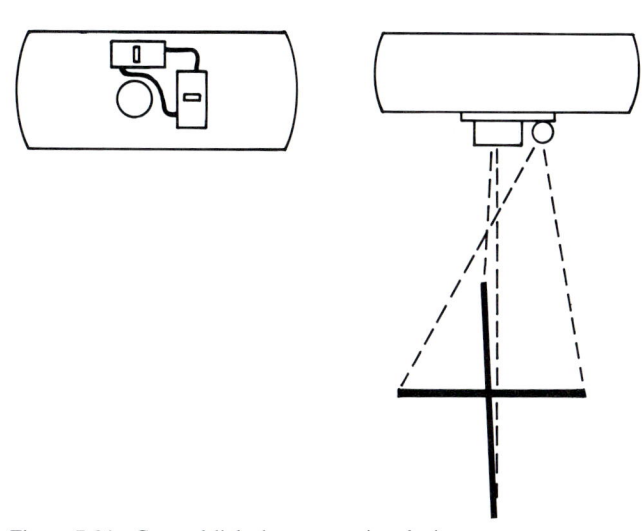

Figure 7.34 Crossed light beam centring device

Light from a focused high intensity lamp is projected through a slit in a metal container, two such containers being mounted at right angles to one another at each side of the tube window (Figure 7.34). Unlike the light beam diaphragm this device does not indicate or control the area being irradiated. As it does not obstruct the X-ray beam it need not be removed during an exposure, and cones may be used in conjunction with it. It is sometimes fitted to mobile units (most now have a small LBD) and skull units. When used with a skull unit these lights are useful as an aid to positioning as well as indicating the centre of the beam (Figure 7.35).

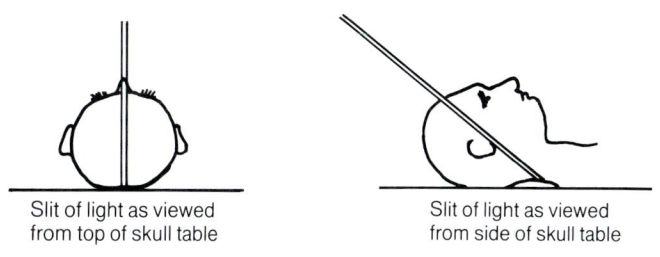

Slit of light as viewed from top of skull table

Slit of light as viewed from side of skull table

Figure 7.35 Crossed light beam centring device used as a positioning aid in radiography of the skull

X-RAY TABLES

The simplest X-ray table consists of a radiolucent top supported on four legs. The plain 'bucky' table also has a moving grid assembly (bucky) and cassette holder which is slung on rails under the table top. The grid and cassette, within the 'bucky' assembly, are thus held parallel to the table top and may be moved along the table under the patient and locked in any desired position (Figure 7.36). The locks are either manually or electromagnetically operated. Provision is made along the edges of the table for the attachment of displacement bands, head clamps, etc.

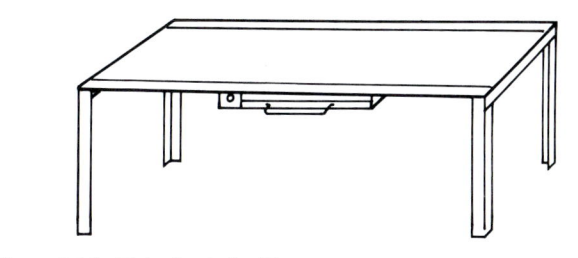

Figure 7.36 Plain 'bucky' table

Floating top table

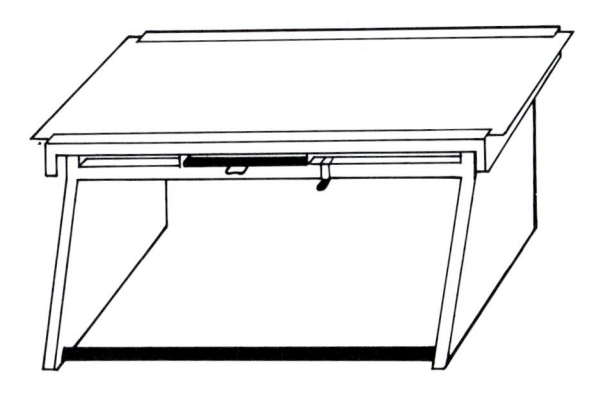

Figure 7.37 Floating top table

The floating top table makes it much easier to position the patient but the provision of a floating top also tends to increase the table top to film distance which also increases the enlargement and geometric unsharpness of the image. The table top may be 'dished' to reduce this effect, or in some models the 'bucky' mechanism is raised after the patient has been positioned. Alternatively the FFD may be increased slightly to minimize the increase in geometric unsharpness.

Longitudinal and lateral movements of the table are controlled by electromagnetic brakes and these are operated from either a full length pedal located at the base of the table or by hand-operated switches at each end of the table (Figure 7.37). The longitudinal and transverse movements may be locked independently of one another.

Variable height table

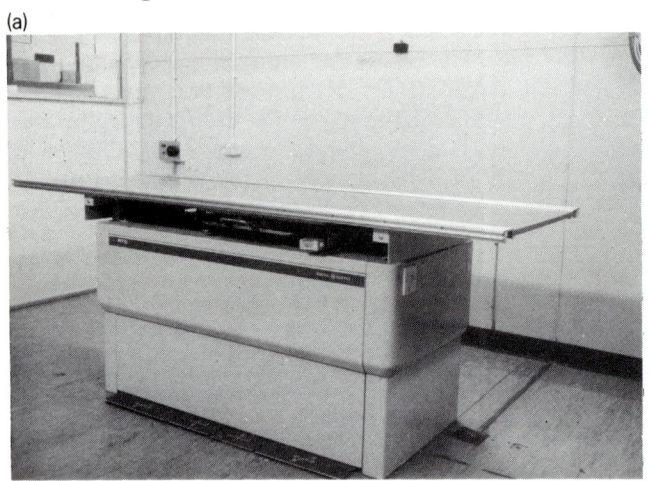

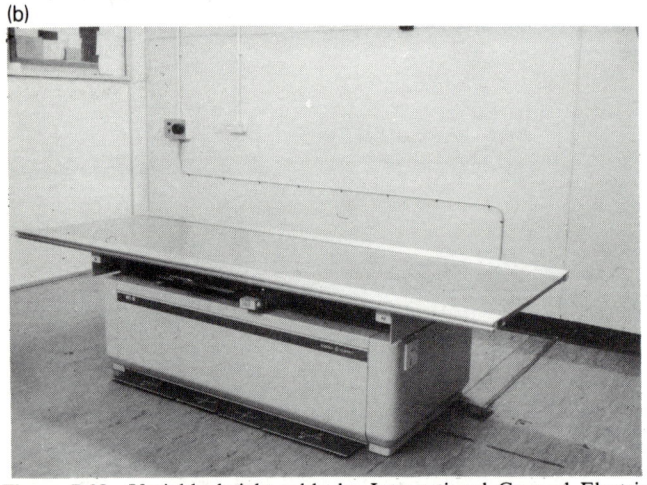

Figure 7.38 Variable height table by International General Electric installed at the Royal Lancaster Infirmary, England, (a) raised (b) lowered

Tables with this facility are very useful, particularly for the elderly or infirm. The table illustrated in Figure 7.38 has a floating top which can be raised from a lower height of 52.5 cm to a maximum height of 85 cm from the floor. The table top can be moved longitudinally or transversely and locked in any desired position by electromagnetic brakes, controlled by foot switches at the base of the table. Other foot switches control the up and down movements of the table. The table is fitted with a moving grid mechanism, the grid having a ratio of 12:1.

The table top measures 220 cm by 81 cm. The wide table which is an advantage to the radiographer when positioning the patient can be a disadvantage for the smaller radiographer when trying to pull a patient on a mattress from a trolley onto the table.

Accessory equipment includes an immobilization band, hand grips, lateral cassette holder and hip clamps.

Other 'bucky' assemblies

Vertical buckies, pedestal buckies and versatilt (variable angle) buckies all have their own advantages in particular situations. As with other 'bucky' systems automatic exposure control is an optional facility.

The vertical bucky

This consists of a counterbalanced moving grid/cassette holder assembly which can be raised or lowered. It is supported on a vertical column and may be locked in any desired position (Figure 7.39). Provision is made for the attachment of a cassette holder to the front of the bucky unit so that it may be used for chest radiography. Provision is also made for the attachment of head clamps and displacement (compression) bands to the front of the bucky assembly. Standard cassettes from 13 × 18 cm may be fitted one way and 18 × 24 cm up to 35 × 43 cm fitted both ways can be accommodated in a tray with self-centring mechanism. The tray can usually be loaded into the bucky from the left or right hand side, according to requirement.

Accessories such as the headclamp and the cassette holder are simply attached to the front of the bucky by means of a single socket and hand-operated lock screw. To ensure continued smooth and easy movement of the bucky carriage when accessories are fitted, trimming counterweights are provided; these are simply added or subtracted by means of a foot-operated control at the base of the vertical column.

The Versatilt bucky (Picker)

The bucky unit is raised or lowered on a single vertical column which may be floor-to-ceiling or floor-to-wall

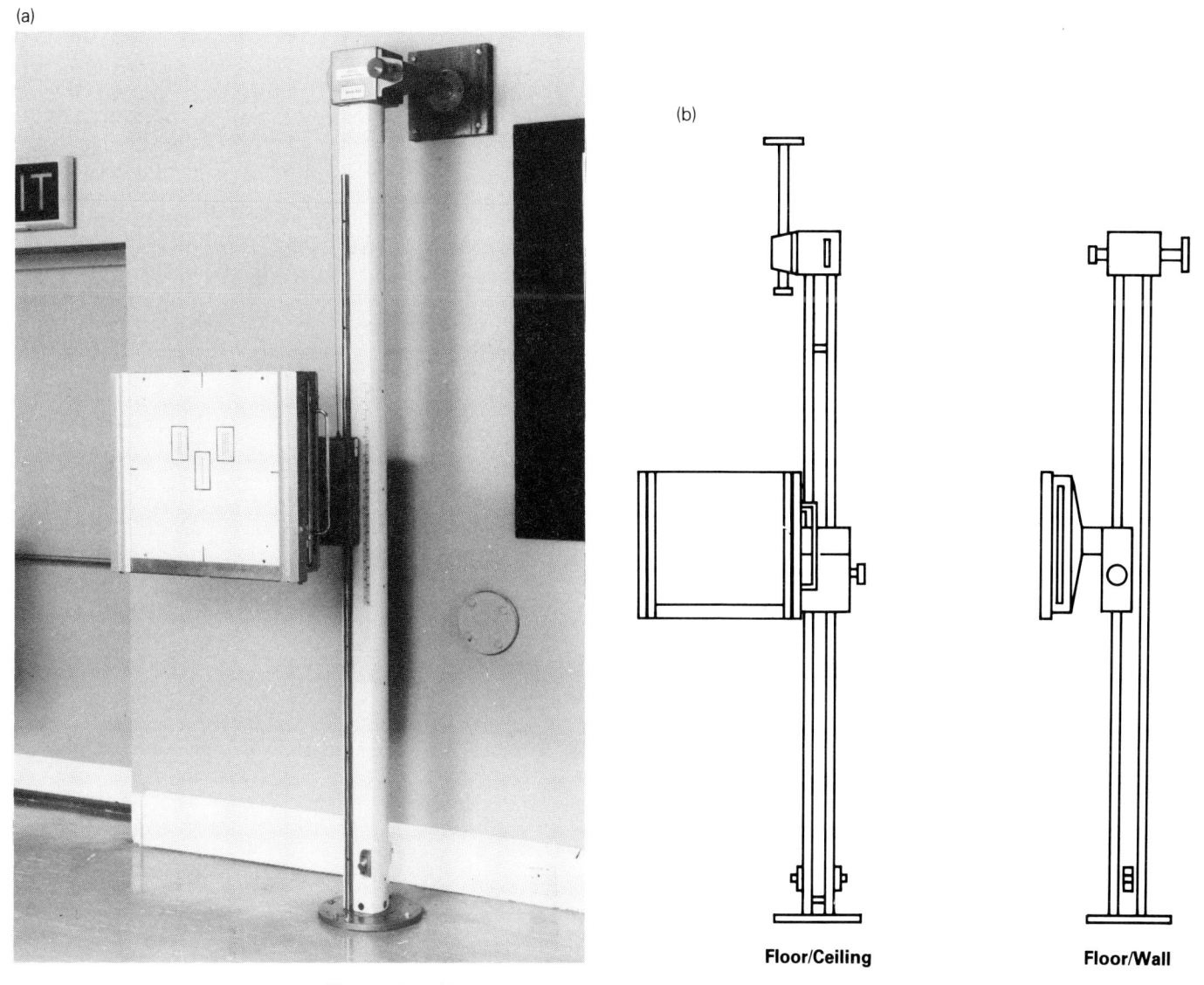

Figure 7.39 (a) Vertical bucky stand (Picker), (b) Alternative mountings

mounted (Figure 7.40b). A scale on the vertical column indicates the bucky centre-to-floor distance. The bucky may be supplied so as to be offset left or right of the vertical column or centred to it. The bucky can be angled through 105° and has automatic check stops in the vertical, horizontal and forward tilt positions.

All movements of the bucky are counterbalanced. It may be rotated through 180° and locked into position automatically at 90° intervals. This is useful when the bucky is being used under a trolley as the bucky can be rotated to enable loading of cassettes from either side. The unit is fitted with a vibrating grid mechanism, the grid having a ratio of 10:1. A self-centring cassette tray accommodates cassettes from 18 × 24 cm to 35 × 43 cm.

A wide range of accessories are available including a lightweight cassette holder which attaches to the front of the bucky unit and which accepts cassettes from 18 × 24 cm to 35 × 43 cm; a headclamp which immobilizes the patient's head between two rubber pads and a nylon immobilization band.

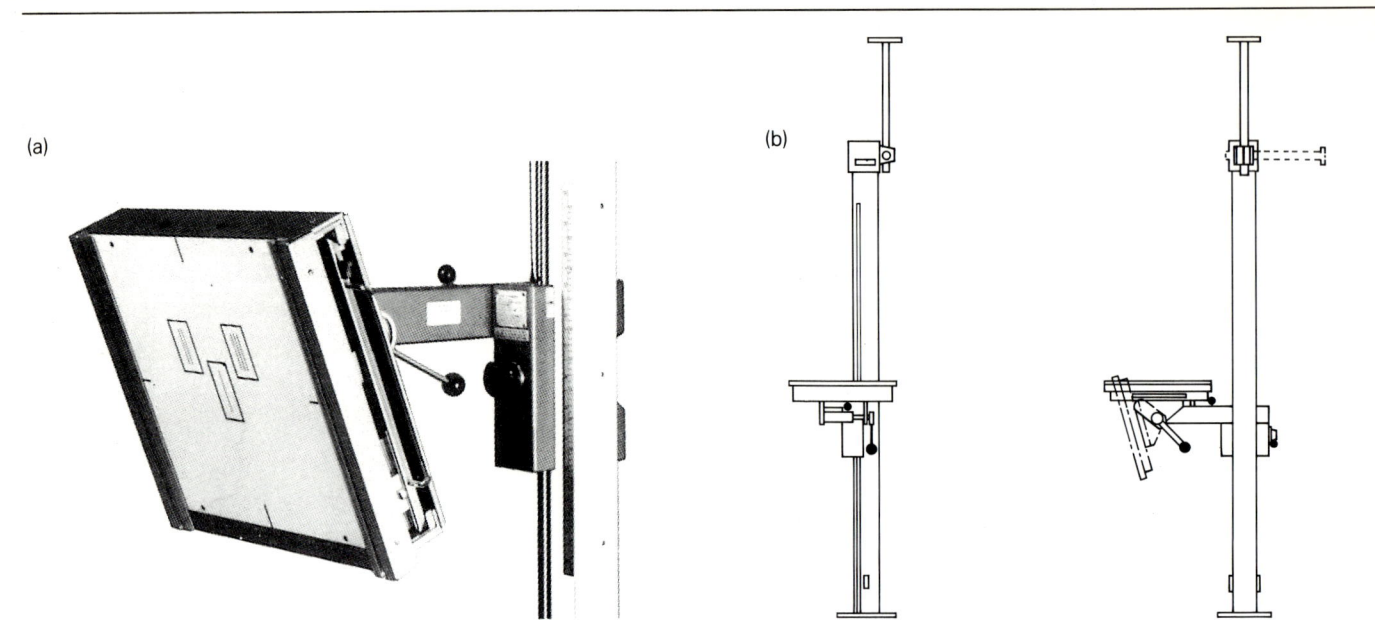

Figure 7.40 (a) Versatilt bucky (Picker), (b) range of movements

8
Equipment for fluoroscopy and fluorography

FLUOROSCOPIC EQUIPMENT	101
The serial changer (spot film device)	103
Remote controlled equipment	103
Changing from fluoroscopy to radiography	103
Fluoroscopic timer	105
Protection	105
Code of practice	105
Measuring patient dose	105
IMAGE INTENSIFIER TUBES	105
Magnification (dual field)	107
VIEWING THE OUTPUT IMAGE	108
Triple field 35 cm image intensifier	108
Fibre optic coupling	109
Television cameras	109
The vidicon camera tube	109
The plumbicon camera tube	110
THE TV MONITOR	110
Mode of action	111
VIDEO TAPE RECORDING	111
Mode of operation	111
Image memory (or retention) systems	112
KINESCOPY	112
Roll and cut film cameras	112
Patient identification	112
CINE FLUOROGRAPHY	112
Mode of operation	113
Cine pulsing	113
AUTOMATIC BRIGHTNESS CONTROL	113
Fluoroscopic density control	114
DIGITAL FLUOROGRAPHY	114
QUALITY ASSURANCE TESTS FOR FLUOROSCOPIC EQUIPMENT	115
kV and radiation output tests	115
Frequency	115
Variation in dose with change in field size	115
Beam alignment and collimation test	115
Mobile image intensifier	116
Frequency	116
Resolution tests	116
Frequency	116
Conversion factor	116
Frequency	117
Video test pattern generator	117
Other tests	117

FLUOROSCOPIC EQUIPMENT

The simplest type of fluoroscopic unit consists of an X-ray table, an undercouch tube and an overcouch 'screen'. The 'screen', consisting of a phosphor such as cadmium zinc sulphide coated onto thin card is sandwiched between a piece of protective plastic on the patient's side and a sheet of lead glass on the observer's side (Figure 8.1). This sandwich is mounted in a metal framework which gives support to the screen and provides a means of attachment for the screen to the undercouch tube, as well as providing a means of keeping the screen parallel to the table top. Whilst such a system of direct viewing is very simple it has many associated disadvantages. For example, viewing is, of necessity, by rod vision (rods being sensitive to poor light conditions) and the X-ray room must, in consequence, be in total darkness and the radiologist's eyes accommodated to such darkness before the examination begins.

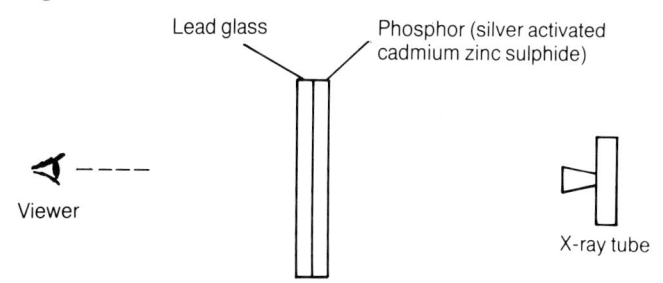

Figure 8.1 Principle of fluoroscopy

Visual brightness of the fluorescent screen may, of course, be increased by increasing the tube current but as this would necessitate an increase in current of some 5000-fold to increase the screen brightness sufficiently for cone vision to be used, it can be appreciated that such an increase would be quite impracticable.

The image intensifier which is now widely used with fluoroscopic equipment gives an increase in image brightness of some 6000 times, without increase in radiation dose to the patient, whilst the use of closed circuit television reduces the dose even further. By using an image intensifier system in conjunction with closed circuit television the output image is made sufficiently bright for cone vision to be used and at the same time radiation dose to the patient is greatly reduced.

Whether the image is viewed directly on the fluorescent screen or via the image intensifier and closed circuit television system, it is clearly essential to ensure that the X-ray tube and recording system are linked so that they move synchronously with one another.

The fluoroscopy table has an undercouch tube which is physically linked to the fluorescent screen (or image intensifier). The essential features are indicated in Figure 8.2.

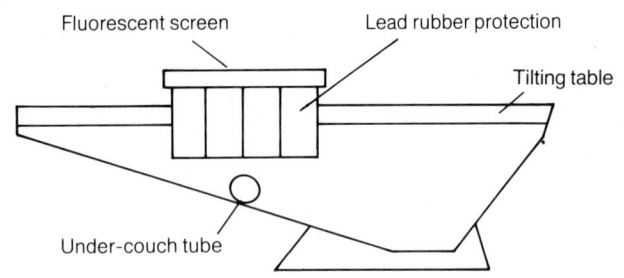

Figure 8.2 Simple fluoroscopy unit

The screen can be raised or lowered, moved longitudinally or transversely and the tube always follows it and is always centred to it. The X-ray tube is supported a fixed distance beneath the X-ray table but the screen may be raised or lowered to accommodate different thicknesses of patient. Provision is made to accommodate a cassette under the screen (or image intensifier) when a radiograph is needed, (Figure 8.4). The table and screening assembly may be tilted into the erect or horizontal positions or at any intermediate angle. The maximum degree of tilt in either direction varies according to the design of the table, some tilting 90° in one direction and 15° or 30° in the other, whilst others have a 90° forward and a 90° adverse tilt (Figure 8.3). The tilting movement is usually provided by means of a two-speed electric motor, although some manufacturers use a hydraulic system.

In addition to the undercouch tube used for fluoroscopy, there is usually an overcouch tube which is used for conventional radiography. When not in use the fluorescent screen assembly may be moved to one end of the table, provision sometimes being made to swing the screen clear of the table top leaving the table clear for conventional radiography. The table is fitted with a moving grid mechanism which is secured at one end of the table when the unit is being used for fluoroscopy.

The table top, in common with most other X-ray tables, is made of a radiolucent material (specially bonded bakelite) with side rails or runners to provide the necessary attachment for accessories such as hand grips, head clamps, displacement bands, nylon harness, foot rest, etc. A foot rest is essential as the table is frequently used in the erect position. The modern table top can be moved in the longitudinal and sometimes transverse directions and locked in any desired position by means of electromagnetic locks. Interlocks ensure that if the end of the table touches anything the electric motor drive is automatically switched off. The extent of the longitudinal movement varies with different models of table, but it is usually possible to extend the table top over a film changer such as the AOT when the occasion demands. The patient can thus be screened and the table top then moved over the AOT for serial films to be taken, see Chapter 11, Figure 11.7.

The screening assembly contains the fluorescent screen, or, alternatively in modern equipment, the image intensifier, the face plate of which is secured in place of the fluorescent screen. The image intensifier unit is counterbalanced, easily movable and is usually parked at one end of the room when not in use. The image intensifier tube will be described later. The screening assembly also has associated with it the controls and switches needed to make radiographic exposures, move the table top, tilt the table, move the undercouch tube and screen holder, etc. It also accommodates the serial changer.

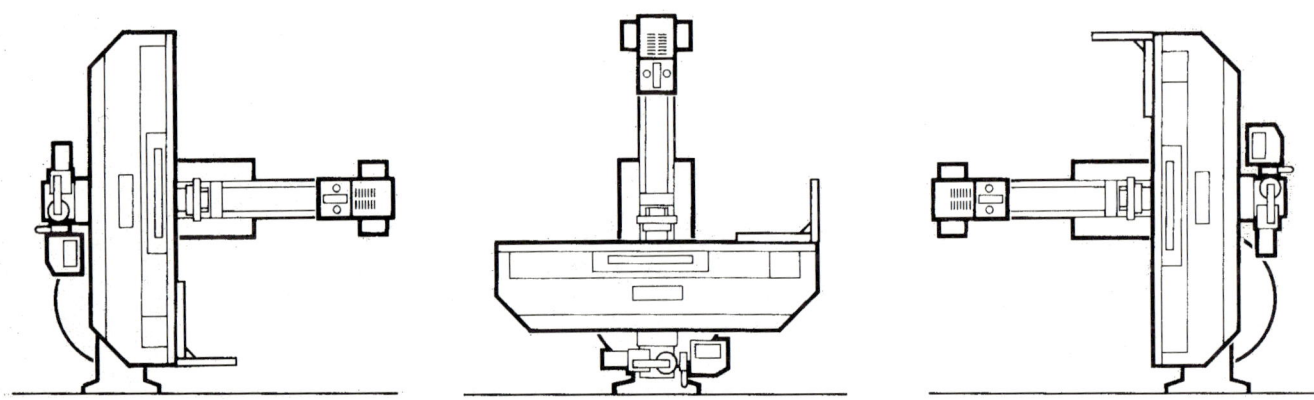

Figure 8.3 The range of forward and adverse tilt possible with a +90° to −90° fluoroscopy table

EQUIPMENT FOR FLUOROSCOPY AND FLUOROGRAPHY

The serial changer (Spot film device)

This is used to bring a cassette into position ready for a radiographic exposure. An interlock ensures that an exposure cannot be made until the undercouch tube has been switched from screening to radiography. The beam of radiation is automatically collimated to a particular area at a particular focal film distance.

By means of a format selector one is able to irradiate any chosen size of film, or alternatively, by means of lead masks, make a number of exposures on different parts of a single film, i.e. the film may be split into two, four, six or eight small areas.

A secondary radiation grid, moving or stationary, may be brought across into the field of radiation, either manually or by motorized drive, when required. Compression devices of different shapes and sizes can be brought across into the field of radiation as required to provide the requisite amount of tissue displacement during fluoroscopic or radiographic examinations.

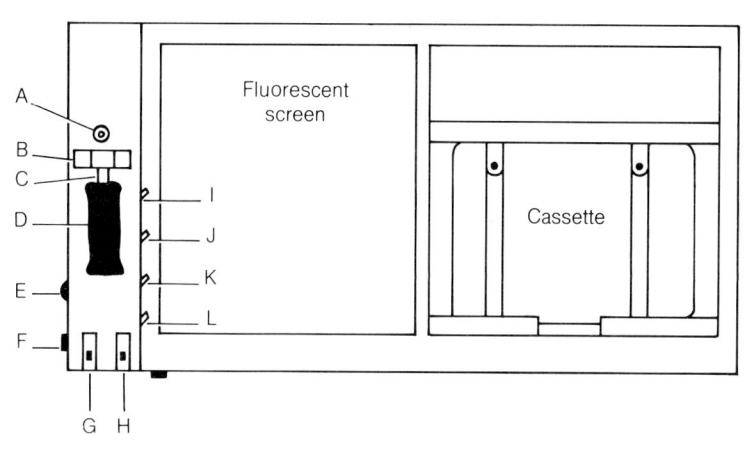

Figure 8.4 Diagrammatic representation of a simple serial changer. A – Diaphragm control; B – Prepare and expose switches; C – Fluoroscopy control; D – Brake and servo drive control handle; E – mask control; F – format selector; G – Table tilt switch; H – Table top movement switch; I – Grid in/grid out switch; J – Compression brake switch; K – Patient light switch; L – White light switch

Remote controlled equipment

Some of the more recent types of fluoroscopic units have the serial changer controls duplicated and mounted on a mobile unit which may then be located behind the lead-lined protective cubicle. All the table movements etc. previously controlled from the serial changer may then be operated from a safe distance or, as stated, from within the protective cubicle itself. An example of such a table is shown in Figure 8.5.

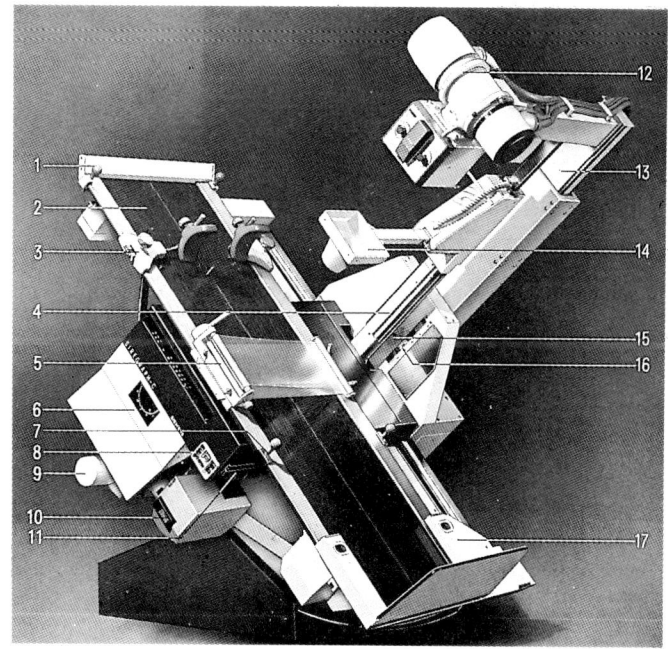

Key:
1. Hand protection bar
2. Patient's table with longitudinal and transverse excursion
3. Shoulder supports with vertical and lateral adjustment
4. Planigraphic attachment
5. Belt compressor
6. Angle indicator for table tilt
7. Adjustable hand-grips
8. Local control panel
9. Undertable spotfilm device with image intensifier and TV camera
10. SIRCAM camera
11. Coupling for film changer
12. Tube assembly with multi-leaf collimator
13. Tube assembly arm with telescopic extension for FFD
14. Removable compression cone
15. Indicator for the oblique beam projection angle
16. Planigraphic height indicator
17. Footboard, height adjustable and removable

Figure 8.5 Siemens siregraphic remote controlled fluoroscopy table

Changing from fluoroscopy to radiography

As previously mentioned the X-ray tube must be switched from fluoroscopy to radiography operation before a radiographic exposure is made. For example, a patient may be screened at 3 mA and 85 kVp (or with image intensifier 0.5 mA and 100 kVp) whilst a radiographic exposure may necessitate 400 mA and 70 kVp for 0.25 s. To switch rapidly from one set of exposure factors to the other, two completely separate sets of controls are provided. The screening kV control taps off a certain number of turns from the autotransformer and can be varied independently of the radiography kV control. The two sets of controls are shown in Figure 8.7. Selection of either set of controls is by means of a changeover switch. It is thus possible to set radiography kV quite independently of screening kV then switch rapidly from one to the other.

In addition, the mA must be raised from the small value used for fluoroscopy to the 400 mA or so needed for radiography. To achieve this a changeover switch is used to switch from the circuit providing the small current needed for fluoroscopy to the circuit providing the high

104   EQUIPMENT FOR DIAGNOSTIC RADIOGRAPHY

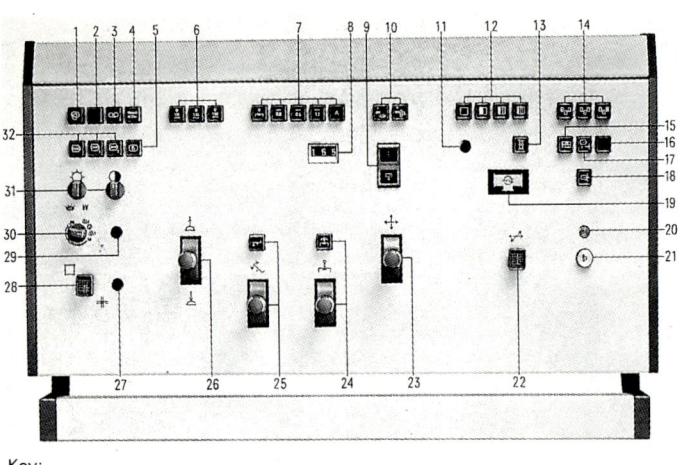

Key:
1 Automatic format collimation
2 Reserve switch
3 X-ray video-recorder
4 TRANSICON
5 TV-image reversal
6 FFD adjustment
7 Operating mode selector switch (routine, tomography, film changer)
8 Planigraphic height indicator, digital
9 Planigraphic height setting
10 Travel of table and X-ray system into angiographic position
11 Signal lamp (green): ready for exposure spotfilm device
12 Selection of cassette programme
13 Rapid series technique with cassettes and indirect camera
14 Selection of the three-field measuring chamber
15 Spotfilm device operation
16 Reserve switch
17 I.-I. fluorography
18 Cassette carriage in/out travel (load/unload)
19 LOADIX indicator (thermal tube assembly monitoring)
20 Signal lamp (yellow): work-station occupied (with OPTIMATIC generators only)
21 Exposure release
22 Patient's table longitudinal and transverse excursion
23 Spotfilm device/I.I.-tube unit, longitudinal movement and patient's table transverse excursion
24 Oblique beam projection with automatic mid-positioning
25 Unit tilting and Trendelenburg
26 Compression
27 Signal lamp (green) multi-leaf collimator closed
28 Multi-leaf collimator open and close
29 Signal lamp (red): radiation
30 Fluoroscopy-kV (7 steps) and automatic dose rate control (2 values)
31 Contrast and brightness (TV)
32 I.I.-format change-over

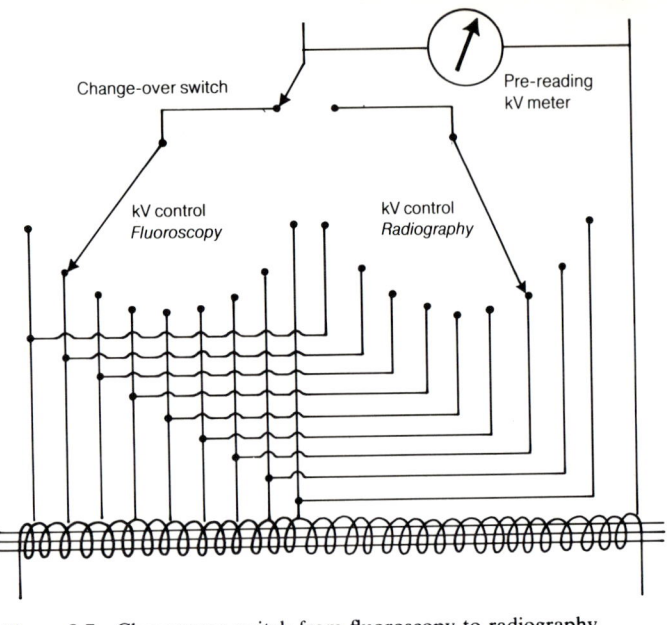

Figure 8.6 Control elements of remote control console

Figure 8.7 Changeover switch from fluoroscopy to radiography

filament current needed for radiography (Figure 8.8). At the same time the speed of anode rotation is increased to that appropriate to radiography. As the radiography mA has been selected previously, changeover to this circuit is rapid, although time is needed (about 1.0 s) for the anode to reach full rotational speed etc.

The following sequence of events takes place when the equipment is switched from screening to radiography.

(1) First pressure on the exposure switch prepares the circuits for the exposure.
(2) The screening circuits are switched out.
(3) Preselected radiography circuits are switched in.
(4) The cassette is moved into the expose position.
(5) Further or continued pressure on the exposure switch causes an exposure to be made.

Removal of pressure from the exposure switch causes the cassette to be moved laterally to the right or left of the serial changer where it can be removed. The preselected screening factors are automatically re-engaged and fluoroscopy continues. For ease of working a foot controlled switch may be used for fluoroscopy.

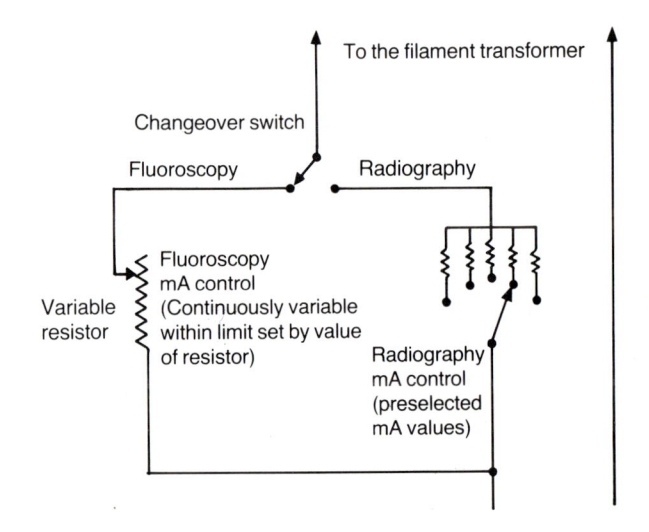

Figure 8.8 Circuit to change over from radiography mA to fluoroscopy mA and vice versa

Fluoroscopic timer

A timer, linked to the fluoroscopic circuit in such a way as to record the screening time of each patient, is now used in most departments. The timer is set by the radiographer, at the start of each examination, for a predetermined length of time, say up to 8 min. The timer is activated whenever the tube is energized for fluoroscopy and stops recording whenever fluoroscopy stops. At the end of the predetermined period of time a buzzer sounds and continues until fluoroscopy stops or until the timer is reset.

Protection

Primary radiation during direct viewing is heavily attenuated by the lead glass which is mounted in front of the fluorescent screen whilst scatter is absorbed by overlapping leaves of lead rubber which hang down from the edges of the serial changer. The metal sides of the table also provide protection against scatter and the aperture along the upper edge of the table, which gives access to the cassette tray used for general radiography is covered by a hinged flap when the unit is used for fluoroscopy.

Code of practice

The overlapping lead rubber leaves which are suspended from the serial changer must be not less than 45 cm × 45 cm and have a lead equivalent of at least 0.5 mm.

Measuring patient dose

Whilst great efforts have always been made to assess as accurately as possible the radiation dose absorbed by each patient undergoing therapeutic examination, it has never, until recently, been common practice to measure the radiation dose applied to a patient undergoing a diagnostic examination. Tables are available, of course, which indicate the average dose administered to a patient for specific examinations and the skin dose for a tube operating at a particular kVp, mAs and FFD and a particular thickness of aluminium filtration can be calculated by using a nomogram. It is only recently, however, that the dose applied to a patient undergoing such examinations as fluoroscopy, cine fluorography, angiography, etc. could be measured during the actual procedure without hindrance to the procedure in any way.

Such an instrument which measures patient exposure dose during diagnostic procedures is the *diamentor*. It consists of a flat ionization chamber, a pre-amplifier and a measuring and display unit. The flat ionization chamber, which is transparent to X-rays and light, is fitted to the front of the light beam diaphragm. All the radiation passing through the light beam diaphragm is measured and it is assumed that all the radiation falls on the patient. The chamber has a filtering effect equivalent to approximately 0.5 mm aluminium.

The radiation dose applied to the patient is recorded visually on the display unit by means of a digital counter. Each unit corresponds to an exposure of 10 R times the irradiated area in square centimetres (10 R cm²). An audio signal in the form of a 'pip', adjustable in volume, is emitted by a loudspeaker with each count. Variation in applied dose due to changes in kVp, mA, exposure time and irradiated area (field size) can thus be not only seen but also heard. This tends to make radiographers, radiologists, cardiologists, surgeons, etc. more conscious of the radiation dose being applied to the patient and indirectly to themselves. This increased awareness frequently leads to a reduction in applied dosage.

When the counter mechanism has registered the applied dose for a particular exposure it may be reset by press button, or left to integrate the dose associated with a series of exposures for a particular procedure or examination.

A higher sensitivity model of the diamentor is available in which each count is equivalent to 1 R cm². This is of practical value when used with image intensifier installations and when small exposure values are regularly used, e.g. in radiography of children, etc.

Dose to the patient can also be measured using thermoluminescent discs as described in Chapter 13.

IMAGE INTENSIFIER TUBES

The image intensifier tube which was mentioned earlier consists of an evacuated hard glass envelope as shown in Figure 8.10. The inner front surface of the tube is coated with a fluorescent material, usually caesium iodide. The photocathode (caesium activated by silver) is coated directly onto the input phosphor. This is done by a special process which ensures that there is no chemical reaction between the photocathode and input phosphor. The input phosphor and the photocathode must be in intimate contact. The result of separation is increased unsharpness and loss of contrast in the output image.

A small area at the other end of the glass tube is coated with an output phosphor (e.g. zinc cadmium sulphide activated by silver). The tube also encloses an electrostatic focusing system and an anode. These also are indicated in Figure 8.9.

The diameter of the input phosphor varies from 12.5 cm to 35 cm according to the manufacturer and the particular model, whilst the output phosphor varies from approximately 1.25 cm to 3.5 cm. (There are some other variations in the case of the 35 cm image intensifier tube but these

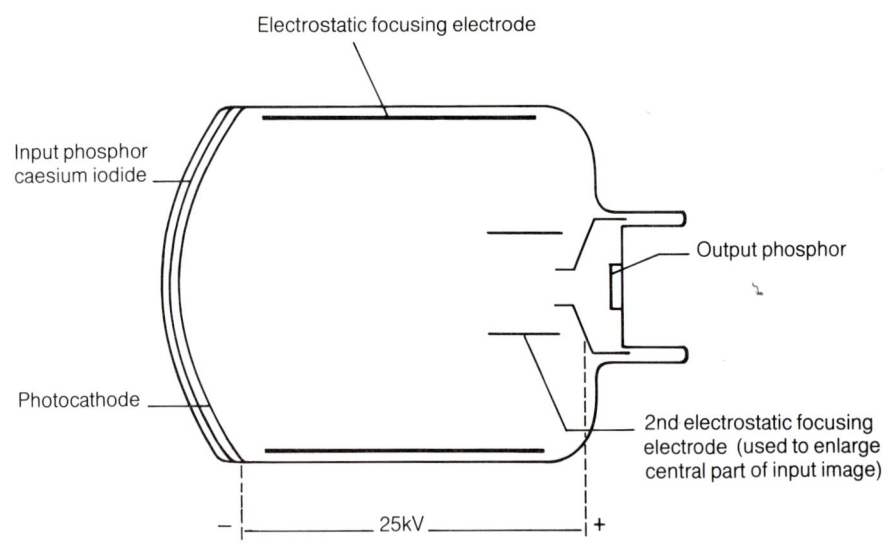

Figure 8.9 Image intensifier tube

will be discussed later.) The image intensifier functions as shown in Figure 8.10.

The body structures attenuate the beam of radiation, the emergent photons forming an invisible image of the structures through which they have passed. The emergent photons may be thought of as information carriers, the total image being composed of countless numbers of such photons. Each of these X-ray photons has its energy converted into photons of light at the input phosphor of the image intensifier tube. This results in a visual image at the input phosphor. The input phosphor must convert as much of the X-ray photon energy as possible into photons of light and, in fact, each X-ray photon produces some 5000 photons of light. The photons of light (constituting the visible light image at the input phosphor) strike the photocathode which is in intimate contact with the input phosphor causing it to emit electrons, the number of electrons produced at any given part of the photocathode being dependent upon the intensity of light at that particular part. An electron image is therefore produced at the photocathode which corresponds to the light image produced at the input phosphor. The electrons constituting the electron image are focused by an electrostatic focusing system and accelerated towards the anode by a potential difference of 25 kV which exists between the photocathode and the anode. On entering the field-free region the electrons diverge and strike the output phosphor where the high speed electrons give up their energy as photons of

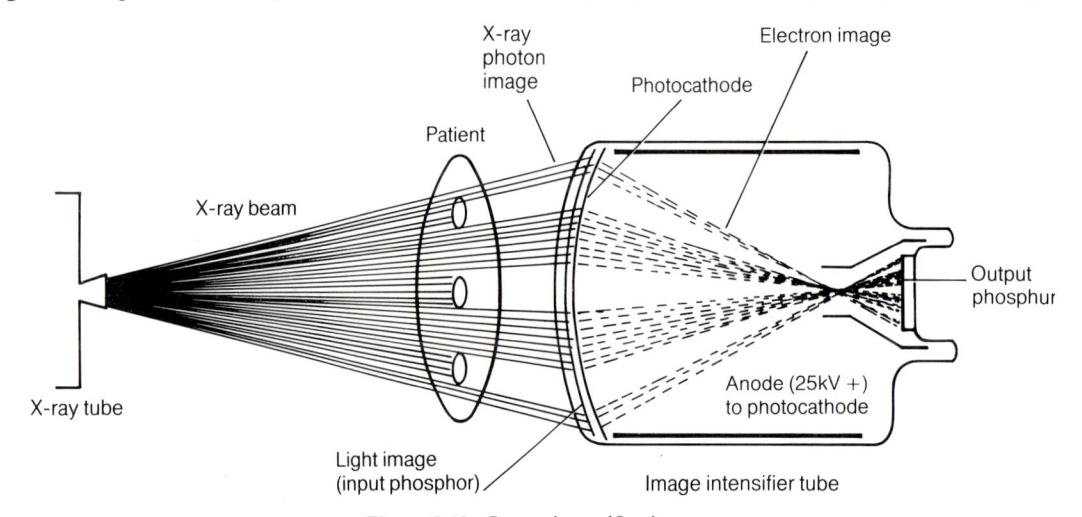

Figure 8.10 Image intensifier in use

EQUIPMENT FOR FLUOROSCOPY AND FLUOROGRAPHY

light. A visual image is thus formed at the output phosphor of the image intensifier which is many times brighter than that of the input phosphor.

The brightness of the image at the output phosphor is increased many times compared with that of the input phosphor. There are two main reasons for this:

(1) The small area covered by the output phosphor compared with that of the input phosphor, the image being much reduced in size.
(2) The energy imparted to the electrons as they are accelerated from the photocathode to the anode by the potential difference of 25 kV.

The image intensifier tube is surrounded by a light-tight protective antimagnetic metal casing (Figure 8.11). A rectangular front plate is used to locate the image intensifier to the screening carriage of the fluoroscopic unit. The front plate and the image intensifier casing must have a lead equivalent of at least 2 mm for 100 kV with an additional 0.01 mm per kV from 100–150 kV (Code of Practice).

To summarize, a weak visible light image (input phosphor) is converted into an electron image by the photocathode. The energy of the electrons is increased by accelerating them through a potential difference of 25 kV. The electrons with their energy much increased strike the output phosphor and produce an image which is many times brighter than the original.

Magnification (dual field)

By energizing a secondary focusing electrode it is possible to enlarge a small area of the input phosphor so as to cover the full area of the output phosphor. This is illustrated in Figure 8.12.

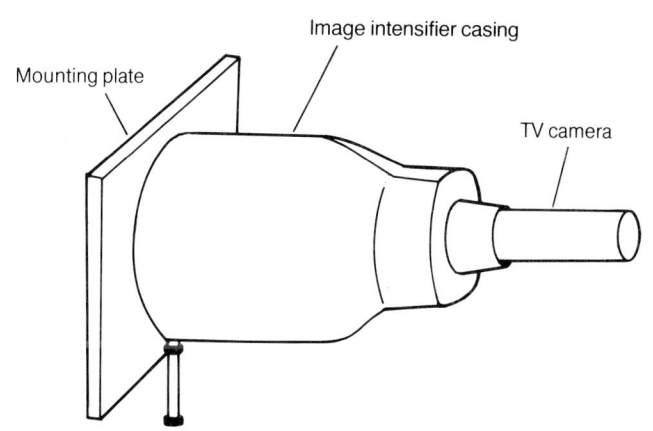

Figure 8.11 Light-tight ray-proof casing for image intensifier and TV camera tubes

Due to the reduction in input field size a smaller number of electrons are available to cover the output phosphor (the area of which remains unchanged). In these circumstances the exposure must be increased (by about 15 kV) if the number of electrons reaching the output phosphor is to remain constant. If the exposure is not increased the quality of the output image will almost certainly be degraded due to quantum mottle.

When enlargement facilities are available, providing two field sizes, e.g. 25 cm and 15 cm, it may be called a 25/15 image intensifier tube. This means that the large field will be 25 cm in diameter and the small field (subsequently enlarged to normal size) will be 15 cm in diameter. Typical brightness gain claimed by the manufacturers for a 25 cm field image intensifier tube is approximately 9000 times with resolution at the centre of the field of approximately 4–5 line pairs per mm.

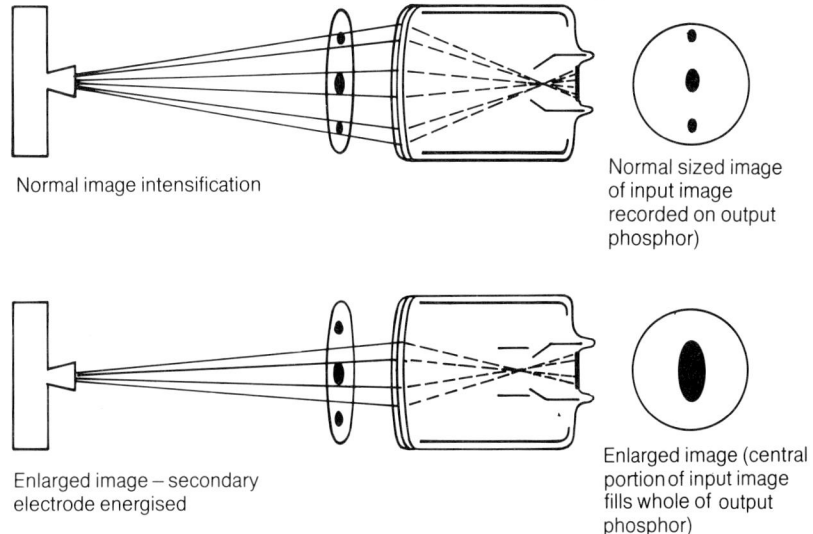

Figure 8.12 Enlargement of the intensified image

VIEWING THE OUTPUT IMAGE

The small output image (approximately 1.25–3.5 cm in diameter) may be viewed or recorded in a number of different ways:

(1) Directly – by means of an optical system (now rarely, if ever, used).

(2) By means of a TV monitor via a closed circuit television chain (the video signal can also be recorded on video tape).

(3) By photography of the image using a cut film or roll film camera.

(4) By recording the image on cine film (either directly using a cine camera or indirectly by filming the image on a TV monitor – called kinescopy.

Triple field 35 cm image intensifier

Recently Philips have introduced a 35 cm image intensifier with a choice of three fields – 35 cm, 25 cm or 16.25 cm (Figure 8.13). Whilst using the same principle of operation as other image intensifier tubes it does have some differences:

(1) The front of the intensifier is made of titanium foil. This metal is very strong and absorbs less primary radiation than glass.

(2) A potential difference of 35 kV, as opposed to the more normal 25 kV, is applied between photocathode and anode.

(3) The output phosphor is in close contact with a planoconcave fibre optic disc. This system increases light transmission, reduces scatter, improves resolution and reduces image distortion.

(4) The tube is shorter than its predecessors although the face of the tube is of greater diameter.

The advantage of the 35 cm image intensifier lies in the fact that it is now possible to image areas comparable to those used for conventional radiography, and to record them on 105 mm roll film or 100 mm cut film. By recording on the smaller film format compared with large X-ray film format it is possible to:

(1) Reduce patient dose (less dose per frame).

(2) Make exposures at a faster rate than possible with, for example the AOT and at short exposure times, with consequent reduction in movement unsharpness.

The disadvantage lies in smaller sized images. Radiologists and surgeons are used to looking at 'normal' sized radiographs and tend to be put off by the smaller image, particularly if measurements are to be made. There is no doubt, however, that the large field image intensifier will have a profound effect on radiography techniques in the future.

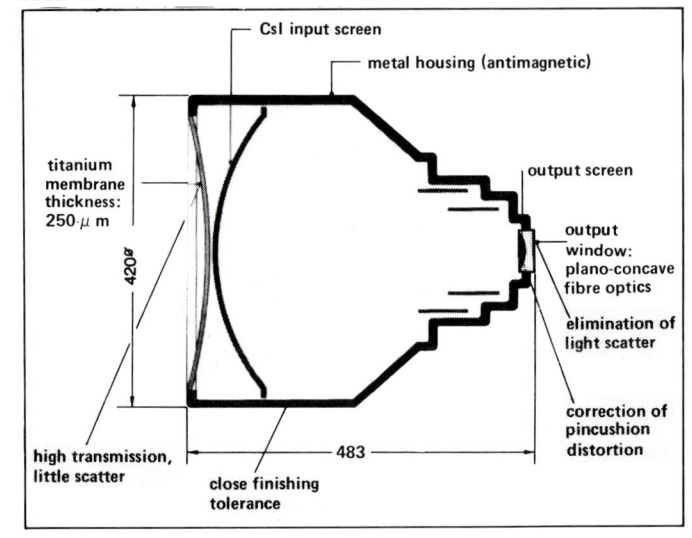

Figure 8.13 Philips 35 cm image intensifier tube

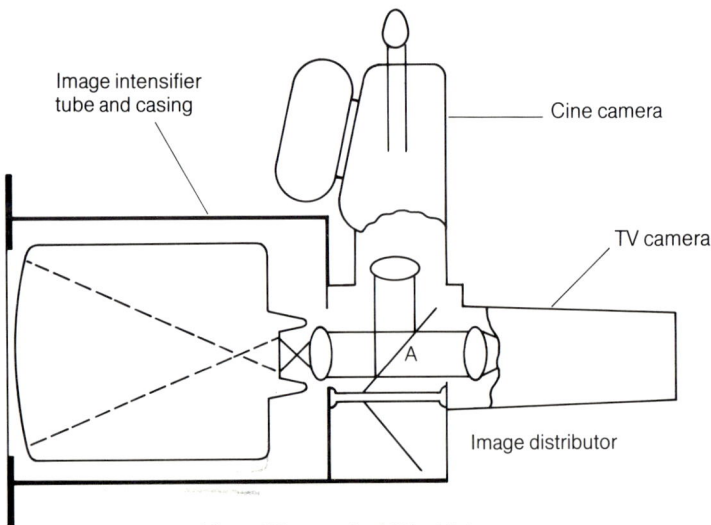

Figure 8.14 Image distributor – 10% of the light is passed to the TV camera and 90% to the cine camera

The output image may be transferred from one imaging system to another, i.e. from the cut film camera to, say, the cine camera, by using an image distributor. This consists of a mirror set at an angle of 45° which directs the image onto the face of the recording system selected. Provision is

EQUIPMENT FOR FLUOROSCOPY AND FLUOROGRAPHY

made around the image distributor for the attachment of a cine camera, cut film camera, television camera, etc. A rotary movement of the mirror (usually motorized) enables any particular system to be chosen at will (Figure 8.14).

A special feature of the mirror is that it is not wholly reflective but transmits a proportion of the light. Approximately 90% of the light is reflected and 10% transmitted. This enables the TV camera to be used at the same time as, say, the cine camera, 10% of the increased dose rate needed for cine being used for the television camera. This is a great advantage as the image may be viewed continuously on the TV monitor whilst the cine film is being exposed. This ensures that the cine run is as short as possible recording only the information needed. The maximum information is thus obtained with a minimum of radiation dose to the patient.

Fibre optic coupling

As mentioned previously, the light image from the output phosphor of the image intensifier tube may be focused by means of a tandem lens system onto the face of a selected recording system. This distribution box, as it is sometimes called, will be described later. If, however, a television camera is to be the only recording system used (i.e. no cine or 100 mm film camera) the output phosphor of the image intensifier tube may be connected *directly* to the face of the camera tube by means of a fibre optic coupling. The fibre optic system consists of a collection of glass fibres which transmit the light more effectively than the lens system. The disadvantage, of course, lies in the fact that where there is *direct* coupling a beam splitter (distribution box) cannot be used. The only means of recording the image is to use kinescopy (described later).

Television cameras

The television camera converts the visual image into a series of electronic impulses called a video signal. The signal is passed through a television chain to a TV monitor. Electronic components within the TV chain ensure synchronization of the image on the TV monitor with that of the original image as viewed by the TV camera. Synchronization ensures that information recorded at, say, the top left hand side of the television camera is recorded at the top left hand side of the TV monitor, so that the image on the monitor is a facsimile of the original.

There are two types of TV camera in general use for medical imaging. One is called a vidicon and the other a plumbicon.

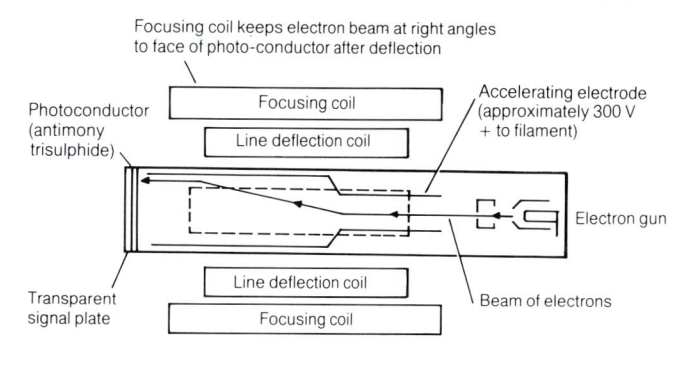

Figure 8.15 Focusing coil keeps electron beam at right angles to face of photoconductor after deflection

The vidicon camera tube

This is an evacuated glass envelope about 15 cm in length and 2.5 cm in diameter (Figure 8.15).

It will be noted that a layer of transparent conductive material is coated onto the inner surface of the tube face. In close contact with this lies a layer of photoconductive material which acts as an insulator unless light falls on it in which case it becomes conductive, the degree of conductivity at any particular point being related to the intensity of the light falling on it at that point. At the opposite end of the tube is an electron gun, the function of which is to produce a beam of electrons which scan the presenting surface of the photoconductor.

The beam of electrons moves across the photoconductor in a similar manner to the eye scanning the pages of a book – reading first the top line from left to right, then moving rapidly back to the left and dropping to the second line, moving again across to the right, dropping back to the left before scanning the third line. This process is repeated until the whole surface has been scanned then the sequence starts again at the top left hand corner.

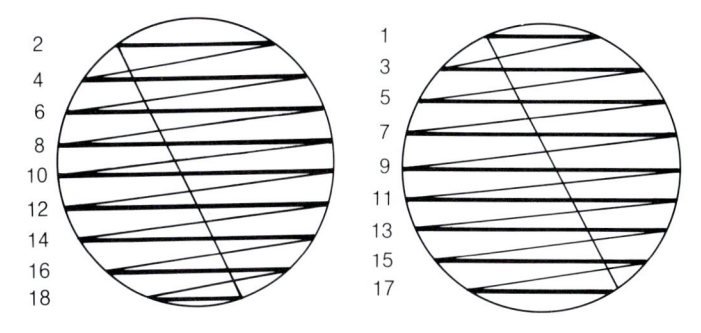

Each scan takes 1/50th s

Figure 8.16 Double interlacing

Double interlacing consists of two scans, the first scan covering the even lines and the second scan covering the odd lines (Figure 8.16). The complete picture made up of two such scans is called a *frame* (Figure 8.17). In the U.K. there are 25 frames per second (each complete scan taking one-fiftieth of a second), each frame comprising 625 lines, i.e. 312.5 lines per scan. After each scan (when the electron beam comes to the end of the last line) the electron beam is moved vertically back to the start of the top line, this vertical retrace taking approximately 10^{-4} seconds.

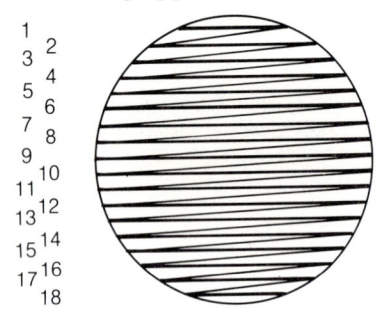

One frame (2 scans combined)

Figure 8.17 One frame (two scans combined)

Triple interlacing is used where maximum resolution (vertical) is required and the frame may be made up of three scans.

Vertical resolution improves with increase in the number of lines per frame.

Horizontal resolution is determined by the number of lines scanned per frame and by the range of frequencies transmitted by the electronic circuit which passes the video signal to the TV monitor.

So much for the electron beam; let us now consider the sequence of events which occur when light from the image intensifier tube is focused onto the face of the TV camera. Photons of light pass through the transparent conductive signal plate to the photoconductive plate. Electrons at that particular point move across from the inner surface of the photoconductor to the signal plate (which is positive) leaving the face of the photoconductor positively charged at that particular point. This occurs whenever light falls on the photoconductor leaving a positive image which is a facsimile of the original light image on the presenting face of the photocathode.

As the electron beam scans the face of the photocathode it neutralizes the positive charges it encounters. A current therefore flows from the negative terminal via the electron gun through the photoconductor and back to the positive terminal having passed through the load resistor marked 'R' in Figure 8.18. Current flows only during those instants in time that the electron beam is scanning a point which is positive. A series of electrical impulses is, therefore, built up over a period of time. Each line or sweep contains some 300 pieces of information.

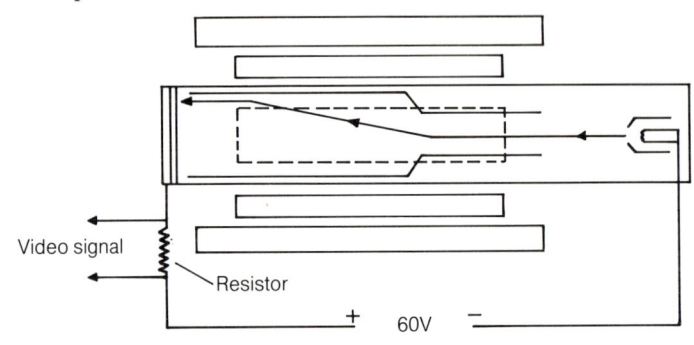

Figure 8.18 Formation of the video signal

The *vidicon camera* tube exhibits a time lag or persistence of image when in use. This manifests itself as a smearing or blurring of the image for a short time when there is movement of the part under investigation. This is due to the fact that the new image is superimposed on the previous image resulting in a mixture of images. Whilst this is a disadvantage when imaging fast moving subjects, e.g. angiocardiography, etc. it is not particularly noticeable with slower moving subjects. An advantage of lag in the vidicon is that, due to the mixing of the images, scintillation noise tends to be smoothed out giving a more acceptable image as signal-to-noise ratio is reduced. A new generation of vidicon tubes produced by Philips have less time lag and greater sensitivity.

The plumbicon camera tube

This is similar to the vidicon, the main difference being in the target material which is *lead monoxide* as opposed to the antimony trisulphide used in the vidicon. The plumbicon has much less time lag than the vidicon resulting in a reduction in image blurring. It is normally used for imaging fast moving subjects e.g. angiocardiography. Because there is very little time lag there is less integration of noise than with the vidicon resulting in a slightly noisier image.

THE TV MONITOR

We have seen the way in which the visual image at the output phosphor of the image intensifier tube is converted into an electronic signal by the TV camera. Let us now consider the way in which the video signal can be reconstituted as a visual image. This function is performed by the TV monitor. This consists essentially of an evacuated glass tube. It has a large face, the inner surface of which is coated with a fluorescent material. At the other end of the tube is an electron gun, an anode, and a grid or modulator (Figure 8.19). The electron gun produces a fine beam of electrons which are accelerated by the anode towards the face of the cathode ray tube causing it to fluoresce. Electrostatic focusing coils are used to make the electron beam scan the face of the cathode ray tube in the same way as the electron beam scans the face of the TV camera tube. Special components within the TV chain synchronize the image on the monitor tube with that of the camera tube, thus ensuring that the TV camera scan and the TV monitor scan each start and stop at the same instant in time, i.e. each scan starts at the top left hand side of the image at the same instant in time, and each scan finishes at the same instant in time.

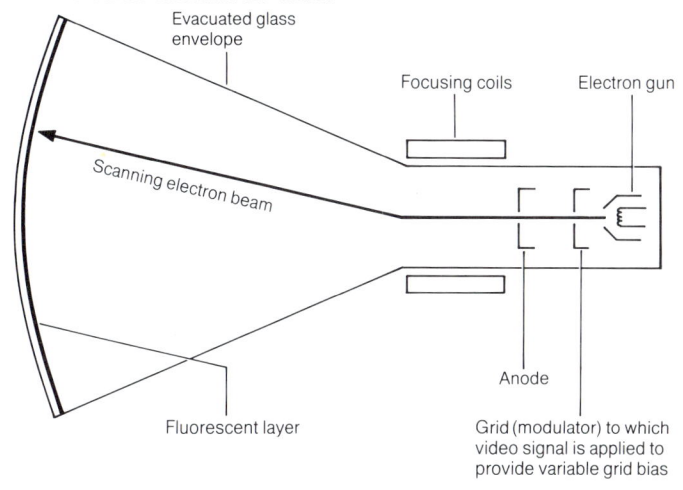

Figure 8.19 Diagrammatic representation of cathode ray tube (as used in TV monitor)

Mode of action

A beam of electrons scans the face of the TV monitor causing it to fluoresce. A grid in front of the electron gun has a varying negative bias applied by the video signal. When the grid has a strong negative bias the number of electrons passing from the gun is reduced and when the negative grid bias is low the number of electrons from the gun is increased. The video signal is therefore used to produce a pattern of fluorescence on the inner face of the tube which matches the pattern of brightness of the original image. As the electron beam scanning the inner surface of the cathode ray tube (monitor) is synchronized to the scanning beam of the TV camera it follows that the time taken for each scan (0.02 s) is the same in each case and as each frame is made up of two scans it follows that the spot of light produced by the electron beam takes 0.04 s to record all the information contained within one frame. When we view the face of the TV monitor screen we are not conscious of a single spot of light moving across the screen but of a complete visual image. This is, of course, due to persistence of vision.

The contrast of the image at the monitor can be varied electronically and the image can be made positive or negative or even inverted.

Note: The electronic circuitry within the TV chain and that associated with the monitor itself produces a lot of heat which must be dissipated. This is achieved by means of ventilation slots which are located in the sides and top of the casings which enclose the TV monitor, electronic rack, etc. It will be appreciated that these ventilation slots must not be covered with towels etc. otherwise the components may overheat.

VIDEO TAPE RECORDING

In addition to giving us an instantaneous visual image at the TV monitor the video signal may be stored on magnetic tape as a series of magnetic impulses. These magnetic impulses can then be changed back into a series of electronic impulses (video signal) at any future time.

Mode of operation

The video tape recorder is similar in appearance to a reel-to-reel audio tape recorder and indeed they both operate on the same principle.

A plastic tape (1.25 cm or 2.5 cm in width) is used to record the video signal, one side of the tape being coated with a thin emulsion containing particles of a readily magnetizable material, e.g. iron oxide. When recording, the tape passes from the full spool to a take-up spool via a recording head. The recording head encloses a coil through which the video signal is passed. The varying magnetic field associated with the video signal is used to magnetize the tape as it passes the recording head.

For 'play-back' the tape is once again passed from one spool to the other via the recording head but this time the moving magnetic tape induces a varying voltage into the coil as it passes the head. This varying voltage (video signal) is applied to the grid of the monitor tube to provide the image on the monitor screen.

Like the audio tape recorder, video tape can be 'wiped' clean and used again and again.

To get an 'action replay' immediately after fluoroscopy or at some later date without the necessity of re-irradiating the patient is, of course, a great advantage. It should be borne in mind, however, that the quality of the monitor image is never as good as that obtained by cine radiography although the latter, of course, necessitates a much increased radiation dose to the patient.

There are two tracks on the video tape which may be used for audio recording, e.g. radiologist's commentary, recording of patient's heart beat, etc.

Image memory (or retention) systems

These are available on most units. They store the last frame, when scanning with the image intensifier, by, for example, recording on a continuous loop of videotape. The image is constantly being recorded and wiped off, retaining only the final image. This provision is extremely useful in the orthopaedic theatre, for example when the surgeon can retain the image of, say, the hip joint in the AP projection on one monitor whilst the image intensifier unit is swung round to give him, say, a lateral image of the hip on another monitor.

It also helps to reduce dose to patient and staff in the theatre.

KINESCOPY

The image from a small TV monitor is photographed using a cine camera. The monitor screen is usually coated with a blue emitting phosphor and the sensitivity of the cine film is matched accordingly.

The camera shutter must be synchronized with the electron beam scanning the TV monitor screen (which in turn is synchronized with the electron beam scanning the inner face of the TV camera tube). The camera shutter must open when the electron beam starts its scan at the top of the monitor screen and close when it reaches the end of a scan at the bottom of the screen. The camera shutter is then closed whilst a new piece of film is pulled down ready for the next exposure.

The advantage of this form of cine recording lies in the fact that the patient need not be exposed to more radiation that that required for TV recording.

The disadvantages include:

(1) Information is lost whilst the shutter of the cine camera is closed and a new section of film being pulled down.
(2) Because of the low dose used each frame of the cine film may show marked quantum mottle.
(3) Horizontal bands may appear on the cine film if the camera and TV system are not accurately synchronized.

Roll and cut film cameras

Such a camera may be mounted on the distributor of the image intensifier as shown in Figure 8.20. The 70 mm or 105 mm roll film cameras can be used for single exposures or for a series of exposures up to a rate of 12 per second. The supply magazine has enough film for 400 exposures and a take-up cassette accommodates up to 70 exposures. The film may be cut at any time and the exposed part of the film which is in a light-tight container can be removed from the camera for processing. Film from the supply magazine is then rethreaded into a new take-up cassette.

The 100 mm cut film camera may be used for single exposures or a series of exposures up to a rate of 6 per second. The supply magazine of the 100 mm camera holds up to about 120 cut films and the take-up cassette a maximum of about 100. The take-up cassette can, of course, be removed in daylight so that the films may be processed and an empty cassette placed in the camera making it once again ready for use.

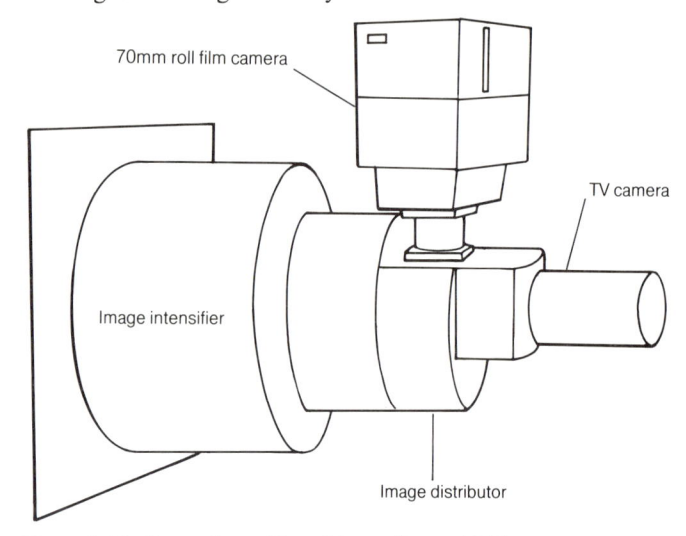

Figure 8.20 Image intensifier with cut film and TV camera

Patient identification

The patient's name, date, etc. is photographed onto each film by placing a card bearing this information into a slot on the film holder.

CINE FLUOROGRAPHY

A cine camera may also be mounted on the image distributor (either permanently or temporarily as the occasion demands), and a run of cine film exposed. The mA/kV must be increased considerably over that required for TV alone but a small portion of the increased dose is usually used to operate the TV system, the remainder being used, of course, to expose the cine film. In this way the image

EQUIPMENT FOR FLUOROSCOPY AND FLUOROGRAPHY

may be viewed on the television monitor at the same time as a cine run is being recorded. This is of great advantage to the radiologist as he is able to use the cine camera only during those periods when useful information is to be obtained, thus reducing radiation dose to the patient to a minimum.

Mode of operation

Within the light-tight camera are two spools, one containing unexposed cine film and the other a take-up spool which accepts the film after it has been exposed. The film passes from the full spool to the take-up spool via the exposure window. This is an aperture in a piece of metal which limits the light to a particular area of film, each exposed area of film being called a frame. A pressure plate holds the film flat whilst the exposure is made. A rotating metal shutter then covers the film for a brief period of time during which it is pulled down. The new section of film is then exposed by rotating the shutter so that it no longer covers the window. Figure 8.21 illustrates the main features of a cine camera.

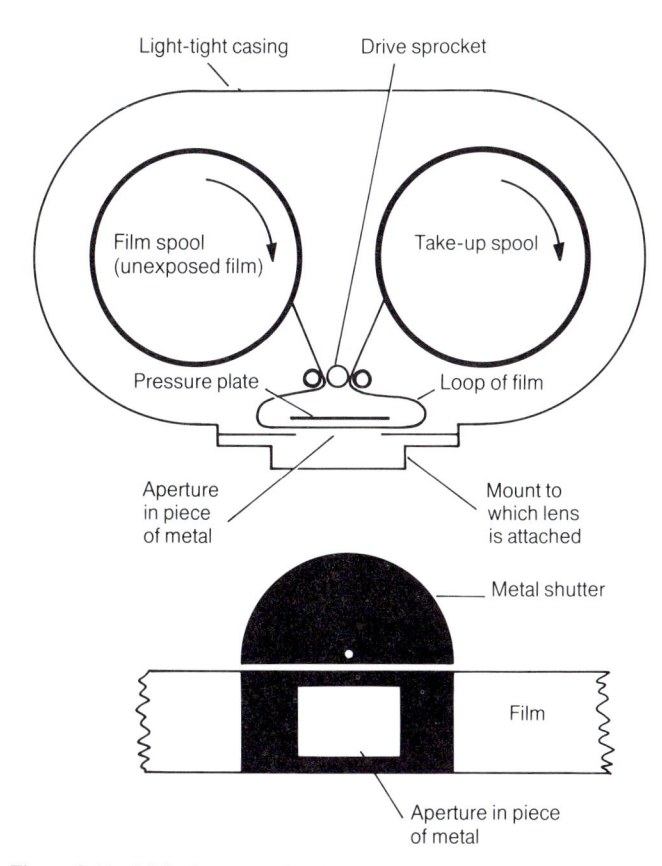

Figure 8.21 Main features of a cine camera

Cine cameras using 35 mm and 16 mm cine film are available. A typical 35 mm cine camera is capable of exposure rates of 12–150 frames per second, whilst a 16 mm camera with speeds of 25–200 frames per second is also available.

High camera speeds of 200 frames per second are of particular value for such examinations as angiocardiography where rapid movement of the heart and vessels can be shown in slow motion by exposing the film at 200 frames per second and projecting it at 16 frames per second.

Cine pulsing

Radiation dose to the patient can be reduced by energizing the X-ray tube only during those instants when the cine film is stationary in the cine camera awaiting exposure (Figure 8.22). Whilst the film is being pulled down ready for the next exposure the X-ray tube is not energized and in consequence the patient is not exposed to radiation. Cine pulsing can be achieved by synchronizing the X-ray exposure to those instants when the shutter is open or by using a camera in which the shutter is permanently open. Each pulse of radiation exposes the film which is then pulled down ready for the next exposure in the time interval before the next pulse of radiation. Such pulsing may be achieved by using secondary switching either with a grid-controlled X-ray tube or by means of high tension triodes.

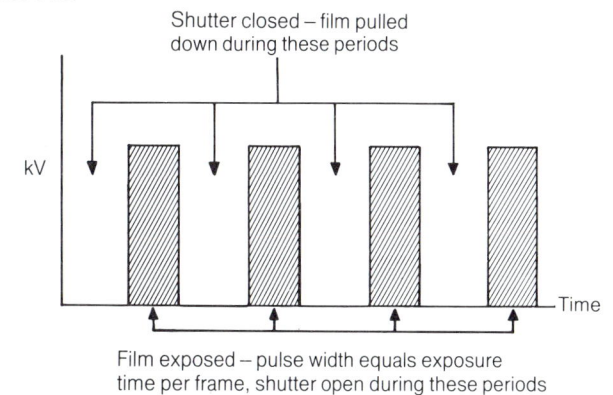

Figure 8.22 Cine pulsing

Short pulses (0.12–4 ms) are used where movement is rapid, e.g. angiocardiography. Long pulses (5–10 ms) are used for examinations of the digestive tract etc. where rapid movement is not such a problem.

AUTOMATIC BRIGHTNESS CONTROL

Automatic exposure control during fluoroscopy, spot filming and cine radiography is available with most modern units. Such a control ensures correct exposure values despite variations in patient thickness, density, etc. Such a device operates by varying kV and/or mA in accordance with the parts under examination so as to maintain a constant radiation dose to the film or a constant dose rate during fluoroscopy.

Fluoroscopic density control

In operation this control compares the maximum value of the video signal (which is proportional to the maximum brightness at the output of the image intensifier tube) to a constant reference value. The tube current and/or kV are then adjusted automatically so as to eliminate variation between peak value of the video signal and the reference voltage.

When a thicker part of the patient is being X-rayed the video signal drops in value. This results in a difference between the video signal and the reference voltage. The mA value is automatically increased which results in a brighter image and an increase in video signal peak value which is now equal to the reference value.

Automatic density control for cut film or cine cameras is operated by a photo pick-up (light sensitive) cell. The signal from this cell is used to determine the exposure time for cut films or the pulse width for cine radiography (Figure 8.23).

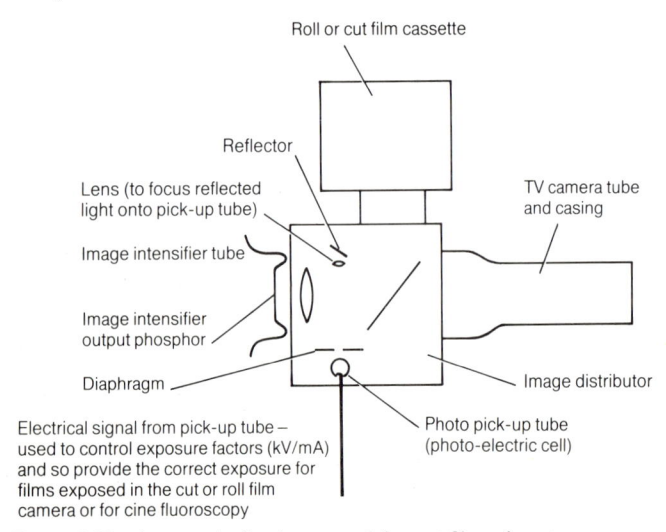

Figure 8.23 Automatic density control for cut film, cine etc.

Although the majority of fluoroscopy units in use today have the image intensifier mounted over the table – using an undercouch X-ray tube – it should be noted that some units use an undercouch image intensifier and an overcouch X-ray tube. In use the image intensifier is held in position closely under the table top for fluoroscopy, 70 mm filming and cine, etc. and moved away from the table to be replaced by the moving grid assembly and cassette holder for large size radiography. This exchange is push button controlled and takes only a few seconds. During fluoroscopy the cassette is protected from radiation. The arrangement is indicated in Figures 8.24 and 8.25.

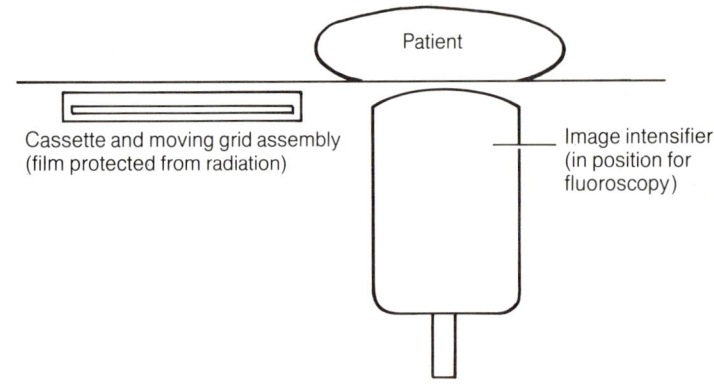

Figure 8.24 Unit used for fluoroscopy

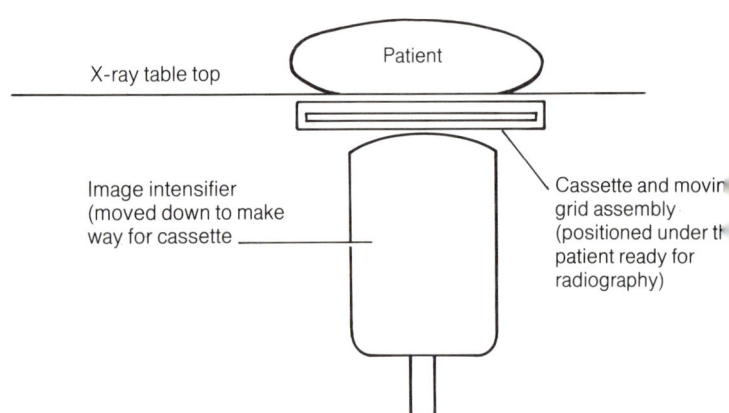

Figure 8.25 Unit used for radiography

DIGITAL FLUOROGRAPHY

Whilst digital imaging is described in detail in a later chapter it is interesting to note at this stage that add-on systems are now available for use with any modern fluoroscopic unit, providing it is coupled with an image intensifier and closed circuit TV. In use the TV output signal is connected via coaxial cable to the digital system. One such system supplied by Micro Consultants Limited has the complete system mounted on a trolley which, with the single coaxial interfacing cable, enables it to be shared between rooms when this is required. Real-time noise-reduced images are recorded on discs, the stored images being retrieved, either immediately or at a later date, for viewing and picture processing. The picture processing functions include integration, subtraction, spatial filtering and matched temporal filtering.

Monitoring of the noise-reduced real-time image is also possible without the need to store the image on discs. Mask images, which are reference pictures for subtraction, can be selected during live study (or retrospectively for stored data). Additionally, a number of frames can be added to produce an integrated mask.

A colour graphics display is also available, with a split screen facility which enables graphics to be displayed at the same time as the image.

A touch sensitive QWERTY keyboard (similar to a typewriter keyboard) is used by the operator to enter patient information and a stylus and control pad enable the user to select any one, of up to six regions of interest, within the picture for analysis.

QUALITY ASSURANCE TESTS FOR FLUOROSCOPIC EQUIPMENT

To ensure that the fluoroscopic equipment is operating to a satisfactory standard at installation and subsequently during its lifetime, it is necessary to carry out certain tests. Tests performed at installation provide a base line against which subsequent performance can be judged. Tests should include some, or all, of the following.

kV and radiation output tests

These use a penetrameter and radiation dosemeter as described in Chapter 15 but this time using fluoroscopic conditions. If the equipment is provided with an area exposure product meter such as the diamentor it is a simple matter to make regular checks on radiation output. A block of aluminium some 4 cm thick can be used to represent the patient and it should be placed about 25 cm above the table top. Using average fluoroscopic factors a meter reading should be taken, over about 30 s, at the centre of the field; at table top level if a dosemeter is being used. The measured dose should be recorded and be reproducible under identical conditions at subsequent tests. When the equipment is fitted with automatic brightness control, a note should be made of the kV set and mA recorded during the exposure.

To check the consistency of the exposure required for spot films the same procedure is carried out but this time a cassette is put into the serial changer and the equipment set for radiography. An exposure is made and the dose measured as before, in the centre of the field. A series of exposures may be made to check consistency in the short term and if the tests are carried out over a period of time they will indicate whether or not the exposure is consistent over a longer period of time. When automatic exposure control is used it is useful to make an exposure as above but this time with the aluminium plate on the table top and with a step wedge and motorized spinning top placed on it. When the exposed film is processed the exposure time can be calculated and the density of a given step on the wedge measured. Ongoing tests will indicate consistency or otherwise of film density and also of the time needed to obtain that density. (Density should be reproducible to plus or minus 2 optical units.)

Similar procedures may be used as consistency tests for cut film and cine camera exposures.

Frequency

The tests should be carried out on installation, after repair and thereafter at weekly intervals.

Variation in dose with change in field size

It is important to ensure that reduction in field size does not result in excessive rise in exposure rate when automatic brightness control is in operation. Such increases in dose should not exceed 100%.

Beam alignment and collimation test

Beam alignment can be checked using the tool and procedure described in Chapter 15. This time, however, it is the image intensifier which is centred over the test tool. In a correctly aligned system the dot should be seen within the hole on the resultant image.

The spot film device can also be checked for alignment using the same procedure.

Correct collimation can be checked using a test tool consisting of an aluminium plate which has four sliding brass strips set into recessed channels (Figure 8.26). Holes drilled at 1.0 cm intervals along each channel are filled with radiopaque material and a plastic cover keeps the brass strips within the channels by limiting vertical movement.

In use the test tool is placed on the table top and the brass strips pushed into their channels until the edge of each strip is just visible at the margin of the image when viewed on the TV monitor. This defines the visual field of the intensifier. The centre of the field is indicated by the central dot and any misalignment of the beam can be checked by counting the number of dots visible in each channel. With a correctly aligned and collimated system the dot at the intersection of the two lines should be at the centre of the image and there should be an equal number of dots visible on each of the channels when counted from the centre.

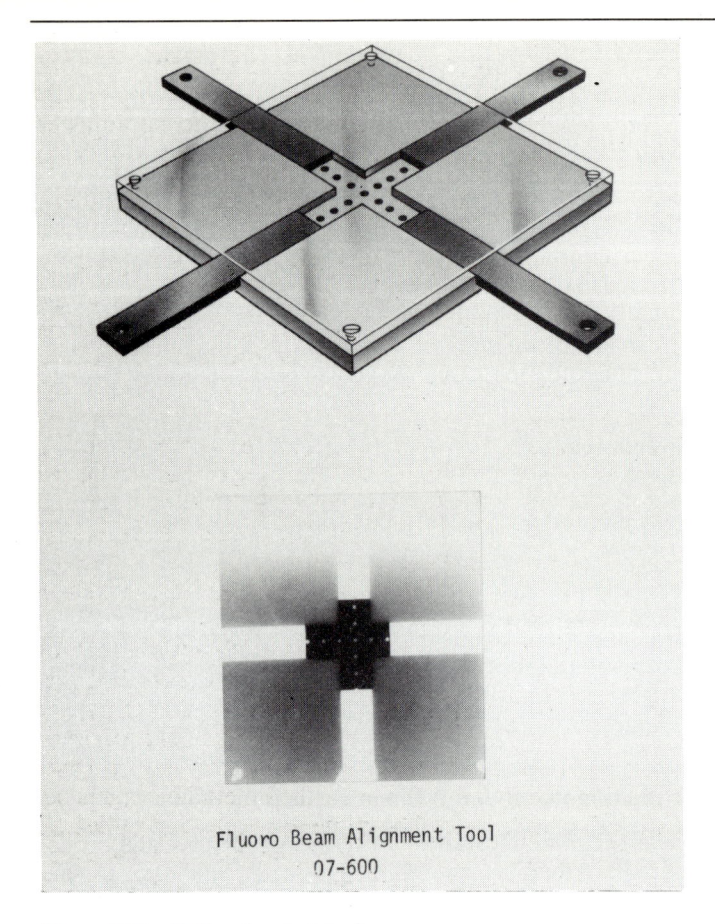

Figure 8.26 Collimation test tool

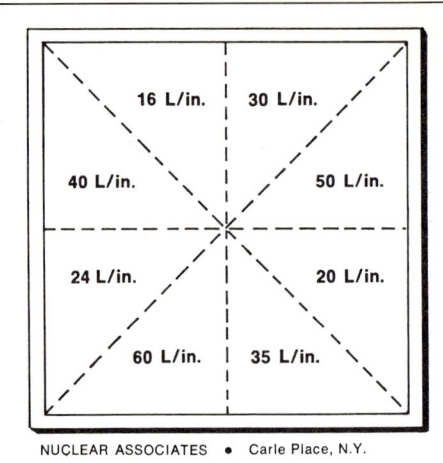

Figure 8.27 Resolution test tool (16–60 lines/inch)

Mobile image intensifier

In the case of a mobile image intensifier checks should also be made to ensure that the central ray remains aligned to the centre of the image intensifier face when the intensifier is rotated on its support to provide a horizontal beam.

Frequency

The tests should be carried out on installation, after repair and thereafter at annual intervals.

Resolution tests

The resolution of the system can be checked by using a test tool made up of a number of segments of copper mesh, as shown in Figure 8.27. Two mesh ranges are available, 16–60 lines per inch and 30–100 lines per inch. To minimize the effect of focal spot size on resolution the test tool should be placed as close as possible to the face of the image intensifier. The image is viewed under appropriate fluoroscopy conditions and a record made of the smallest mesh that can be visualized. If the image is viewed on closed circuit TV and a deterioration in resolution is observed over a period of time, it will be necessary to isolate the part of the system responsible. This may well involve the removal of the camera system to allow direct viewing from the output phosphor of the image intensifier. As this can be a tricky procedure it is best left to the service engineers.

The same procedure as above may be carried out but this time with the test plate sandwiched between two plates of aluminium each about 1.5 cm in thickness. This simulates clinical conditions and the image of the test plate, which has been positioned on the table top may be viewed as a fluoroscopic image or, alternatively, a spot film may be taken. In either case the smallest mesh that can be visualized should be recorded and compared with tests taken before that time. The record also allows comparison with future tests.

If a small test plate is used the resolution at the edges of the field should be checked as well as that in the centre. The mesh size that can reasonably be expected to be resolved by an image intensifier/TV system is about 24 at the centre of a 9 inch field and 20 at the edge.

Frequency

The testing should be done on installation, after repair and thereafter at weekly intervals.

Conversion factor

The conversion factor, which assesses the efficiency of the image receptor to convert X-rays to light, should be calculated at installation, annually or at any time there is felt to be a loss of efficiency in the system. This ensures that image quality is maintained without excessive dose to the patient. To calculate the conversion factor it is necessary to measure the luminescence of the output phosphor and the radiation dose rate at the input phosphor. The ratio of the two is the conversion factor.

$$\text{Conversion factor} = \frac{L}{R}$$

where L = light output of output phosphor in candela per square meter (cd/m²),
and R = radiation at the input phosphor in milliroentgens per second (mR/s).

This test would normally be carried out by a physicist or engineer.

Frequency

Tests should be carried out on installation, after repair and thereafter at annual intervals.

Video test pattern generator

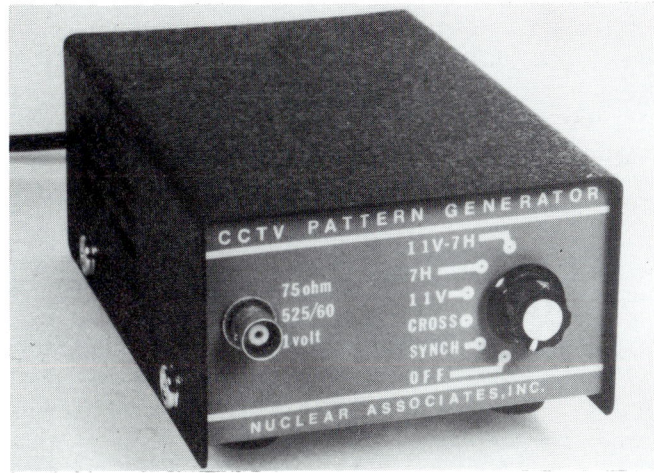

Figure 8.28 Video test pattern generator

The test pattern generator (Figure 8.28) is connected directly to the video input and the resultant pattern on the TV monitor enables the synchronization stability, raster centre, height and vertical linearity, etc. to be adjusted with great precision without the use of X-rays.

Other tests

Tests, for example, to check the ability of the system to resolve low contrast subjects etc. may also be required from time to time. Whatever tests are undertaken, however, it is essential that comprehensive records are kept so that subsequent tests can be carried out under identical conditions.

In addition to the tests described, it is important that the mechanical stability of the equipment be checked at installation and subsequently during its lifetime to ensure that all movements are free and that all locks are operational etc. Safety interlocks should be checked at regular intervals and the grid, if focused, should be checked to ensure that it is correctly fitted etc.

Meters should be checked to ensure they are reading correctly and that glass coverings are not cracked or broken. Meters should also be zeroed at regular intervals. Regular inspection should also be made of the covering of shockproof cables to ensure that they are in good condition and to see that the earthed metallic braid is not exposed. Checks should be made to ensure that cables are not unduly stressed or twisted. The high tension cable retaining screws at the tube head and high tension transformer tank should be checked periodically to make sure they are not loose.

Many of these checks can, and should, be made by radiographers as they use the equipment, any minor faults being either corrected or recorded in the 'faults' book which should be kept with the equipment so that they may be corrected by the service engineer at his next visit.

9
Equipment for mobile, dental, accident and skull radiography

PORTABLE AND MOBILE X-RAY EQUIPMENT	118
Portable X-ray units	118
Mobile equipment	118
Provision of adequate power supply	119
Supply cable resistance compensation	119
Capacitor discharge unit	119
Cordless mobiles	121
Siemens Mobilett mobile unit	121
Mobile image intensifier	122
Image retention systems	123
EQUIPMENT FOR DENTAL RADIOGRAPHY	123
Simple self-rectified unit	123
The orthopantomograph (OPG) unit	123
The cephalostat	124
Philips Cephalix unit	124
EQUIPMENT FOR ACCIDENT RADIOGRAPHY	125
Picker 'Care' system	126
Advantages of the 'Care' type system	126
Disadvantages	126
THE SKULL UNIT	127
Grid rotation	128
Choice of generator	128
Attachments	128
Spring-loaded manually operated cassette changers	128
Patient trolley	129
Bipod tube support	129

PORTABLE AND MOBILE X-RAY EQUIPMENT

Portable X-ray units

X-ray equipment may be considered as being portable when it can be packed into a small carrying case and carried from place to place by one person. Such equipment is particularly useful for domiciliary radiography or when X-ray equipment needs to be transported from hospital to hospital to take the occasional radiograph. Whilst its principal advantage is mobility its main disadvantages are lack of power, lack of stability and lack of precision.

It consists essentially of an oil-filled lead-lined tank or casing which houses the tube insert, high tension transformer and step-down filament transformer. A small control unit which accommodates the main switch, rheostats (variable resistors) is used to vary the mA and kV, and a clockwork timer built into a portable handset also accommodates the exposure switch. The maximum output of such equipment is usually in the order of 75 kVp at 15 mA.

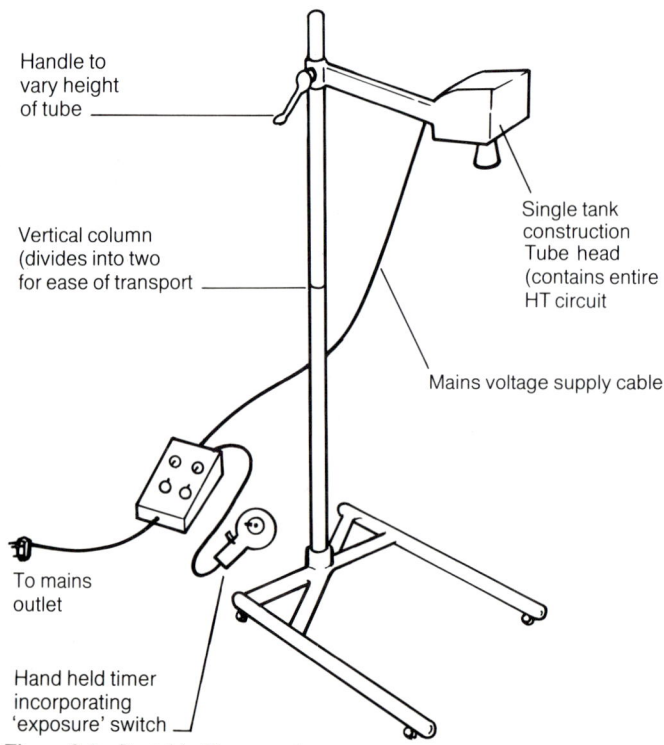

Figure 9.1 Portable X-ray equipment

Mobile equipment

Mobile equipment is much heavier than portable equipment and offers greater stability, increased power and a wider range of kV and mA values. It may be moved about the hospital, movement being either manual or by means of a motorized drive. Mobile equipment varies from self-rectified equipment operating at a maximum of 25 mA and 90 kV to fully rectified units operating at 125 kVp and 300 mA. The use of solid state rectifiers has led to the introduction of full-wave rectified high tension circuits contained, with the X-ray tube, in a single casing.

One of the greatest difficulties associated with the use of high powered mobile equipment is the provision of the necessary electrical power supply in the wards, theatre, etc. where the unit is to be used.

Provision of adequate power supply

Assume that an exposure is to be made with a mobile unit using 300 mA at 100 kVp. This would involve an expenditure of energy by the secondary circuit of approximately

$$300\,mA \times 100\,kVp \times 0.707\,(r.m.s.) = \frac{300}{1000} \times 100\,000 \times 0.707 = 21\,000\,W$$

Such an energy expenditure in the secondary circuit requires an equal energy in the primary circuit. A power supply of 21 000 W is therefore required, assuming 100% conversion of energy. Now 21 000 W = primary voltage × primary current. Assuming a primary voltage of 240 V, then:

21 000 = 240 × primary current

Therefore primary current = 21 000 ÷ 240 = 87.5 A.

In theory the wards, theatre, etc. should therefore be provided with electrical outlets capable of carrying 87.5 A at 240 V. However, the largest power outlet generally available in wards or theatre is 30 A and it therefore follows that we must either use less energy in the secondary (lower exposure factors) and thereby reduce the current drawn from the primary, or, alternatively, replace the 30 A fuses with others capable of withstanding 87.5 A. This latter course has been adopted in some hospitals. It is a cheap way round the problem and some electrical engineers would argue that such a course of action is acceptable as the diagnostic exposures are very short and conducting cables are unlikely to overheat during the short periods of time that current is flowing. It cannot be denied, however, that the replacement of existing fuses with heavier ones can result in a fire hazard and the conducting cables must be inspected by competent engineers before such action is undertaken. For the reasons indicated, radiographic staff should not, in any circumstances, replace fuses with a heavier variety. Another solution adopted by some engineers is to use slow acting fuses. These will burn out if a long exposure is made but not for a short one, thus protecting the conducting cables from the effects of overheating.

Supply cable resistance compensation

The voltage available at a particular electric point is determined by the resistance of the cable supplying the point and the current flowing. The further the point is from the mains supply cable the greater is its resistance and the greater will be the voltage drop for a given current (Figure 9.2). To achieve greater constancy in the voltage applied to the mobile unit it is common practice to add resistance when the resistance of the cable is low (short run of cable from the mains supply) and to remove resistance when the resistance of the cable is high. The unit is thus always provided with the same supply voltage irrespective of cable length. It should be noted that a constant value is achieved by considering maximum cable resistance and making all other points comparable with this (Figure 9.3).

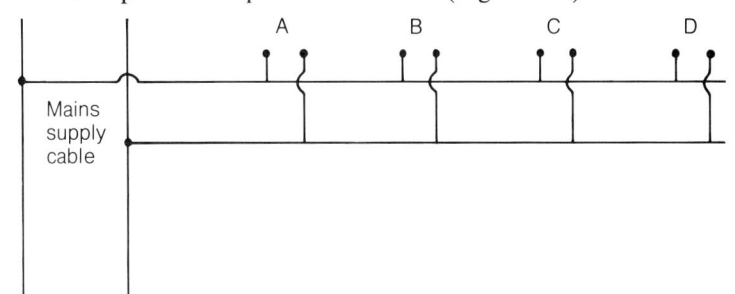

Figure 9.2 Resistance of hospital cables increases with distance from the supply, i.e. electrical socket D may be 100 m from the supply cable and have a resistance of say 'X' ohms whilst electrical socket A being much closer to the supply is shorter and therefore has a lower resistance of say 'Y' ohms

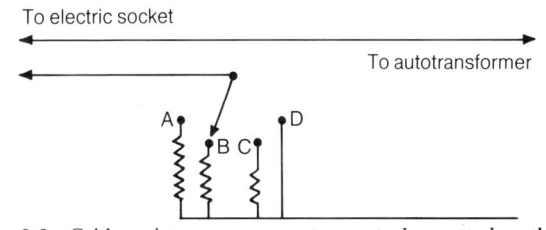

Figure 9.3 Cable resistance compensator control mounted on the control panel of the mobile unit

Capacitor discharge and cordless mobile units go some way to overcoming the problem of inadequate power supply. Let us consider them individually.

Capacitor discharge unit

The capacitor discharge unit is connected to the available mains supply (say 5 A outlet) which is used to charge a high tension capacitor (Figure 9.4). The charging of the capacitor may take place over a period of say, 10 seconds. When the capacitor is fully charged the secondary circuit is disconnected from the primary and the capacitor is discharged through the grid-controlled X-ray tube.

A 1 μF capacitor charged to a voltage of 100 kV would store the following charge:

Charge in coulombs = voltage × capacitance

$\therefore$ charge in coulombs (A s) = $100\,000 \times 10^{-6}$

$\therefore$ charge in coulombs = 0.1

$\therefore$ charge in mA s (mC) = $0.1 \times 1000 = 100$ mA s

A charge of 100 mA s is therefore available providing the capacitor is completely discharged.

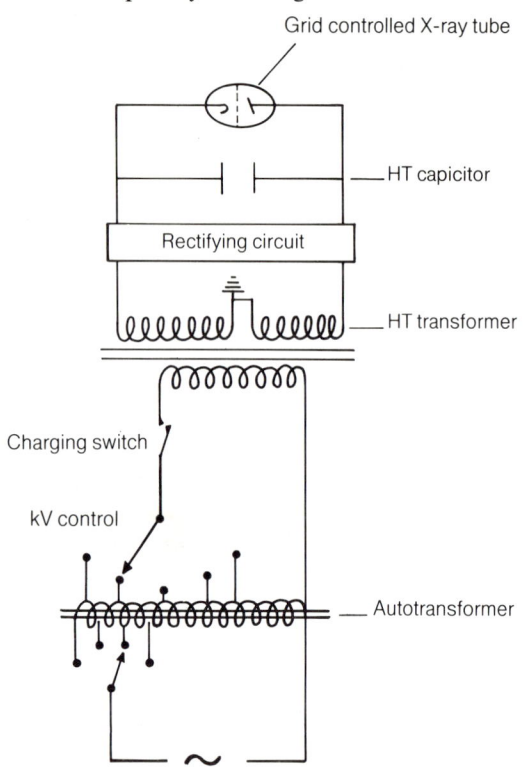

Figure 9.4 Simplified circuit for capacitor discharge unit

To operate, the capacitor discharge unit is plugged into the mains supply and kV and mA s are selected (Figure 9.5). The 'charge' button is pressed and the capacitor begins to charge up to the selected value. The capacitor cannot discharge as the grid of the tube is held negative and acts as an open switch.

Whilst the capacitors are charging, the grid of the X-ray tube has sufficient negative bias to keep the circuit open (tube acts as an open switch). When the capacitor is charged to the required kV a green light indicates that the exposure can be made. The exposure is initiated by removing the negative bias from the grid of the tube. The tube now acts as a closed switch and the capacitor begins to discharge. Any desired mA s (up to full discharge of the capacitor) may be obtained by reapplying the negative bias to the grid of the tube after an appropriate time.

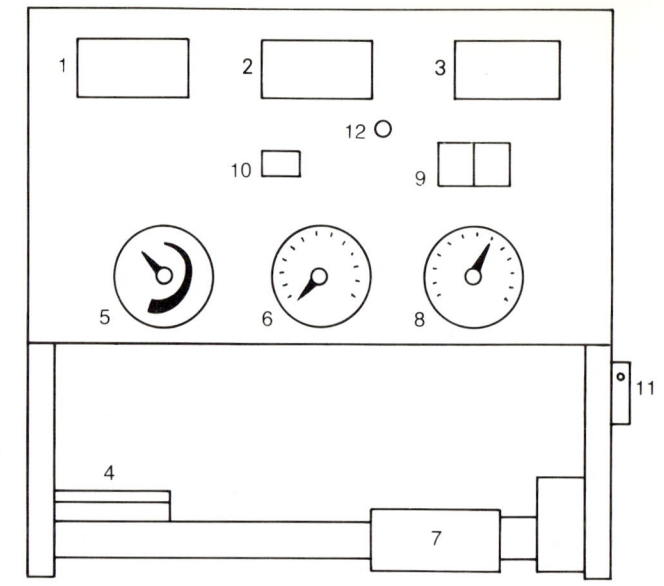

Figure 9.5 Control panel of capacitor discharge unit. (1) line voltmeter; (2) tube voltage meter – indicates voltage to which the capacitor has been charged; (3) battery voltmeter – indicates state of battery which drives the unit; (4) handbrake; (5) line voltage compensator control; (6) tube voltage control; (7) motor drive – twist grip control; (8) mA s control – two scales, one 4–50 mA s for ordinary radiography and the other up to 5 mA s for instantaneous exposure; (9) technique selector – for ordinary or instantaneous exposures; (10) charging stop/discharge button – capacitor charging is interrupted by depressing button. When continuously pressed, condensor is discharged without emission of X-rays; (11) exposure handswitch; (12) exposure indicator lamp

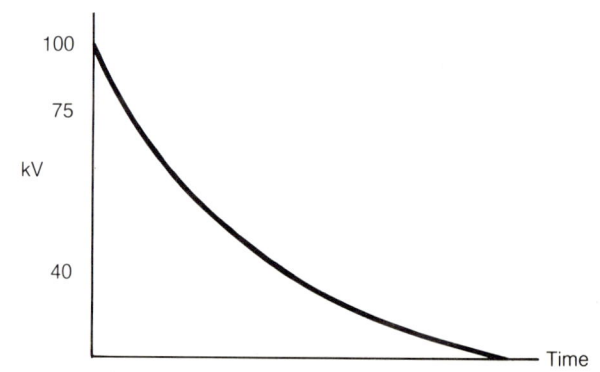

Figure 9.6 Capacitor discharge with time

If, for any reason, the exposure is not made as soon as the green light comes on, the capacitors begin to lose charge and if the kV drops to 2 kV less than the selected value the green light goes out and no exposure can be made until the capacitors are recharged to the selected value. This 'topping-up' of kV is done automatically.

If the exposure is terminated when the capacitor has discharged say 25 mA s through the tube, the voltage across the plates of the capacitor will have dropped from 100 kV to 75 kV, i.e. most of the radiation is produced at high kV (Figure 9.6). If, however, an exposure of 75 mA s is made, the voltage drops from 100 kV to 25 kV during the exposure and some of the exposure is made at low kV value. If an exposure of 100 mA s (full discharge) is made then the voltage drops from 100 kV to zero and a lot of very soft radiation is produced.

To overcome this problem some manufacturers provide automatic cut-off of the exposure when the kV drops to a particular value; others operate cut-off when the kV has dropped to a selected percentage of the chosen value. A separate switch usually provides for full discharge when this is required.

Some manufacturers claim that the exposure is made at virtual constant potential. This is true and of great practical value but *only* when a small mA s is used. As we have seen, if the capacitor is fully discharged the kV drops to zero. This, however, is not as disastrous as it may sound. Remember that in a two-pulse generator the kV drops to zero after each pulse.

Some capacitor discharge units have a separate switch to provide small mA s values at very short exposure times. For example, mA s values between 0.5 and 5.0 are provided with a higher filament temperature then those between 5.0 and 50. A lower filament temperature is necessary when using the 5.0–50 mA s values to prevent overload of the tube.

Capacitor discharge units are particularly useful when small mA s values are used because the mA s is obtained in a very short time and the kV is almost constant. The unit is therefore ideal for chest radiography (especially babies), paediatric radiography and for use in intensive care units.

Used within the limits set, i.e. the charge that can be stored on the plates of the capacitor, the mobile capacitor discharge unit has an important part to play in mobile radiography.

This unit should not be confused with the cordless mobile which is completely independent of mains electric supply. The capacitor discharge unit is independent of mains supply during the exposure only. The capacitor must be charged *immediately* before use. It is not possible to charge the capacitor in the X-ray department then take it out to the ward for subsequent use, as the charge would rapidly leak away from the capacitor.

Cordless mobiles

The cordless mobile unit is completely independent of the mains supply as it draws its power from batteries usually built up from lead or nickel cadmium cells.

One such unit draws its power from three 40 V batteries. This power is used to propel the unit and to provide the necessary energy for the X-ray exposures. Current from the batteries is, of course, d.c. but this is used to power a rotary converter which generates a polyphase supply which is stepped up by the high tension transformer to provide the necessary kV for application to the X-ray tube. The applied kV is claimed to be near constant potential.

The rotating anode X-ray tube insert is contained within an oil-filled casing which also incorporates the high tension transformer and solid state rectifiers which provide a unidirectional current through the X-ray tube. The tube is mounted on an extendable cross-arm which, in turn, is secured to a vertical support on which the tube and cross-arm may be raised or lowered. The tube may be angled for oblique projections and locks are provided to stabilize each of these movements. A light beam diaphragm is mounted on the X-ray tube casing. A timer provides a range of exposures typically in the range from 0.4 to 5.0 s with a maximum tube voltage of 100 kV at 15 mA and 60 kV at 25 mA.

The great advantage of such equipment is its independence from mains supply and within its limitations it provides a useful addition to the range of mobile equipment used in the hospital.

Note: The batteries are recharged from the mains supply by means of a battery charger. All that is normally necessary is to connect the charger, which is an integral part of the X-ray unit, to the mains supply each evening. The unit is then ready for use the following morning. Charging time is 8 hours. This is the length of time required to fully charge the battery after it has been completely discharged. The state of charge of the battery may be indicated by a meter which records the degree of charge and is calibrated in terms of adequate or inadequate charge. Alternatively, a green light may be used to indicate adequate charge and a red light to indicate insufficient charge for efficient operation of the equipment.

Siemen's Mobilett mobile unit

This mobile unit (Figure 9.7a) is mains operated and uses a medium frequency generator similar to the one described on page 122. The high tension circuit is contained within a single tank structure tube head and is microprocessor controlled. The tube has a focal spot of 0.8 mm × 0.8 mm, an anode angle of 15° and an anode rotational speed of 8500 r.p.m. It can give 1.6–200 mA s at 55 kV, 1.2–120 mA s at 77 kV, and 0.5–20 mA s at 133 kV. It has a shortest exposure time of 3 ms.

Figure 9.7b illustrates the main parts of the circuit. The mains voltage is rectified and smoothed to provide a near constant voltage which is then interrupted, during an exposure, by trigger pulses from the microprocessor, to produce a varying voltage of 3000 H. This high frequency voltage is stepped up by the high tension transformer, smoothed and applied as constant potential to the X-ray tube. A feed-back circuit to the microprocessor enables it to maintain the kV and mA at the set value, during the exposure. The control panel is shown in Figure 9.7c.

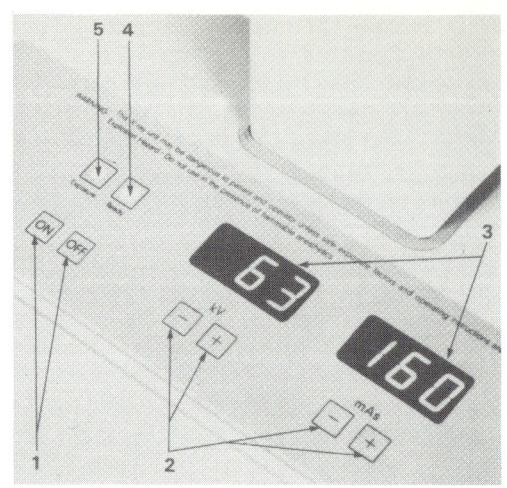

Figure 9.7c (1) power supply on/off; (2) touch controls for free setting of kV and mAs; (3) display of set kV and mAs values or of coded information for the operator; (4) ready for exposure; (5) light and audible tone indication of exposure release

Mobile image intensifier

In addition to its use with a major installation the image intensifier can also be used to good effect with mobile units. Its main application is in theatre radiography. The range of movements are as indicated in Figure 9.8. It is almost always used with a closed circuit TV system nowadays.

Provision is made on the underside of the image intensifier casing for the accommodation of a cassette so that a film may be exposed. A grid may also be accommodated.

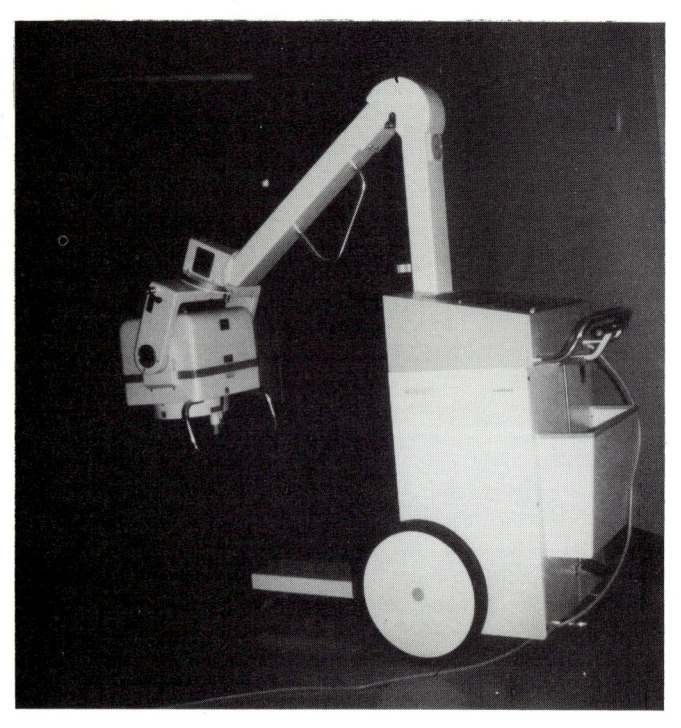

Figure 9.7a Siemens Mobilette mobile unit

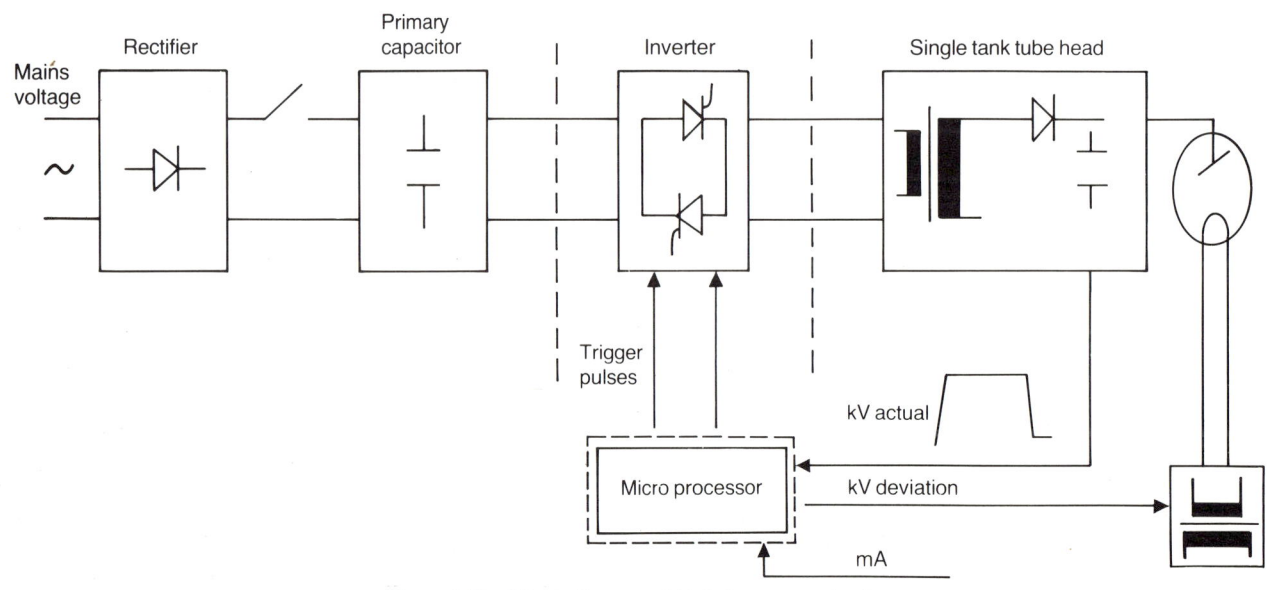

Figure 9.7b Block diagram of high-frequency circuit

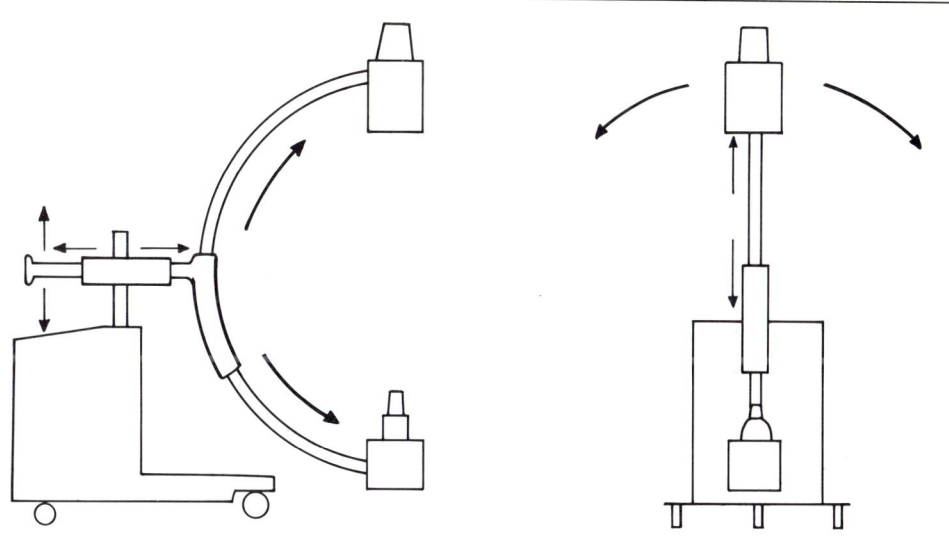

EQUIPMENT FOR MOBILE, DENTAL, ACCIDENT AND SKULL RADIOGRAPHY 123

Figure 9.8 Range of movements of mobile image intensifier

Image retention systems

As previously described, image retention systems may also be usefully employed with mobile image intensifier units, particularly when they are to be used in the orthopaedic theatre. During fluoroscopy of a hip pinning, for example, rather than expose the patient and staff to continuous radiation whilst the image of the hip and pin are displayed on the television screen, fluoroscopy can be restricted to a short period of, say, 1 s, after which the radiation is switched off, whilst the image continues to be displayed on the monitor screen.

EQUIPMENT FOR DENTAL RADIOGRAPHY

Such equipment includes a simple self-rectified unit, the orthopantomograph unit (OPG) and the cephalostat or craniostat. Each will be considered separately.

Simple self-rectified unit

The dental unit, used mainly for intraoral radiography of teeth, consists essentially of a single structure, self-rectified tube head. The tube is mounted in such a fashion as to provide a high degree of manoeuvrability. The unit may be either wall mounted or mobile. Whilst the power of such a unit is low, e.g. 12 mA at 55 kVp, it is adequate for radiography of teeth. The focal spot size is small, e.g. 0.8 mm. The timer may be of the clockwork or electronic variety and has a range of times from zero up to 5.0 s in steps of 0.1–0.25 s. The range of movements of such a unit are indicated in Figure 9.9.

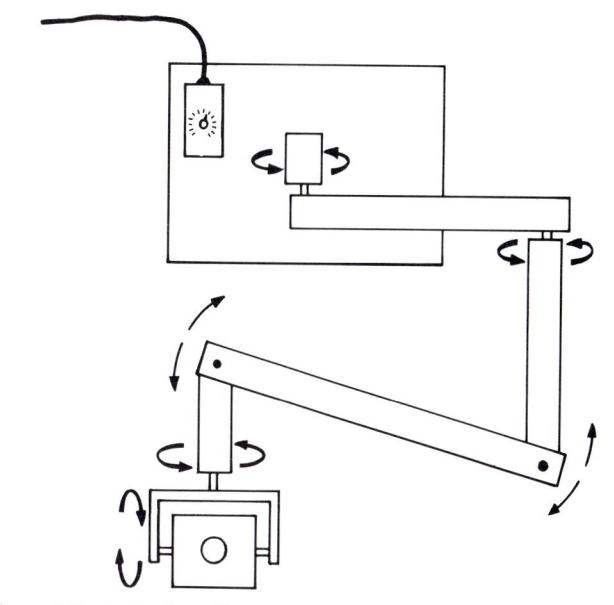

Figure 9.9 A simple wall mounted dental unit

The orthopantomograph (OPG) unit

This unit provides a panoramic view of both jaws during a single excursion of tube and film.

The patient is positioned with his chin resting on a plastic support, the head being held in the correct plane by means of plastic ear pieces. Surrounding the head is a plastic guard. During the exposure the curved cassette rotates around the patient's head whilst the X-ray tube moves in the opposite direction. The cassette also rotates about its own axis as it moves around the patient. The beam of radiation is collimated into a narrow slit by means of a diaphragm at the X-ray tube and by another directly in front of the cassette. The incident beam is thus always passing through the structure of interest at an angle of 90° (Figure 9.11).

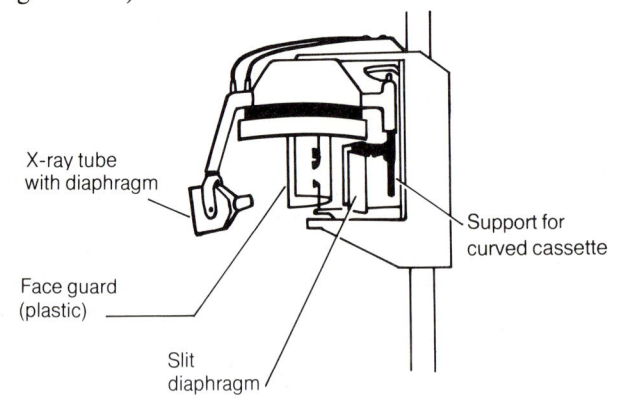

Figure 9.10 Dental tomograph unit

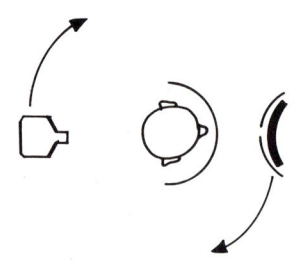

Figure 9.11 Diagram showing the tube rotating in one direction whilst slit diaphragm and cassette rotate in the opposite direction. The patient is immobilized and cassette rotates about its own axis in addition to rotating round the patient

The X-ray tube changes its axis of rotation during the exposure (Figure 9.12), passing through point 3 at the start of the exposure then through point 2 and finally through point 1. Axes 1 and 3 are the same whilst axis 2 is closer to the front teeth. Two different axes are needed to ensure that the slit of radiation always passes through the teeth at right angles.

At the beginning of an exposure the slit of radiation passes through point 3 and records on the film an image of that part of the left side of the face and jaw through which it is passing. As the tube arcs in one direction the film arcs in the other and due to the rotation of the cassette about its own axis it presents a fresh section of film to the slit of radiation at each successive instant in time. A tomographic image is thus built up of the structures on the left side of the jaw. The axis of rotation is now smoothly changed to point 2 and a similar sequence of events occur,

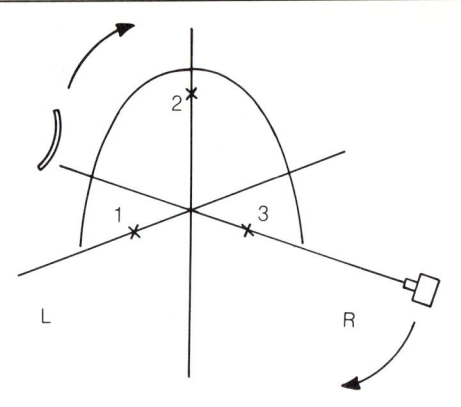

Figure 9.12 Two different axes used to ensure correct projection of beam through teeth

this time recording a tomographic image of the teeth in the front of the jaw. The axis finally changes to point 1 and an image is built up of structures on the right side of the face.

Secondary shadows can be formed as some parts of the right and left sides of the jaw are scanned twice during each exposure. Component parts of the unit itself, i.e. chin support, ear pieces, etc. may also present confusing images.

The great advantage of the OPG is that it gives a panoramic view of the face and jaws and shows the relationships of one structure to another. Definition is obviously inferior to that obtained with an intraoral dental film and the OPG film shows a relatively high degree of enlargement. Distortion is, however, minimized, as the beam of radiation always passes through the point of interest at 90°. The level of radiation dose to the patient is relatively low, which is attributable largely to the restriction of the radiation to a narrow slit and to the use of intensifying screens.

The cephalostat

The cephalostat, or craniostat, as it is sometimes called, provides a means of accurately localizing the patient's head so that comparable views of the patient's skull and facial bones can be obtained at subsequent examinations. This is an essential requirement for good orthodontic radiography.

Philips Cephalix unit

This unit is wall mounted, for rigidity, and has an f.f.d. of 1500 mm. The cross-arm which supports the tube at one end and the head clamp/cassette holder at the other is adjustable in height so that patients of different heights, standing or sitting can be accommodated.

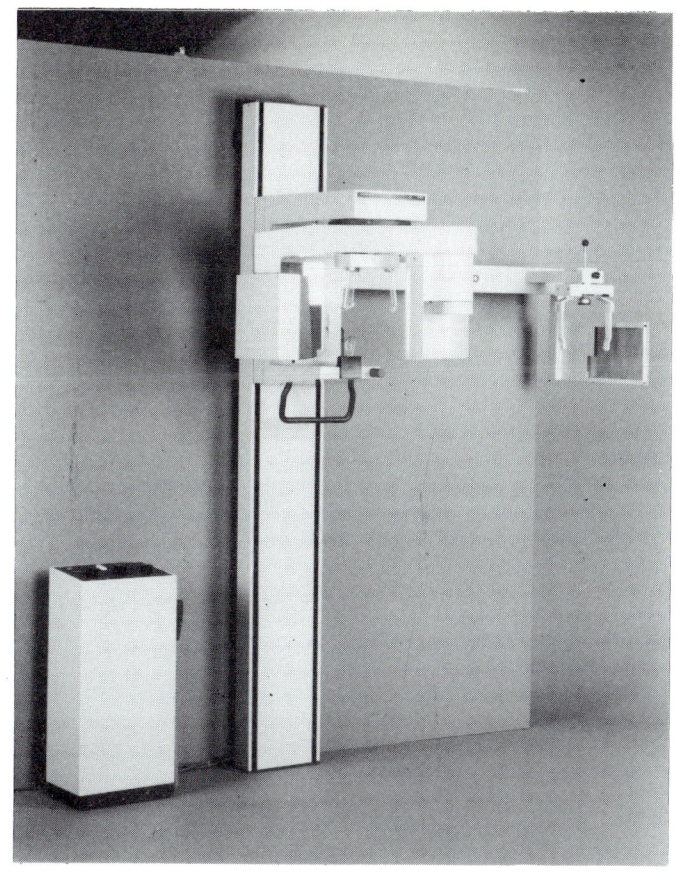

EQUIPMENT FOR MOBILE, DENTAL, ACCIDENT AND SKULL RADIOGRAPHY 125

Figure 9.13 Philips Cephalix CX 90/20 unit

A long cone is used at the end of which are fitted crosswires. These, in conjunction with the light beam, provide a cross of light which facilitates accurate centring. Slide-in diaphragms may also be fitted to the end of the cone to delineate the beam to the required area.

The head clamp (Figure 9.14) can be rotated with stops at every 90° and with provision for stops at intermediate angles.

The right hand bracket (one of the ear localizers) hinges upwards to allow access for the patient's head into the clamp.

The X-ray tube is of single pulse tank structure. The control panel is illustrated on page 55 (Figure 4.22).

EQUIPMENT FOR ACCIDENT RADIOGRAPHY

The examination of accident patients, whether clinical or radiographic, should be carried out with as little movement of the patient as possible so as to reduce discomfort and minimize aggravation of the patient's injuries.

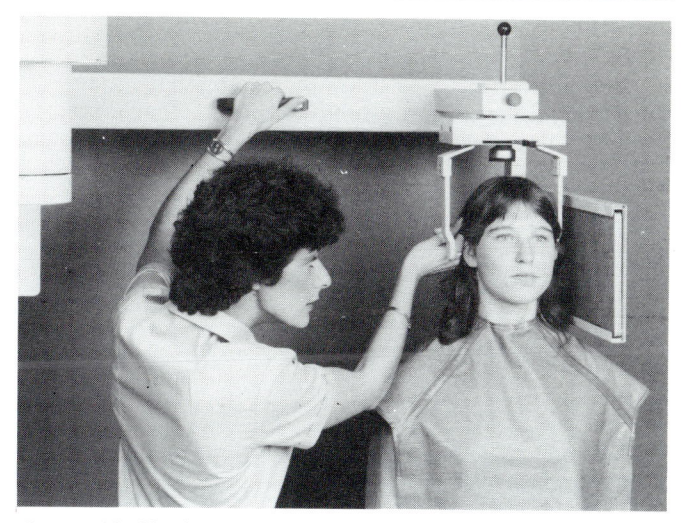

Figure 9.14 Head clamp and cassette holder. The bracket is raised to allow the patient's head to be inserted into the clamp

Different hospitals have different ways of achieving this objective. Some use trolleys, the tops of which are the same height as the X-ray table and pull the patient across on a radiolucent mattress (Figure 9.15). Other departments use accident trolleys of one form or another and some use specialized systems. Whatever method is used it should be simple and uncomplicated in operation and

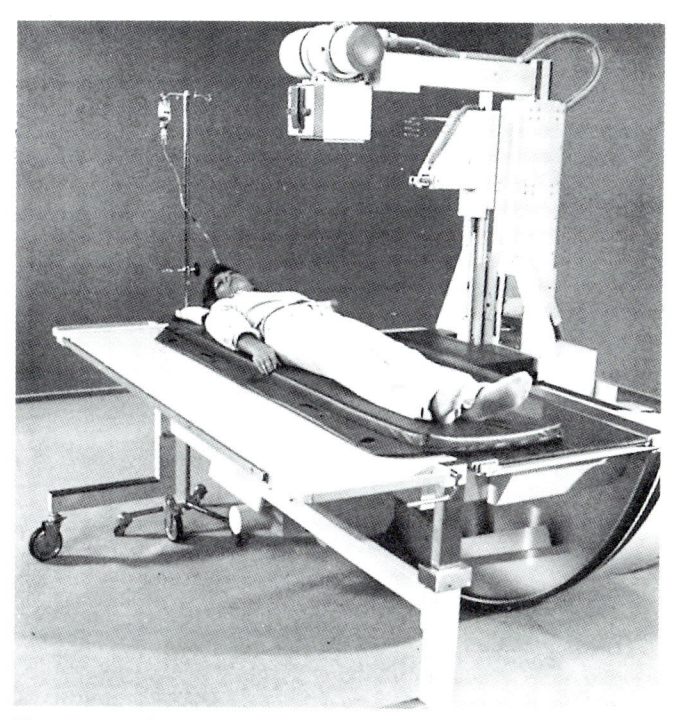

Figure 9.15 Siemens adjustable height trolley

capable of being used by inexperienced staff. If special trolleys are used there should be enough of them to meet the hospital's needs. This usually means that the cost of each trolley should not be excessive.

Most of the major firms produce accident systems, but only one will be described. It is in fairly wide use and is called the 'Care' system.

Picker 'Care' system

The 'Care' system consists essentially of a special patient trolley (Figure 9.16) and a mobile cassette carrier (Figure 9.17). The special trolley, which is lightweight, has lockable wheels and an X-ray transparent top which can be tilted 15° in the Trendelenburg position. A shelf under the table top accommodates the cassette tray. The trolley has an adjustable back rest, cot sides and facilities for fitting a drip. The base of the trolley accommodates an oxygen cylinder and a removable wire tray in which to store the patient's clothes etc.

Two versions of the trolley are available, one of fixed height and the other adjustable so that the table top (and patient) can be raised or lowered.

The patient, having been transferred to the 'Care' trolley on admission to the hospital, need not transferred to any other couch or table for clinical or radiographic examination. This ensures that the patient is not moved unnecessarily, reduces the patient's discomfort and avoids aggravation of injuries.

A plain mattress, some 5 cm thick, which may be slotted to accept cassettes, is available for use with the trolley. Provision is also made for the attachment of a lateral cassette holder to either side of the trolley and for a cassette holder used for radiography of the skull.

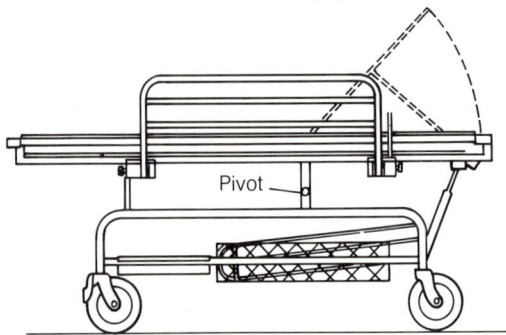

Figure 9.16 'Care' patient trolley type STC

The 'Care' cassette carrier is a ray-proof mobile box, kept in the X-ray room and used to store cassettes (Figure 9.17). The upper surface of the box accommodates a cassette tray and grid which can be slid into position under the trolley top. Alternatively, the cassette tray and grid can be tilted into the vertical position for lateral projections.

When the patient is brought into the X-ray room, the trolley wheels are locked and the mobile cassette carrier is brought up to the side of the trolley opposite the part to be examined. The cassette tray is slid under the table top and the X-ray tube positioned. To facilitate centring of the tube to the grid and film two light beams are projected from the side of the light beam diaphragm. These light beams are quite separate from the beam which delineates the X-ray field but as they are connected in parallel they switch on at the same time. Whilst the normal light beam indicates the field covered by radiation the two positioning lights are projected towards the handle of the cassette tray where they form a cross when the tube is centred to the grid and film and when the tube is at the correct FFD.

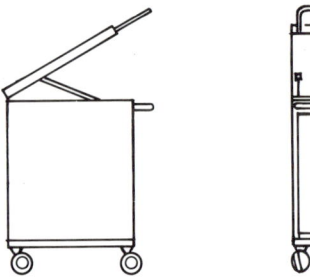

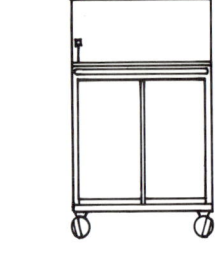

Figure 9.17 Care cassette carrier

Advantages of the 'Care' type system

(1) The patient need not be transferred from the trolley to the X-ray table for examination.

(2) Using a ceiling-suspended tube AP radiographs or laterals can be taken from either side of the trolley without undue disturbance of the patient.

(3) Centring of the tube to grid and film is simplified by the use of the light beam centring system.

(4) Cassettes are readily available from the mobile cassette box.

(5) Simplicity of the system ensures rapid examination of the patient.

Disadvantages

(1) Large object–film distance due to the thickness of the mattress and the distance between the trolley top and cassette tray.

(2) Difficulty in obtaining good lateral films due to patient 'sinking' into the mattress.

(3) Only two sizes of film format available, i.e. 35 cm × 43 cm and 24 cm × 30 cm which can lead to film wastage.

EQUIPMENT FOR MOBILE, DENTAL, ACCIDENT AND SKULL RADIOGRAPHY

(4) Sufficient numbers of trolleys must be available in the casualty department to ensure availability of a trolley for each serious casualty. This may lead to difficulty in striking a balance between the need for a large number of trolleys and their cost.

THE SKULL UNIT

As the name implies this unit is designed specifically for radiography of the skull. There are two basic systems namely the *Lysholm* system and the *Dulac* system.

In the Lysholm system the centre of rotation between the film and the X-ray tube lies at the centre of the film whilst in the Dulac system the centre of rotation lies at a point in space corresponding to the centre of the patient's skull as illustrated in Figure 9.18.

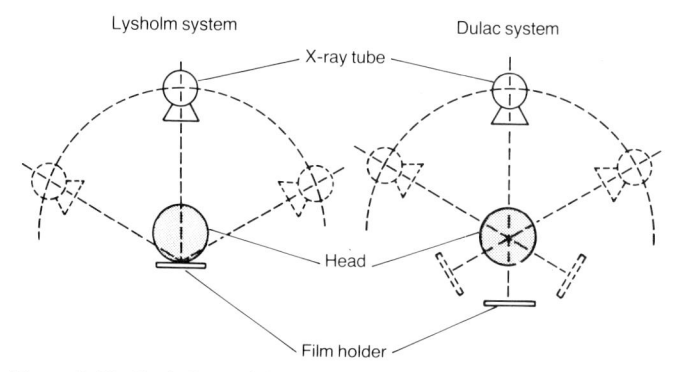

Figure 9.18 Lysholm and Dulac systems

The Dulac system is used in sophisticated skull units designed for specialized techniques. These will be described later.

In general use many of the skull units use the Lysholm system. Such a unit consists of an X-ray tube supported on a counterbalanced 'C' arm which can be rotated in any direction (Figure 9.19). The table is small in comparison with the conventional X-ray table and accommodates cassettes up to 18 cm × 30 cm in size. The table incorporates a moving grid mechanism which is removable. The table and tube support can be raised or lowered and the table can be tilted independently of the tube. The tube itself can be angled in any direction.

The primary movements of the tube are such that however it is angled the central ray always passes through the centre of the table. By using secondary movements the tube can be off-centred.

The moving grid mechanism can be withdrawn from the table completely or made to hang down by the side of the table. With the grid mechanism removed or pulled out in this fashion the patient's skull is resting on a piece of clear perspex; the perspex is marked with lines radiating outwards from the centre point. A periscopic mirror device and light which are positioned under the table enable the radiographer to see the patient's skull through the mirror of the periscope. By using this mirror in conjunction with the lines marked on the perspex it is relatively easy to position the patient accurately for such views as Stenvers, optic foramina, etc. Of equal importance is the fact that it is also possible to obtain relatively easily comparable views of each side. The range of movements of the skull unit is indicated in Figure 9.19.

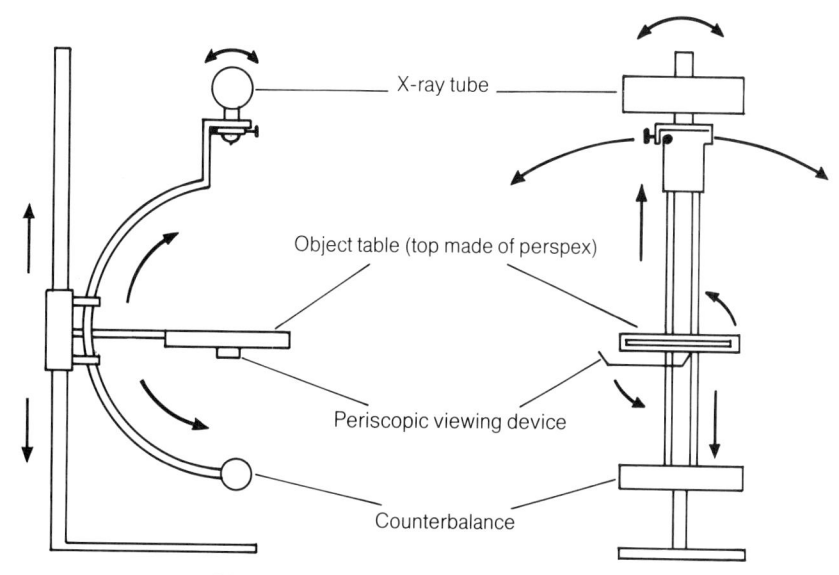

Figure 9.19 Skull unit using Lysholm principle

Grid rotation

It has been mentioned that the tube may be angled in any direction. If a double angulation of the tube is used the beam would be directed into the lead slats of the grid. Figure 9.20 should illustrate this point. With the moving grid mechanism in position (1) it can be seen that the X-ray beam B is parallel to the grid lines which is normal and satisfactory. If, however, a double tilt is used the X-ray beam is now directed as in arrow C and the beam is directed into the grid lines. As this is obviously unsatisfactory, provision is made to rotate the grid assembly as shown in (2) so that the grid lines and X-ray beam are once again parallel.

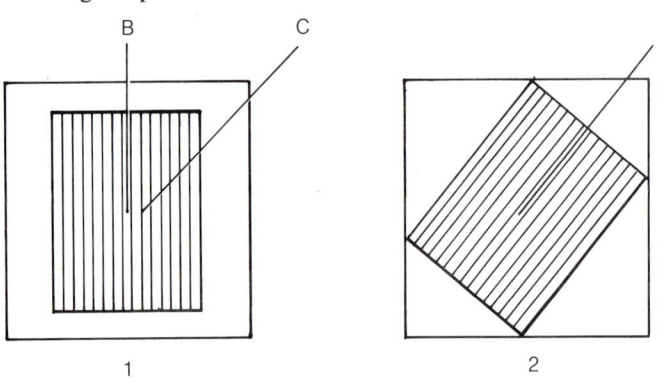

Figure 9.20 The central ray is kept parallel to the grid lines by rotating the grid

Choice of generator

The skull unit should be used in conjunction with a high powered generator so that a series of exposures can be made in rapid succession, as in examinations such as cerebral angiography. Such a generator may be used to power other tubes in the same room or in an adjacent room, the appropriate tube being selected by means of a changeover switch located in the high tension transformer tank.

The skull unit tube should, of course, be fitted with a narrow angle anode so that geometric blurring is reduced to a minimum.

Attachments

Various attachments are available for use with the skull table. An immobilization band may be fitted and provision is made for the attachment of a lateral cassette holder. Cones, plate diaphragms or a light beam diaphragm may be fitted to the tube, a light beam centring device sometimes being fitted as an alternative to the light beam diaphragm. The light beam centring device is particularly useful when used with the skull unit as the intersecting white lines help not only in centring but in assessing the degree of rotation of the patient's skull. The white line also gives a visual indication of tube angulation.

Spring-loaded manually operated cassette changers

These may be used to expose a series of films in rapid succession for examinations such as cerebral angiography. The cassette changers, each consisting of a metal box holding a number of lead-lined cassette trays, are illustrated in Figure 9.21.

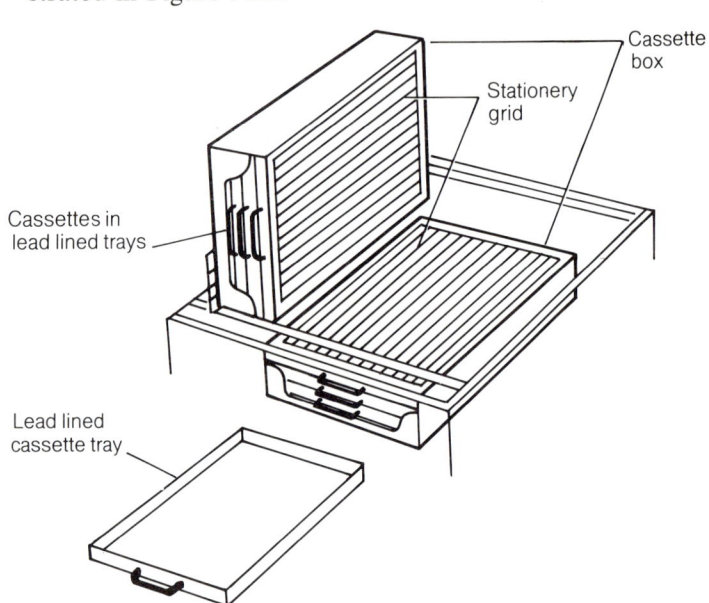

Figure 9.21 Spring-loaded manually operated cassette changer

In operation the moving grid assembly is removed from the skull unit table and the metal container inserted in its place. The container is locked in position. The upper surface of the container is formed by a stationary grid and in the base are two strong leaf springs. The cassettes placed in the lead-lined trays are inserted in the box one on top of the other, the container usually holding up to three cassettes.

When the first film in the upper cassette has been exposed it is pulled out and the second cassette which has been lying under the first and protected from radiation by the lead lining of the upper tray is pushed up by leaf springs into position ready for the next exposure. This sequence is repeated until all the cassettes have been exposed.

A similar procedure is adopted for the lateral projection but this time the metal container is locked in position, vertically by the side of the patient's head. The tube is rotated into a horizontal position, radiographs exposed, cassettes pulled out, etc. as previously described for the AP projection.

Provision must be made for the anode to rotate continuously once the exposures are being made. This is usually achieved by fitting a separate anode switch. Care must be taken to ensure that it is switched off as soon as the series of exposures has been completed otherwise the life of the tube will be shortened.

Note: Manually operated changers such as described above can represent a serious radiation hazard for staff unless effective lead or lead rubber shielding is provided and used. Counterbalanced lead rubber screens can be raised or lowered, are frequently used during cerebral angiography procedures and are shown in Figure 9.22.

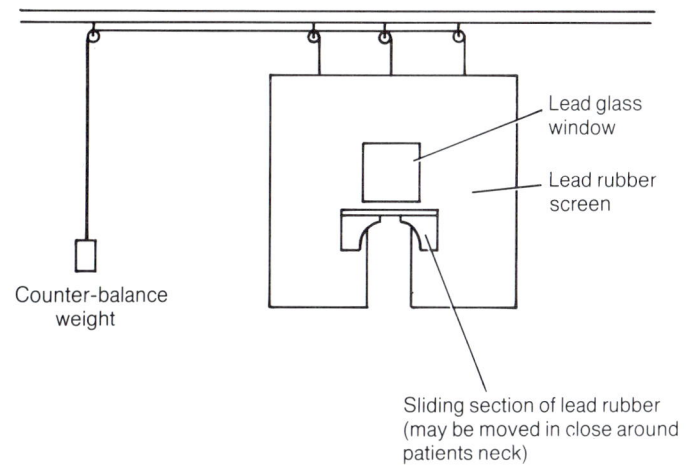

Figure 9.22 Counterbalanced lead rubber screens used in cerebral angiography

An automatic changer such as AOT biplane equipment overcomes the problem of excessive dose to staff and also provides a programme which is exactly reproducible. The relatively long exposures and time intervals between exposures means that the outline of the vessels is, of necessity, 'traced' onto the radiograph. Much more information is gained from a rapid series of short exposures. For this reason digital radiography is the method of choice in most major neuroradiology centres. This technique is described later.

Other accessory equipment for use with the skull unit includes the following.

Patient trolley

This should have wheel locks which make the trolley absolutely steady and secure. It should preferably be possible to raise or lower the table and it should be capable of moving and locking in both longitudinal and transverse directions.

Bipod tube support

This can be used to hold the tube steady when exposures are made with the tube in the horizontal position. As the tube is supported on a metal arc it can easily vibrate and if this happens the quality of the films is impaired. The bipod tube support reduces such vibration.

Other types of unit using the Dulac system provide an even greater degree of precision and refinement. Such units include the Siemens Angioscop or the Philips Diagnostic units. The main features of the Angioscop are indicated in Chapter 11, Figure 11.5. It has facilities for macroradiography, image intensification and tomography. It will frequently be used in conjunction with an AOT or Puck film changer for angiography. 100 mm or 105 mm film cameras may be used in conjunction with the image intensifier, but as previously stated digital imaging would now be the method of choice.

10
Tomography – theory and equipment

TOMOGRAPHIC ATTACHMENT	130
Sequential tomography	131
Simultaneous multisection tomography	131
Inclined plane tomography	133
TOMOGRAPHIC UNITS	133
Philips BTS4 (Bucky Tomographic System)	133
Philips Polytome U	134
X-ray generator and tube	135
The Polytome U3	135
AUTOMATIC EXPOSURE CONTROL	136
How is this achieved?	136
QUALITY ASSURANCE TESTS	137
Checks	137
Tests	137
Accuracy of layer height indication	138
Fan test	138
Frequency of testing	139

Unlike a normal radiograph where the degree of radiographic unsharpness throughout the part of the body being radiographed remains more or less constant, a tomogram has one selected plane in which the degree of unsharpness is less than that of the planes above and below it. That is to say, the planes above and below the selected plane in the body become progressively more and more blurred as the distance increases above and below the selected plane.

This is achieved by moving the X-ray tube in one direction and the film in the opposite direction whilst the exposure is being made (Figure 10.1). For effective tomography the tube/film movement should be across the long axis of the object of interest and not in line with it. This minimizes the build-up of linear shadows on the radiograph and produces an effective 'cut' through the object.

This may be difficult to achieve, however. When taking tomograms of the sternum, for instance, the patient is positioned with the sternum (and the patient's body) along the long axis of the table. It is difficult to do otherwise as the patient's head gets in the way of the tomographic equipment if he is positioned across the long axis of the table! The difficulty may be overcome by using either a transverse linear movement, or a complex movement which will be described later.

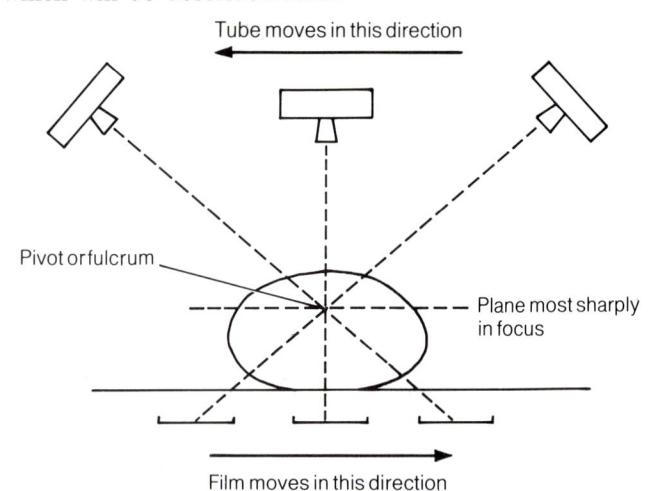

Figure 10.1 Line to line tomographic movement

The linear movements of tube and film are described as line-to-line, line-to-arc, or arc-to-arc (Figure 10.2). The tube and film may also make reciprocal movements in elliptical, circular, hypocycloidal, spiral or lassijous fashion (Figure 10.3).

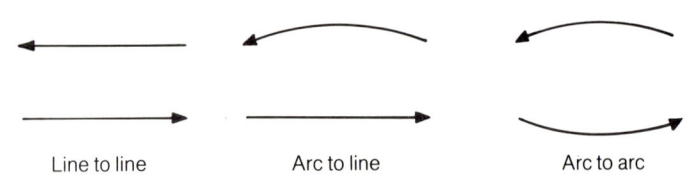

Figure 10.2 Linear and arcuate movements

TOMOGRAPHIC ATTACHMENT

This is the simplest form of tomographic equipment and may be attached to a conventional X-ray table and tube. The attachment consists essentially of a metal bar which connects the X-ray tube and moving grid assembly (Figure 10.4). It pivots about a fulcrum which can be raised or

130

TOMOGRAPHY – THEORY AND EQUIPMENT

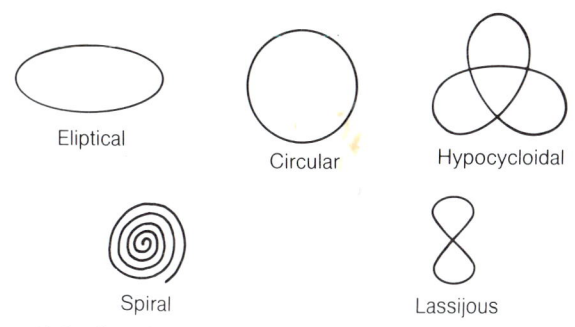

Figure 10.3 Complex movements

lowered in relation to the table top. The X-ray tube moves in one direction at a fixed distance from the table top whilst the cassette and moving grid assembly moves in the opposite direction. Switches operated by the connecting arm ensure that the exposure starts after the X-ray tube has started its movement and that the exposure is terminated before the end of its movement. The distance of the fulcrum from the table top is the same distance as the section in focus from the table top. The angle of exposure determines the thickness of section to be sharply in focus. We can thus select any particular plane to be most sharply in focus whilst the planes above and below the selected plane become progressively more and more blurred.

If, for example, a plane 15 cm above the table top is to be sharply in focus we would set the fulcrum to a height of 15 cm above the table top, the fulcrum–table top distance being indicated on a scale.

The greater the angle of exposure the thinner is the section sharply in focus whilst the smaller the angle of exposure the thicker is the section most sharply in focus.

The level of 'cut' may be varied by changing the fulcrum level or, alternatively, the patient may be raised or lowered.

When assembling a tomographic attachment, care must be taken to fasten securely all clamps, wing nuts, etc. used to secure the connecting bar to the moving grid assembly at one end and to the tube at the other. The tube must also be secured at the appropriate FFD and the tube locked on the transverse arm in such a manner that it is centred to the midline of the table. The tube rotational lock must be released so that it can rotate freely. The tube must also be free to move in the longitudinal direction, so any longitudinal locks must also be freed. The floor track should also be free of dirt or debris so that the movement of the tube is smooth and without hindrance. The wheels on which the vertical tube support trolley is mounted and their bearings must be in good order to minimize any vibrations which might take place as the tube is moved along the floor track. The bucky must also be free to move easily during the exposure.

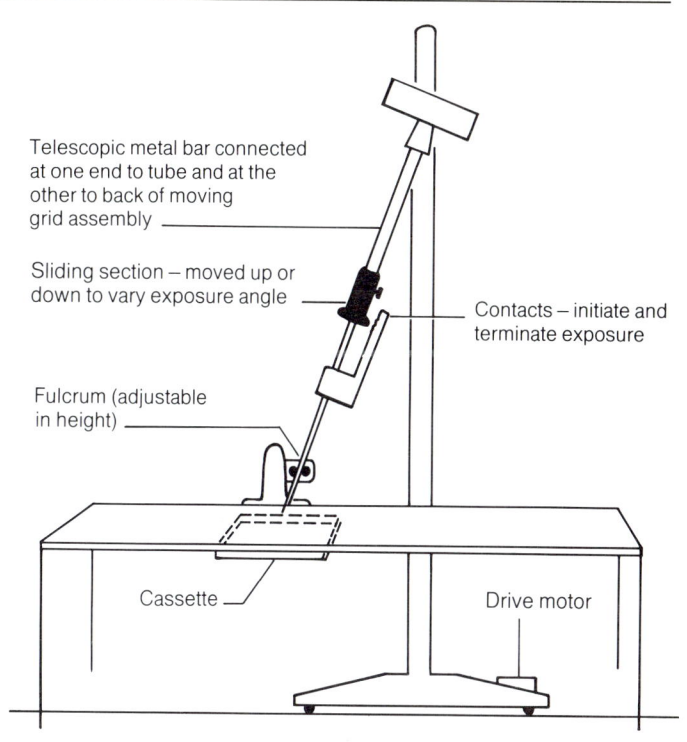

Figure 10.4 Tomographic attachment

Movement of the tube and film during the tomographic exposure may be achieved in a number of different ways. A spring may be tensioned by moving the tube and its support along the floor track prior to the exposure, pressure on the exposure button releasing the spring and causing the tube to move in the opposite direction. In all but the simplest tomographic attachments, however, the tube will be moved by means of a variable speed motor drive unit which is mounted on the base of the tube stand or by means of a motorized overhead tube support.

Sequential tomography

This means the exposure of individual films one for each 'cut' required, the fulcrum–table level distance being adjusted for each exposure. This probably gives the best quality for each individual radiograph, but, of course, necessitates a number of separate exposures.

Simultaneous multisection tomography

Up to seven 'cuts' on seven different films may be recorded with a single exposure. Multisection tomography is of particular value in chest radiography as all films are exposed during the same respiratory phase. There is a saving in time and some reduction in patient radiation dose although the exposure for seven films will always be greater than that required for a single exposure with a conventional cassette. The multisection cassette is essentially a box made of aluminium which accepts up to seven films and seven pairs of screens, each film and screen combination being separated from its neighbour by radiolucent material such as polyfoam, balsa wood, etc. (Figures 10.5 and 10.6). The distance between films is dependent on the thickness of the spacer, some manufacturers providing a number of 0.5 cm spacers and others providing 1 cm spacers. The multisection cassette fits under the table so that the top film in the cassette occupies a plane exactly the same as that which would be occupied by a single cassette in the cassette tray. The cassette tray must, of course, be removed before fitting the multisection cassette.

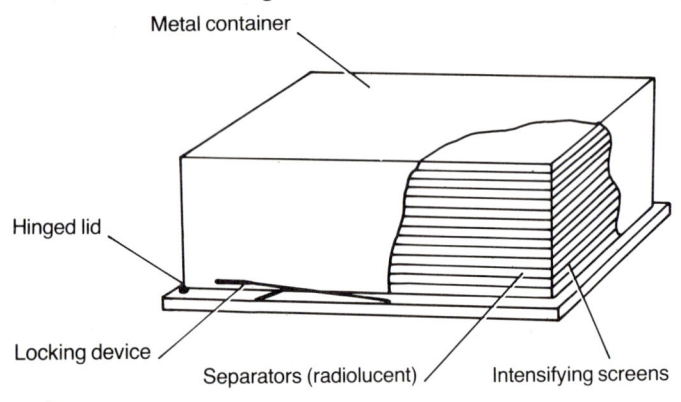

Figure 10.5 Multisection cassette

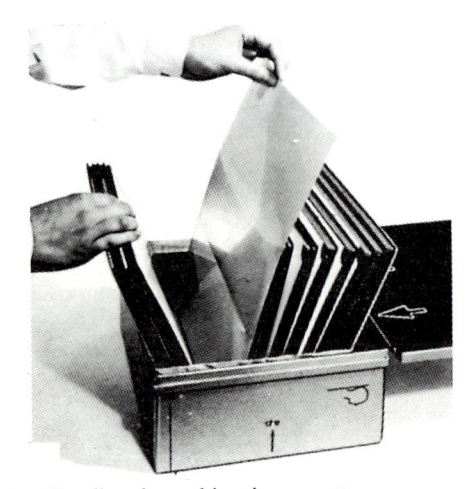

Figure 10.6 Loading the multisection cassette

The multisection cassette houses a number of pairs of screens with radiolucent separators, different manufacturers making cassettes accepting up to three, five, or seven pairs of screens. The speed of each pair of screens is different, the fastest screen combination being at the bottom of the cassette, and each pair of screens becoming progressively slower as they approach the top. The top pair are obviously the slowest. This ensures that although the radiation is attenuated as it passes through the cassette, an even density is maintained for all the films in the pack.

If there are five films in a multisection cassette each 1 cm apart and the fulcrum is set at, say, 10 cm, the top film in the box is in the same plane as would be occupied by film in a conventional cassette. The top film in the multisection cassette therefore records a plane sharply in focus which is 10 cm above the table top. The remainder of the films in the box, if they are 1 cm apart, will record sections in focus which are approximately 9, 8, 7, 6 cm etc. above the table top (Figure 10.7).

Note: The recorded sections are not exactly 1 cm apart as the beam of radiation is diverging.

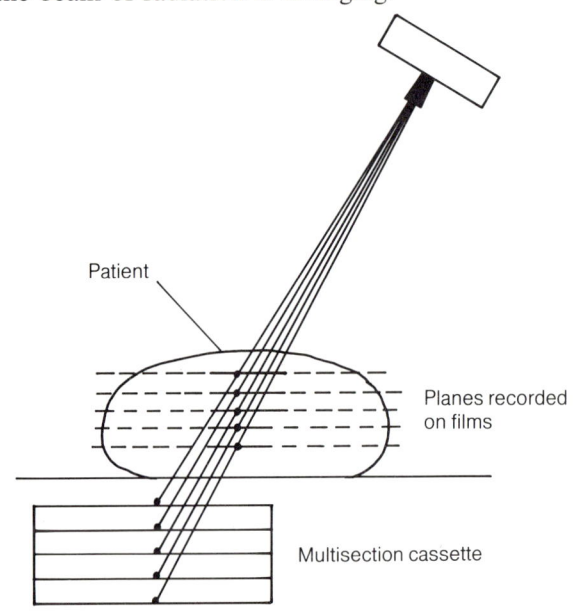

Figure 10.7 Multisection tomography

Although radiation dose is reduced when a multisection cassette is used to produce a series of radiographs with a single exposure, the quality of the resultant radiographs is inevitably poorer than those taken sequentially with a series of exposures. This is mainly due to the fact that screen contact is poorer in a multisection cassette compared with a single film cassette of conventional design. This is because of the difficulty in achieving good screen pressure without unduly squashing the interspacing material which must be radiolucent and about 0.5 or 1 cm thick. The disadvantage of poorer screen contact may, however, be outweighed by the advantages in the case, for example, of chest tomography as all the radiographs in a series are taken in the same respiratory phase.

A special cassette holding three films and screens approx-

TOMOGRAPHY – THEORY AND EQUIPMENT

imately 1 mm apart may be used for tomography of the middle ear or any other technique requiring a very thin section.

A wide angle of exposure is, of course, essential for such an examination (hypocycloidal movement is frequently used).

Zonography is the production of a thick 'cut' tomograph i.e. a relatively thick section of the body is sharply defined. This is achieved by using a narrow angle of exposure, angles of 5° ~ 8° being typical.

Inclined plane tomography

As the plane most sharply in focus is parallel to the plane of the film, it is necessary only to incline the film to produce an inclined plane tomograph (Figure 10.8).

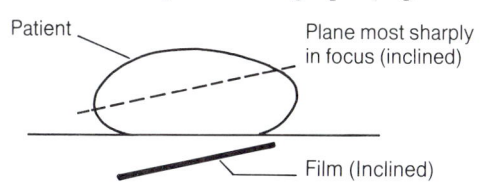

Figure 10.8 Inclined plane (oblique) tomography

TOMOGRAPHIC UNITS

Whilst the tomographic attachment previously described may produce reasonably good tomograms, better results can be obtained with equipment designed with tomography as a major function. Best results of course will always be obtained when using equipment dedicated specifically to tomography.

A good example of the latter is the Philips Polytome U, first produced some 20 years ago, continuously improved over the years and still a leader in its field. Another unit from the same company designed for tomography, but which is readily adaptable to general radiography, is the Philips BTS4.

Each of these units will be described, starting with the BTS4.

Philips BTS4 (Bucky Tomographic System)

This is a system designed to accommodate conventional bucky techniques as well as tomography and zonography. The main features of the unit are indicated in Figure 10.9.

The table top is adjustable in height, making for easy patient transfer from trolley to table and its floating top facility simplifies positioning of the patient. The flat table top is a useful feature when positioning patients for lateral projections. A foot-operated locking bar is readily accessible from either the front or ends of the table.

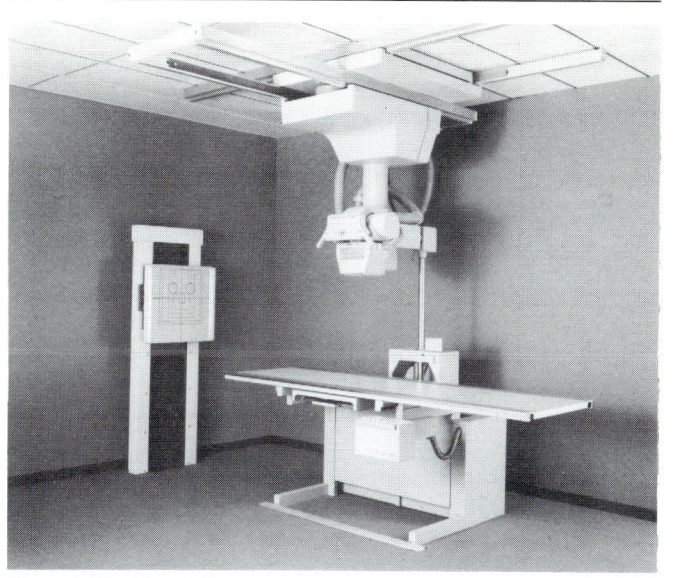

Figure 10.9 The Philips BTS4 tomographic and general unit

The X-ray tube which is ceiling suspended is connected to the bucky by means of a telescopic bar, which provides a firm and stable attachment whilst allowing easy decoupling when the tube is to be used in other parts of the room. The longitudinal, transverse and vertical movements of the tube are push-button controlled. The push buttons, located on a handlebar control, are colour coded for ease of operation and a light beam diaphragm ensures adequate collimation and accurate centring of the beam.

The tomographic drive mechanism is located in the ceiling suspension unit.

The unit has a fixed fulcrum so layer height is selected by raising or lowering the table top.

A control box is mounted on a telescopic bar under the table top. It moves with the table top when it is raised or lowered and can be either pulled out to a convenient position when in use or pushed in under the table top when transferring patients from trolley to table. It has push buttons which control the change over from tomography to general radiography, table height, floating top movement, type of tomographic movement and exposure time, etc. A test button enables the tube to move through a selected trajectory without radiation being produced; this is a useful facility as it enables the patient to experience the tube movement etc. before the actual examination takes place. There is thus less chance of the patient moving when the actual exposure is made. Each button is labelled with the function it represents and lights up when depressed. A microprocessor tests all functions when the equipment is switched on prior to it becoming available for use.

The blurring movements available are elliptical, spiral and linear. Elliptical movements are available with a choice of exposure angles, i.e. 36° or 18° and an exposure time of 2.5 s. The spiral movement has an exposure angle of 30° and an exposure time of 5.5 s. The linear movement has a 30° angle of exposure and a choice of exposure times of 0.8 or 2.5 s

Zonography can be performed with elliptical or linear movements, an angle of 8° or 5° being available with the elliptical movement and an exposure time of 2.5 s, whilst the linear movement has an exposure angle of 8° and an exposure time of 2.5 s.

An undercouch image intensifier coupled with closed circuit television and image storage (memory) facility is available for use with this unit. It enables patient positioning to be checked using a very small dose of radiation prior to the radiographic or tomographic exposure being made.

Philips Polytome U

This is a system designed specifically for tomography. The equipment is mounted on a rigid cast iron pedestal which ensures complete stability and freedom from vibration during the exposure, providing of course that the floor of the room in which the unit is installed is itself rigid and vibration free (Figure 10.10).

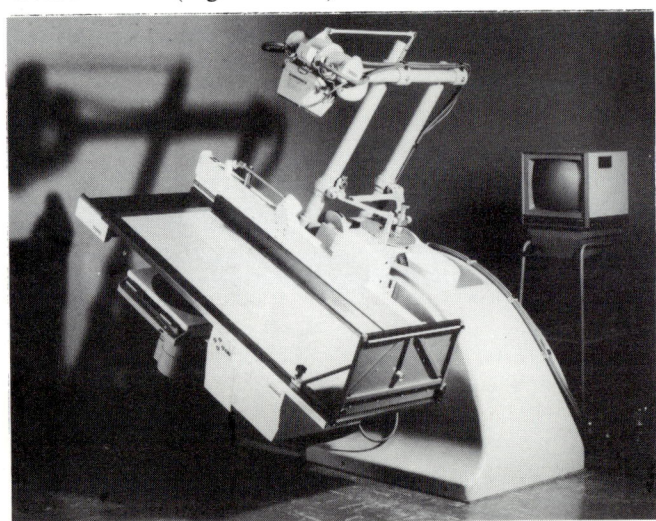

Figure 10.10 Philips Polytome U, a dedicated tomographic unit

The tube and bucky mechanism are supported on either end of a parallelogram which is always in equilibrium and which moves smoothly over the point of balance. The parallelogram is motor driven and the required movement, e.g. linear, circular, hypocycloidal, etc. is selected by means of a programme disc which is fitted on a support at the rear of the unit (Figure 10.11). As the fulcrum is fixed, layer height is selected by raising or lowering the table top, the selected height being indicated on a scale graduated in mm; the scale has a digital readout.

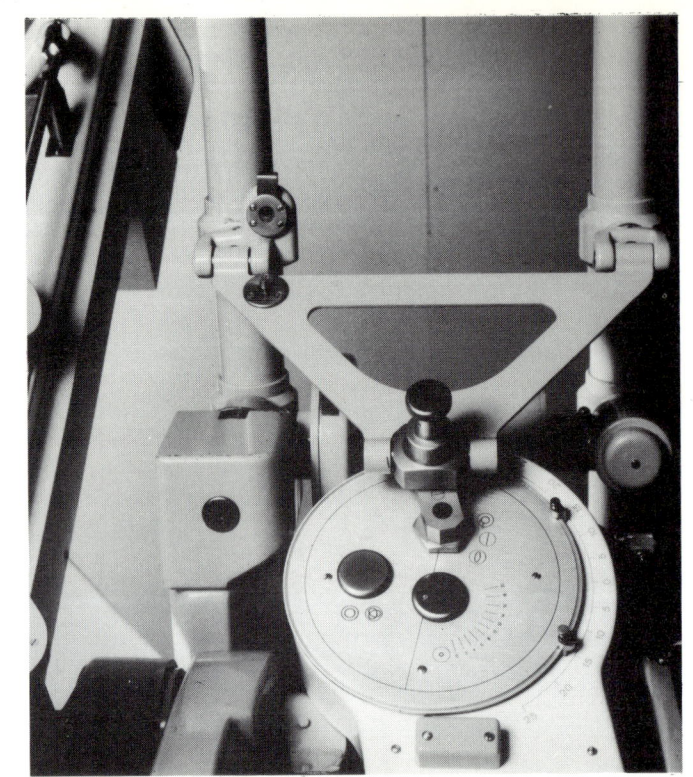

Figure 10.11 The movement required is selected by means of the program disc. This not only provides the correct blurring pattern but also, where applicable, the appropriate movement angle setting

The table can be tilted through any angle from vertical to 15° Trendelenburg and as the parallelogram tilts with the table, the unit is ready for use as soon as the table has been tilted to the required angle.

The table top can be moved longitudinally over a distance of 90 cm and vertically through 23 cm for layer height adjustment. Push button controls for these movements are located on the front of the table unit. Linear, circular, elliptical and hypocycloidal movements of tube and bucky are available in addition to circular or linear zonography.

Movement	Angle	Exposure time
Linear	Selectable between 10° and 50°	Between 0.15 and 0.9 s depending on exposure angle
Elliptical	40°	3.0 s
Circular	29° or 36°	3.0 s for 36° angle
Hypocycloidal	48°	6.0 s
Zonography		
Linear	10°	0.15 s or 0.9 s with speed reduction unit
Circular	up to 20°	3.0 s

TOMOGRAPHY – THEORY AND EQUIPMENT

Whilst the tube and film are making multidirectional movements during an exposure the grid is rotated ensuring continuous alignment of the beam to the grid. Blurring of the grid lines is achieved by rotation and angulation of the grid during the exposure.

For linear movements, in any direction, the grid is aligned to the beam and blurring of the grid lines is achieved by giving it a slight transverse movement during the exposure. The tube and film perform an arc-to-arc movement (Grossman principle) during the exposure (Figure 10.12).

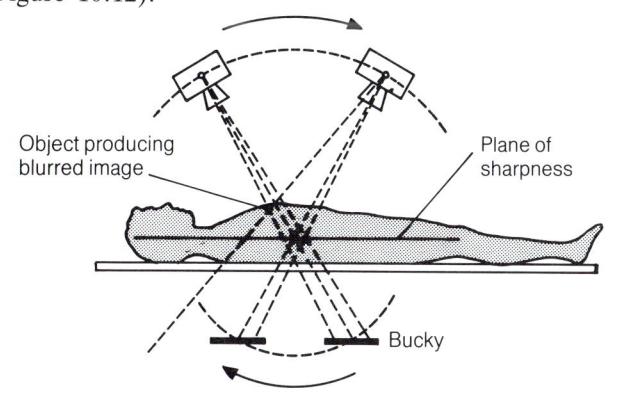

Figure 10.12 Grossman principle (arc to arc movement of tube and film)

This type of movement in conjunction with the fixed fulcrum ensures a constant FFD during the exposure, constant enlargement for a given layer height, constant definition and constant layer thickness.

Enlargement techniques are made possible by the provision of a second cassette tray which is positioned below the primary cassette tray, this facility providing an enlargement factor of 1.6. The tray may also be tilted for oblique tomography.

An *image intensifier* and television camera can be mounted in place of the second tray. This facility enables television fluoroscopy to be carried out. An image retention (memory) system ensures accurate positioning and tight collimation with minimal radiation dose to the patient.

The *cassette holder* accommodates cassettes ranging in size from 13×18 cm to 35×43 cm which can be positioned in either direction. By using a plate diaphragm the 35×35 cm cassette can be split longitudinally to record two exposures on one film.

A single 24×30 cm film may be split into either four or six when a number of small format exposures need to be made in sequence. This results in a saving in time and film as all exposures are recorded on the one film. It also simplifies viewing and is more convenient so far as filing and storage are concerned.

Four exposures can be recorded simultaneously with a *multilayer cassette*, each exposure recording a different layer height; the distance between recorded layers being determined by the spacing of the films in the cassette.

Whilst this unit has been designed specifically for tomography, provision has been made for conventional *bucky radiography* when required. This facility enables preliminary radiographs to be taken when necessary prior to tomography, the conventional moving grid mechanism being brought into position automatically when required.

Automatic exposure control is available for both tomography and conventional bucky radiography.

Other *accessories*, in addition to those so far mentioned include ratchet compressor; head clamps; shoulder rests; patient stool; speed reduction unit (especially for zonography) which reduces the speed of the tube/film movement and conversely increases exposure time; Myelography harness.

X-ray generator and tube

A three-phase generator in conjunction with a heavy duty tube is essential for use with a dedicated tomography unit of this type. The anode should have a small focus (0.3 mm when enlargement techniques are contemplated), large heat storage capacity, and be capable of high speed rotation.

The Polytome U3

This is an automated version of the Polytome U. Prime controls such as table movements, light beam collimation, orientation of tube direction, etc. are all push-button controlled from a recessed control panel at the front of the table as well as from the control desk (Figure 10.13).

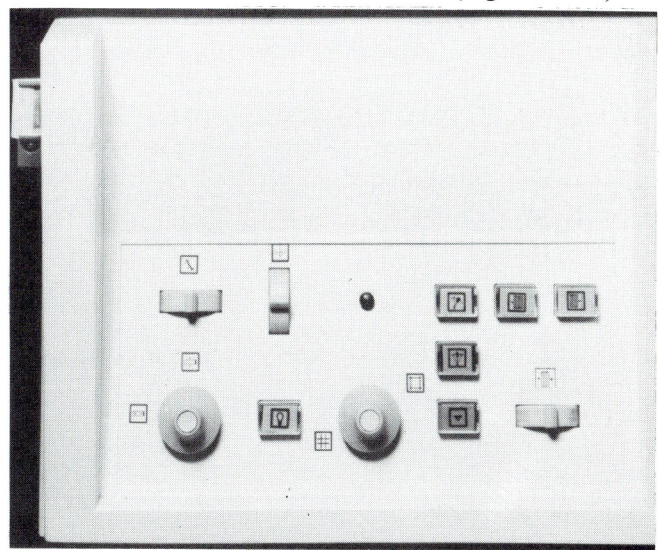

Figure 10.13 Polytome U3 table controls

The blurring movements, linear, elliptical, circular and hypocycloidal are push-button controlled from the control desk. The available range of movements, exposure angles and exposure times are as follows:

Movement	Exposure angle	Exposure time
Linear	10°	1.0 or 0.15 s
	30°	1.0 or 0.5 s
	40°	1.4 or 0.7 s
Elliptical	20° or 36°	3.0 s
Circular	7°, 10° or 36°	3.0 s
Hypocycloidal	34° or 48°	6.0 s

Layer height from 0 to 25 cm is by stepless control from the control desk. The selected layer height is indicated by a digital read out scaled in mm on the control desk.

Linear and elliptical movements of the tube and film may be orientated in any direction by means of controls mounted on the control desk. An automatic serial changer may be used to subdivide the film into either two, four, six or nine rectangular or circular fields, by means of the appropriate masking plate. Placement of the masking plate into the serial changer also adjusts the collimator to the area of the chosen subdivision. An ionization chamber incorporated into the changer provides automatic exposure control. The distance between tomographic layers can be selected at the control desk and the various tomographic 'cuts' will then be made automatically.

When the unit is switched from tomography to the *conventional radiography* mode an auxiliary bucky, which may be fitted with an ionization chamber for automatic exposure control, is automatically brought into position and the tube centred to it. The tube can be tilted along the longitudinal axis by remote control when oblique projections are required and collimation of the beam to a particular sized cassette or to a subdivided film area is automatic in operation.

As with the Polytome U an undercouch image intensifier can be fitted and facilities are also available for enlargement techniques and oblique tomography. The comprehensive list of *accessories* also includes an isocentric chair for neuroradiography, myelography harness, head clamps, etc.

AUTOMATIC EXPOSURE CONTROL

Automatic exposure control for tomography units ensures that the radiation dose to the film is maintained at a constant value throughout the exposure and that the total dose is that required to produce a given film density. It will be recalled that conventional automatic exposure control devices terminate the exposure when a given dose of radiation has reached the film, e.g. a longer exposure time is required for a thick part than is needed for a thin part, all other factors remaining constant. In short, it is the exposure time that is the variable factor. In the case of tomography however, the exposure time, i.e. the time taken for the tube to move through a given exposure angle, is fixed and cannot therefore be the factor which is varied. As the exposure time is fixed and the film dose is also of a fixed value for a given film density, it follows that the mA must be the variable factor, all other factors remaining constant. Automatic exposure control for tomography therefore provides a given film density at a given kV by varying the mA.

How is this achieved?

At the beginning of the tomographic exposure the radiation reaching the film is sampled by a measuring device for a brief period of time, i.e. for a fraction of the exposure time. Let us say that the sampling time is 1% of the exposure time, then it follows that the sample dose should be 1% of the total film dose (which is a known constant value). If the sampled dose is less than 1% of the total film dose the mA is automatically increased. This ensures that over the whole exposure the film dose is constant and the correct amount of radiation reaches the film to give the desired film density.

It should be noted, however, that although the film dose remains constant during the exposure the same is not necessarily true of the mA. Let us consider one exposure made with a linear tube movement (Figure 10.14).

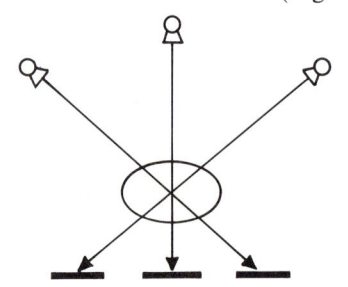

Figure 10.14

At the beginning and end of the exposure the beam of radiation is passing obliquely through the patient and traversing a greater thickness of tissue than it does when the tube is passing centrally over the patient midway through the exposure. To ensure a constant film dose the mA is therefore higher at the beginning and end of the exposure, than it is half-way through the exposure, as the beam is then passing through a thinner section of patient.

Continuous variation in mA throughout the exposure ensures that a constant dose rate is administered to the

TOMOGRAPHY – THEORY AND EQUIPMENT

film during the exposure and that the total dose is that required to produce a correctly exposed tomogram.

QUALITY ASSURANCE TESTS

Tests on tomography equipment should be carried out at installation of the equipment, after repair and at fixed intervals thereafter to confirm that initial and continuing performance is satisfactory.

Checks

In the case of floor mounted tube supports it is important to check that floor tracks are clean as foreign bodies, dirt, etc. may cause uneven movement of the tube. Likewise, check that the tube movement is smooth as worn bearings can cause uneven movement of the tube with consequent increased unsharpness in the tomograph. Worn bearings should, of course, be replaced.

Check all locks to ensure that they are not worn as insecure locks will allow movement to occur during the exposure which will result, once again, in loss of definition in the finished tomograph.

Tests

The accuracy of the reciprocal movement of the tube and film during the exposure when using a linear movement can be checked by stretching a piece of thin wire along the centre line of the X-ray table. A cassette is placed in the bucky tray with one half covered by lead rubber and the tube positioned as it would be at the start of a tomographic exposure (Figure 10.15(a)) and an exposure made (with the tube stationary). The tube is now moved to the position it would occupy at the end of a tomographic exposure, the lead is moved to the other half of the cassette and a second exposure is made, once again with the tube stationary (Figure 10.15(b)).

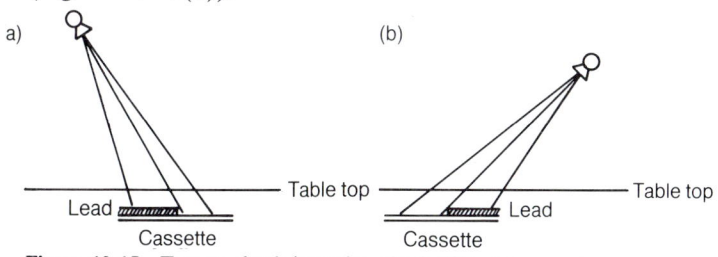

Figure 10.15 Test to check integrity of tube/film movement

When processed the film should show an image of the wire as a continuous line (Figure 10.16(a)).

If, however, the movement of the tube and cassette are not exactly in line, the image of the wire will be separated

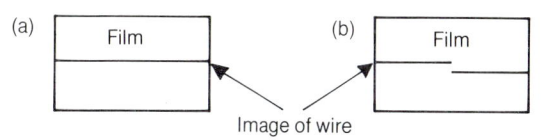

Figure 10.16 Test film (a) satisfactory (b) fault in tube or film movement

at the centre as shown in Figure 10.17(b). This would indicate transverse movement of the tube or film relative to one another during the exposure with consequent loss of definition in the selected plane.

Whilst this test is useful *only* for a linear movement of the tube, irregularity in the movement of tube and/or cassette when using other movements such as circular, elliptical, hypocycloidal, etc. can be checked by means of a pin hole in a sheet of lead. This lead sheet with a pin hole of about 1.0 mm is placed on supports about 12 cm above the table top (Figure 10.17). A film is placed on the table top under the pin hole and the layer height set at twice that of the lead sheet, in this case 24 cm. A tomographic exposure is made and the film processed. The resultant image should show the tube movement used, e.g. circular, hypocycloidal, etc. without irregularities. If there are any irregularities indicated they should be corrected as they will lead to loss of definition within the selected plane.

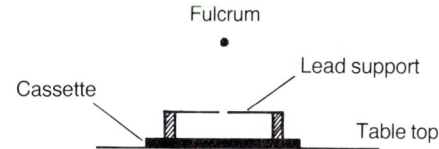

Figure 10.17 Test to check integrity of tube movement

To check that the film is also moving in a smooth trajectory during the exposure, the cassette is now put into the bucky tray and an exposure made as before. A smooth image of the movement of the film, traced out by the radiation passing through the pin hole, will indicate that the movement of the film during the exposure is satisfactory.

When a tomogram is made using a two-pulse generator and a short exposure time the pin hole may trace out the image as a series of pulses, which is, of course, to be expected. If, however, there are some parts of the image which are much darker than others it may be an indication of uneven exposure due to varying velocity of the tube during the exposure.

Even when the image is smooth and of equal density it is important to note whether or not the image is complete. If, for example, only three-quarters of a circle is present this would indicate a fault in the exposure switching whereby the exposure is terminating before the tube has completed its full movement. Such faults should, of course, be rectified.

Accuracy of layer height indication

A number of test tools are available commercially to check that the layer height obtained during a tomographic exposure agrees with the layer height indicated on the scale. One such tool consists of a circular block of plastic in which are embedded 12 lead numerals in the form of a spiral, each number being placed 1.0 mm above its predecessor (Figure 10.18). Other plastic blocks without numerals are provided so that the test tool can be raised to the appropriate height for the test.

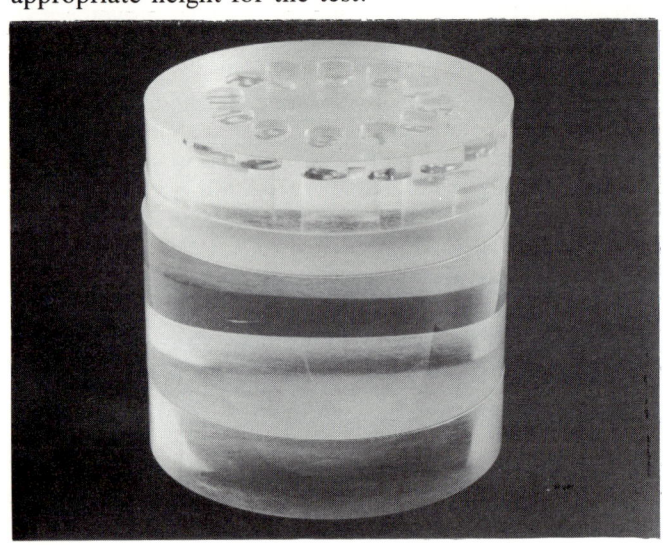

Figure 10.18 Test tool for layer height

In use the layer height scale is set to say 10.5 cm and the test tool, placed on a 10 cm block is centred on the table top. A tomographic exposure is made and the film processed. If the image of the lead numeral 5 is most clearly defined and the numerals 4 and 6 show progressive blurring then the scale is accurate. If not, then the scale should be adjusted followed by tests at other heights. The test may be repeated at all four corners of the field to demonstrate whether or not the image plane is parallel with the table top.

Where no commercial test tool is available it is easy to construct one by pushing pins into a block of polystyrene (or an old film box). The pins should be positioned one centimetre above each other as shown in Figure 10.19.

In use the test tool is positioned on the table top with the long axis of the pins placed transversely to the long axis of the table. The layer height indicator is set at say 6.0 cm and a tomographic exposure made. On the resultant tomograph the 6 pin should be sharply defined with the image of the 5 and 7 pins showing increased blurring. The thickness of the selected layer can also be assessed with this test.

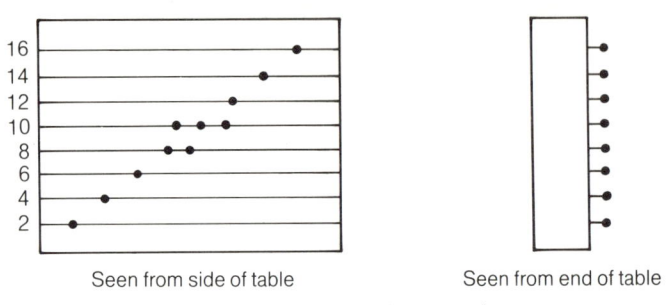

Figure 10.19 Test tool for layer height (using pins)

Fan test

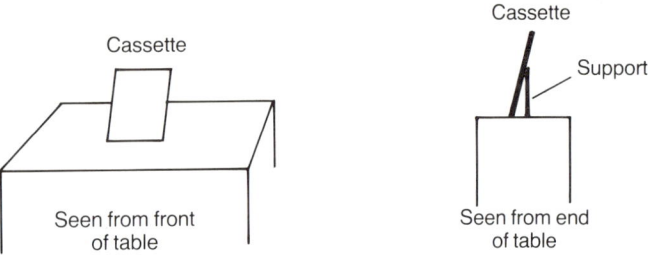

Figure 10.20 Fan test

In this test a film is placed on the table not more than 15° from the vertical (Figure 10.20). The layer height is set to the centre of the film and the light beam diaphragm adjusted so as to give a narrow transverse beam of radiation. A tomographic exposure is made and the film processed. This should show a fan-shaped image of even density (Figure 10.21). To measure the exposure angle it is necessary to either measure the obtuse angle 'x' as shown and subtract it from 180, e.g. if measured angle was 140° then $180 - 140 = 40$. Therefore exposure angle = 40°.

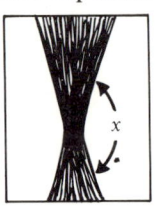

Figure 10.21 Fan test image

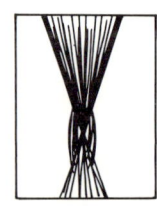

Figure 10.22 Measuring tomographic exposure angle

Alternatively the lines A and B can be extended by drawing them on the radiograph (Figure 10.22) and measuring the exposure angle directly from the film.

If there are streaks of varying density on the film it indicates uneven exposure which may be due to variations in the angular velocity of the tube during the exposure. If the film is placed centrally this film will also indicate whether or not the exposure angle is equal about the midline.

Frequency of testing

This is determined, to a large extent, by the amount of use to which the equipment is subjected. However, it is highly desirable that the tests should be carried out at installation, after repair, and thereafter at quarterly intervals.

11
Organ (anatomatically) programmed units, automatic film changers and other specialized X-ray equipment

ORGAN PROGRAMMED UNITS	140
CASSETTE AND CUT FILM CHANGERS	141
Manually operated cassette changers	141
Automatic cut film changers	141
The film magazine	141
The receiving box	141
The exposure area	141
The motor drive	142
Mode of operation	142
Punch card control of AOT	142
Simultaneous biplane operation	143
The AOT roll film changer	143
Puck film changers	143
EQUIPMENT FOR ANGIOGRAPHY	144
Contrast medium injectors	145
MAMMOGRAPHY UNIT	145
Generator	147
X-ray tube	147
Xeroradiography	147
Siemens Mammomat B	147
Quality assurance tests for mammography equipment	148
Checks	148
Tests	148
Frequency of tests	148
Equipment for paediatric radiography	149
CASSETTELESS RADIOGRAPHY	150
Automatic film transport systems, using magazines	150
Chest stands using film magazines	153

ORGAN PROGRAMMED UNITS

As we have seen, some X-ray units permit individual control of kV, mA and time (called three knob control) others of kV and mAs (two knob control) and others, where the exposure is automatically controlled, of kV only (single knob control). Again, with respect to focal spot size, some equipment permits free selection of focal spot size, within its rating, whilst other equipment is designed on the basis that the smallest focal spot should always be used and automatically selects the smallest focal spot size for a given kV and mAs. Free choice of all exposure parameters leads to great flexibility in the use of equipment and excellent radiographs can be regularly produced by staff who are well trained, who fully understand the equipment they are using, and who use the same equipment over a long period of time. Free choice can, however, lead to repeat exposures if the equipment is used by inexperienced staff or by radiographers who are not familiar with the equipment, as for example when staff operate on a rota basis and do not spend very long in any one room. The use of automatic exposure control goes some way towards overcoming this problem but an extension of this concept in terms of organ programmed units has much to commend it.

An organ programmed (or anatomically programmed) unit has all the exposure factors relevant to a particular examination, e.g. kV, focal spot size (not mA since a falling load generator would normally be used) and appropriate sensor for automatic exposure control programmed into it. All the radiographer needs to do to recall this information is press the appropriate symbol which relates to the required body part then press the exposure switch.

Many radiographers dislike the idea of organ programmed units as they feel the lack of flexibility relegates them to the role of 'button pushers'. It cannot be denied, however, that such units can be useful in situations where there is a rapidly changing staff and they may be looked upon with increasing favour as time goes by. Free choice of exposure factors can be selected when desired by switching out the organ programmed facility.

The unit is programmed with the exposure factors appropriate to a particular examination by a member of staff who selects the factors by free control then programmes them into the unit by pressing a switch or button, usually concealed so that the programme is not changed inadvertently. Any programme can, of course, be subsequently changed by making another selection of factors on free control and pressing the concealed programming button.

Organ programmed units can lead to a speed-up in patient turnover, reduction in film rejects and a reduction in radiation dosage to patients and staff.

CASSETTE AND CUT FILM CHANGERS

Some radiographic examinations necessitate the exposure of several radiographs in rapid succession. Films may be taken in a single plane, i.e. using one tube only, or biplane equipment may be used which enables AP and lateral projections to be taken simultaneously. It may be necessary to expose radiographs in rapid succession at a rate of up to say six per second, more slowly at a rate of say one per second, or even one every 5 seconds. Alternatively, it may be necessary to make some very rapid exposures followed by others at longer intervals. We call this series of intervals a programme which may be manually or automatically controlled.

Manually operated cassette changers

The manually operated changer used for cerebral angiography has already been described. Similar arrangements for use with plain radiographic tables using cassettes in trays have been in use in many departments for a number of years. This type of equipment has a number of disadvantages associated with it, i.e. difficulty of reproducing with accuracy a particular programme of exposures and, secondly, the radiation hazard to the individual pulling out the cassettes.

Automatic cut film changers

The AOT is probably the most widely used cut film changer. It is available in two sizes, one for 24 cm × 30 cm films and the other for 35 cm × 35 cm films. Exposures can be made at a rate of six per second and a maximum of 30 films may be exposed at one examination. A diagrammatic representation of the AOT indicating its main features is shown in Figure 11.1.

The film magazine

The film magazine (A) is loaded up with films (maximum 30), each film being placed between wire separators. Care must be taken not to force the films into position and not to get more than one film between each pair of wire separators.

The sliding lid at the top of the box is closed and locked in position against the side section of the container. The magazine is located on runners and then pushed gently into the changer. A peg (B), shown in Figure 11.1, engages with the projection on the side of the film magazine and a similar engagement takes place between a peg at the back of the changer and the back of the lid (C). When the magazine has been fully inserted into the changer the hinged door is closed, making it light tight.

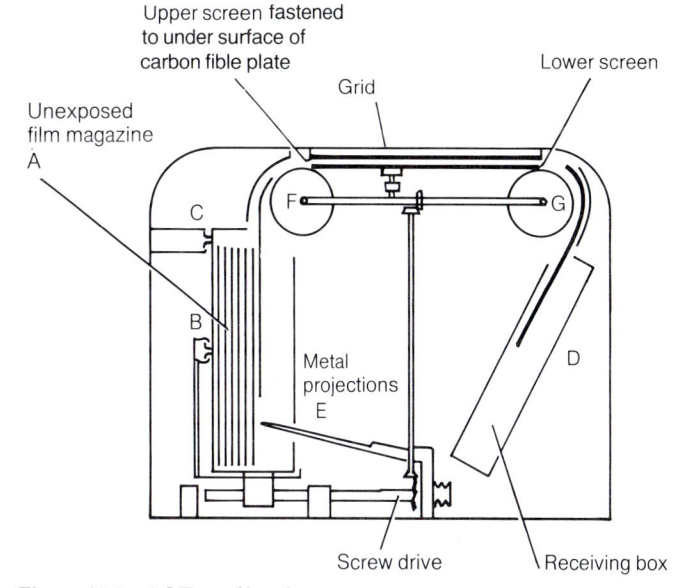

Figure 11.1 AOT cut film changer

The receiving box

The receiving box (D) is a metal box, narrower than the unexposed film magazine, which accommodates up to 30 exposed films. This is placed in the changer as shown in Figure 11.1 and when in position its lid is opened automatically so that films may be received after exposure. An interlock ensures that the magazine drive motor cannot be energized if the receiving box is not in position or if its lid is not opened. A button on the outside of the changer is used to close the lid of the receiving box when the examination is completed so that it may be removed from the changer to be taken to the dark room.

The exposure area

The exposure area is formed by a stationary grid clipped in position on the upper surface of the changer. An intensifying screen mounted on the lower surface of a carbon fibre plate lies under the stationary grid. One edge of the screen has a portion cut out into which projects an arc of thin strong wire This functions as an interlock and ensures that an exposure cannot be made unless a film is between the screens, in which case it compresses the piece of wire and operates the necessary interlock switch, which allows an exposure to be made. The lower intensifying screen is mounted on a metal plate backed with lead. The lower plate and intensifying screen are held in close contact with the upper intensifying screen by two strong springs, whilst an exposure is being made, then lowered by means of a cam when the exposure is ended.

The motor drive

In operation the exposed film magazine is moved to the right by means of a screw drive which is operated by an electric motor. The power to the motor and therefore its speed of rotation is controlled electronically. One rotation of the screw drive moves the unexposed film magazine forward sufficiently to allow a new film to be flicked up for transmission to the exposed area.

Mode of operation

When the 'camera' button on the hand switch is depressed then released, the motor in the changer causes the film magazine to move to the right. Movement of the magazine to the right causes the lid of the magazine and two small apertures at the base of the magazine to be opened. Two metal projections (E) (Figure 11.1) enter the holes and lie under the first film. A cam causes the fingers to flick the film up to roller (F). It is then guided into the exposure area, the lower screen being held down at this stage. When the film comes to a stop the lower screen is moved up, compressing the film tightly between the upper and lower screens. The motor now stops and the changer is ready for the first exposure. Pressure on the hand switch 'start' button now puts the X-ray equipment into 'prep'. Release of the button reactivates the changer motor which operates contacts causing an exposure to be made. After the exposure the lower screen and its support is lowered and the film is taken by roller (G) for onward transmission to the exposed film container. This sequence of events is repeated when the motor screw drive moves the film cassette to the right, bringing a new film into position ready for flicking up to the rollers, and onward transmission to the exposure area.

If the magazine has not been fully loaded with films the changer motor should be allowed to carry on moving the magazine to the right even though the X-ray examination has been completed. No further X-ray exposure can be made as the spring of wire is not depressed unless a film is in the exposure area. When the motor finally stops it is put in reverse by operation of the appropriate push button and the magazine is driven back to the left to its original starting position. It may then be removed from the changer.

Punch card control of AOT

The AOT cut film changer is controlled by means of a punch card Figure 11.2(a) which is programmed by punching out prepared holes in a card. Speeds of 6, 4, 3, 2 or 1 films per sec. can be programmed as well as the desired exposure frequency, activation of the injector and any table top shift that may be required. The program may be stopped automatically at any point by programming 'stop'. The sequence is started by means of a hand switch and the entire program is then carried out without any further action on the part of the radiographer. In the event of emergency the radiographer can stop the program by pressing a button on the hand switch. The precisely controlled programme enables subsequent examinations to be carried out, on the same patient, with exact reproducibility.

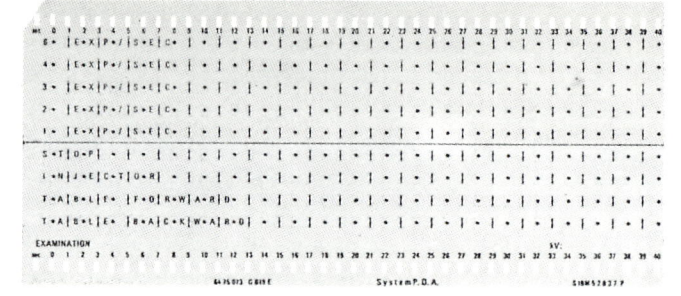

Figure 11.2(a) Punch card which, when inserted in the control box(b) controls the injection time, movement of the table and exposure sequence

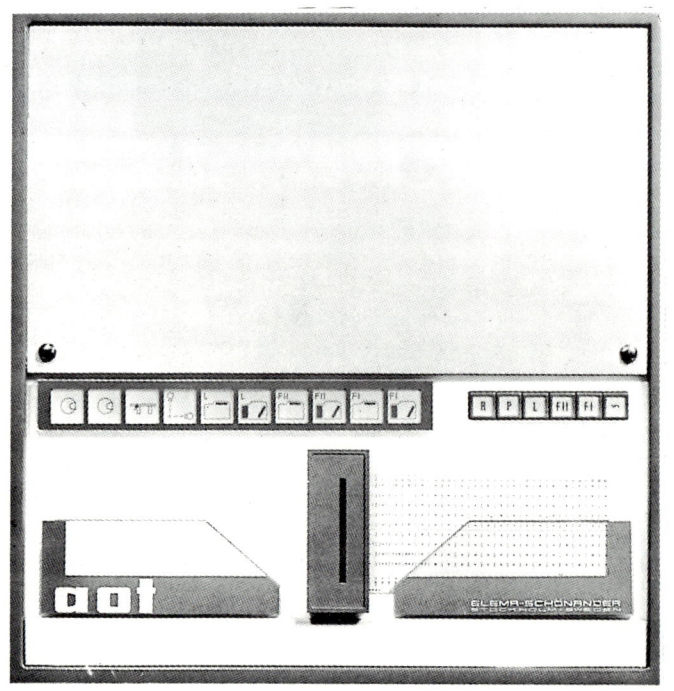

Figure 11.2(b) Control box AOT

ORGAN PROGRAMMED UNITS, AUTOMATIC FILM CHANGES AND OTHER X-RAY EQUIPMENT 143

Simultaneous biplane operation

When required two AOT changers may be used for simultaneous biplane operation as shown in Figure 11.3.

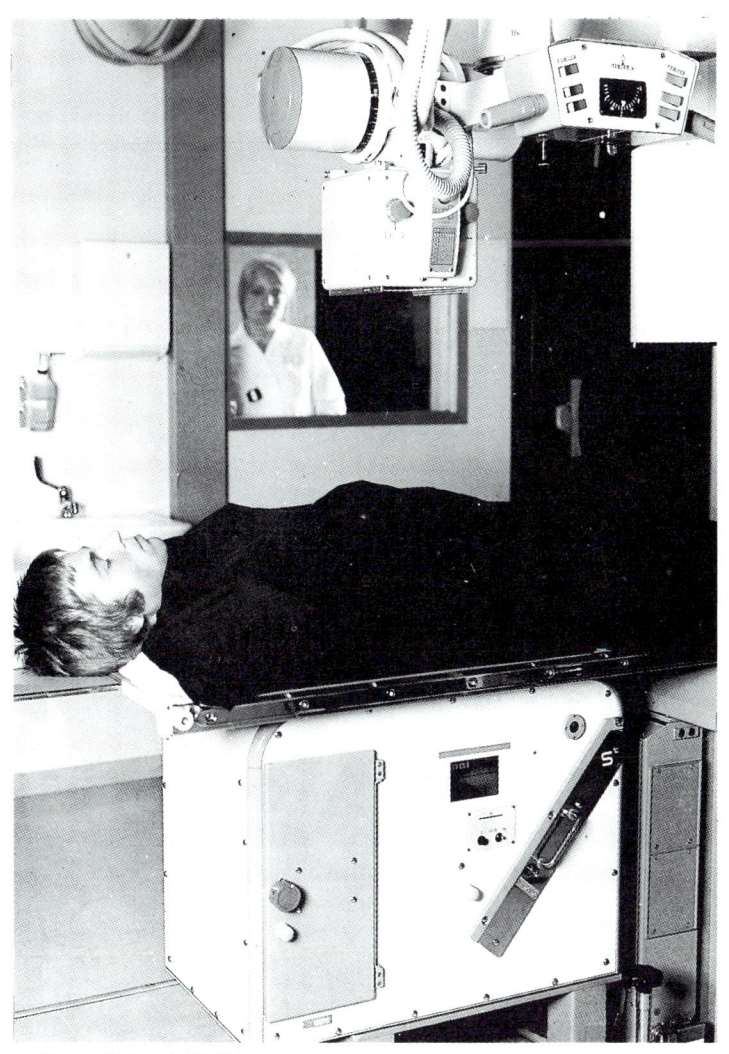

Figure 11.3 AOT-S in use

The AOT roll film changer

This kind of changer is now rarely used. In operation it is similar to the AOT cut film changer just described. The roll film is ordinary x-ray film, double coated, and supplied in rolls up to 25 m in length. The unexposed roll of film passes between a pair of intensifying screens to a take-up spool. Whilst the film is moving, i.e. being wound on, the screens are separated but when the new section of film is in place, the screens are automatically clamped tightly together. Whilst in this position the exposure is made. At the end of the exposure the screens separate and the appropriate length of film is wound on to the take-up spool. This sequence is repeated until all the exposures have been made, the appropriate intervals between exposures having previously been set on the programme selector. The advantage of the roll film changer over the cut film changer is that exposures can be made at a rate of 12 per second as opposed to six per second with the cut film changer. This was mainly the reason for its use for examinations such as angiocardiography but most major departments doing this type of work now favour cine radiography which provides exposures at a rate of 200 per second when a fast repetition rate is required to 'freeze' the movement. The AOT cut film changer is used where large film radiography is required and a slower exposure rate is acceptable.

Puck film changers

The Puck U35 film changer accepts up to 20 films of 35 cm × 35 cm format and the Puck U24 up to 20 films of 24 cm × 30 cm format (Figure 11.4). The maximum exposure time is 100 ms (0.1 s). The Puck D for use with multidirectional stands such as the Angioscop can be used with the X-ray beam in any direction, even upside down (Figure 11.5).

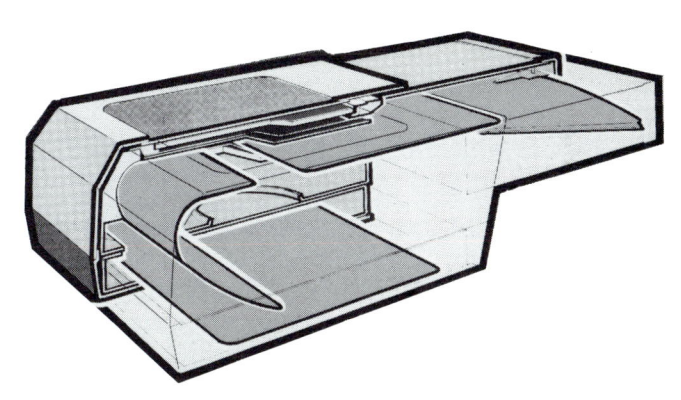

Figure 11.4 Puck film changer

Any two Puck changers can be combined for biplane radiography. Like the AOT all Puck changers are programmed by means of a punch card and when used in the biplane mode the timing of exposures can be programmed to be simultaneous or alternating. Puck changers can be used on a special stand called a Puckwop which provides motorized vertical movements and the facility to use the Puck in the vertical or horizontal positions. Two such stands can be used for biplane work.

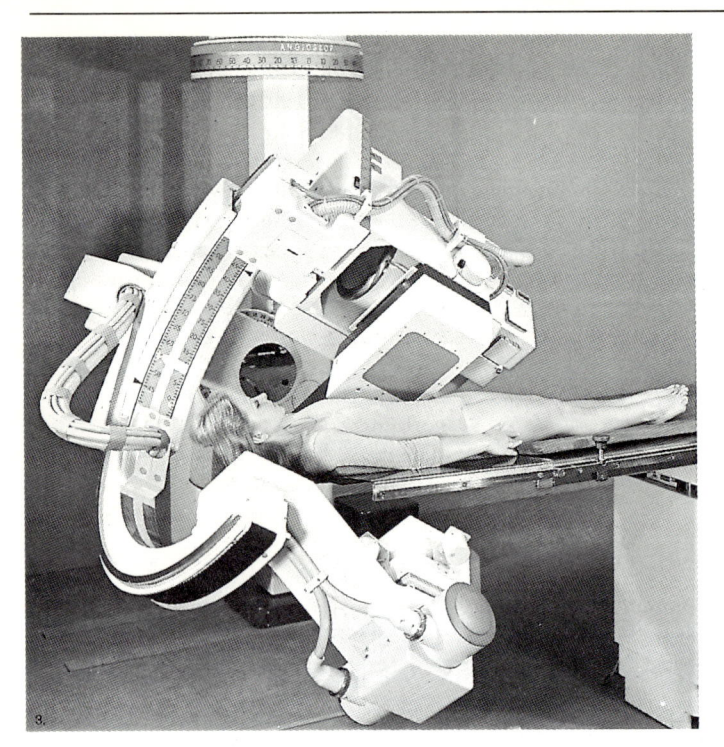

Figure 11.5 Puck UD mounted on a Siemens 'Angioskop' unit

We have now considered different kinds of film changers. Let us now see how they, along with other equipment may be used in angiography examinations.

EQUIPMENT FOR ANGIOGRAPHY

Angiography is the demonstration of vascular structures following the injection of a contrast medium. The rate at which blood vessels in different parts of the body pulsate and the diameter of the blood vessels determine the type of equipment to be used. For example, in angiocardiography, a cine camera is usually used to record a rapid series of exposures, up to 200 frames per second being commonplace. Obviously, equipment capable of providing short exposure times (1–4 ms) is required if time is to be allowed for the shutter of the camera to close and the film to be transported ready for the next exposure when 200 exposures are made each second. Exposure times must not only be short, however, they must also be accurate and reproducible. To meet these requirements the generator must produce constant (or near constant) potential for the X-ray tube and the tube itself must be capable of withstanding heavy loads for relatively long periods. A small focal spot is also needed to provide the necessary resolution for visualization of fine blood vessels of small diameter.

These are demanding requirements and most manufacturers supply a complete system for specialized examinations such as angiocardiography. It is generally unwise to marry up different pieces of equipment from different manufacturers as any faults which may arise are difficult to isolate. Time and money may be wasted by having to call in engineers from different firms to locate the fault.

Cerebral angiography is still performed in some areas using a manually operated cassette changer as previously described, other centres use an AOT, Puck or other automatic cut film changer but most major centres now use digital imaging techniques which are described later.

The needs of *abdominal* and *peripheral angiography* are less demanding and an AOT or Puck cut film changer, capable of operating at up to six exposures per second is adequate for abdominal angiography, whilst peripheral angiography can be performed quite satisfactorily with films taken at a slower rate, say one or two exposures per second. Although most centres use an automatic film changer and a stepped moving top table for abdominal and peripheral angiography, some hospitals still use manually operated cassette changers or long cassettes for peripheral angiography. Whilst the radiographs may be satisfactory so far as diagnostic information is concerned, any manually operated system should be viewed with some concern if it leads to increased radiation dose to staff, which it usually does.

A six-pulse generator and heavy duty tube is satisfactory for most abdominal and peripheral angiography and a tube with a 0.3 mm focus will enable magnification techniques to be used. The equipment should be capable of providing automatic kV reductions for use with a stepped moving top table.

The stepped moving top table makes a series of programmed longitudinal movements during the course of the examination (Figure 11.6). The patient is positioned on the table, over an automatic cut film changer such as the AOT or Puck and the catheter is inserted under fluoroscopic control. The patient's identification and punch cards are inserted into the changer. The punch card carries information which determines the timing of the injection, the initiation of the first exposure, the rates at which the exposures are to be made and the kV drop which is to take place following each movement of the table. The first exposure may, for example, be of the abdominal region, the table top (and patient) then moves automatically so that the femoral region is centred over the changer, another exposure is made at a reduced kV and the table

ORGAN PROGRAMMED UNITS, AUTOMATIC FILM CHANGES AND OTHER X-RAY EQUIPMENT 145

is moved again this time bringing the popliteal region over the changer and so the sequences continue until the lower extremities have been exposed. In this way the patient's vascular system can be imaged from abdominal region to lower extremities.

A stepped moving top table usually provides up to four steps allowing five different areas to be examined in sequence. The table top movements are motorized and each movement of the table initiates a kV drop so that the exposure is automatically adjusted as different areas are brought into the examination field. Reduction in kV at each step is adjustable usually within the range of 5–40 kV per step.

at body temperature (37°C) by means of an electrically heated pad or collar which fits over the syringe. The required flow rate is set prior to the examination at a selectable value between 59 ml/s and 1.0 ml/h. A flow rate meter records the maximum flow rate achieved during the injection.

The timing of the injection, the timing of the exposures at a selected rate and the timing of the table top movements with consequent reduction in kV are all programmed by means of a punch card (Figure 11.2). Pressing one button sets the whole sequence into operation.

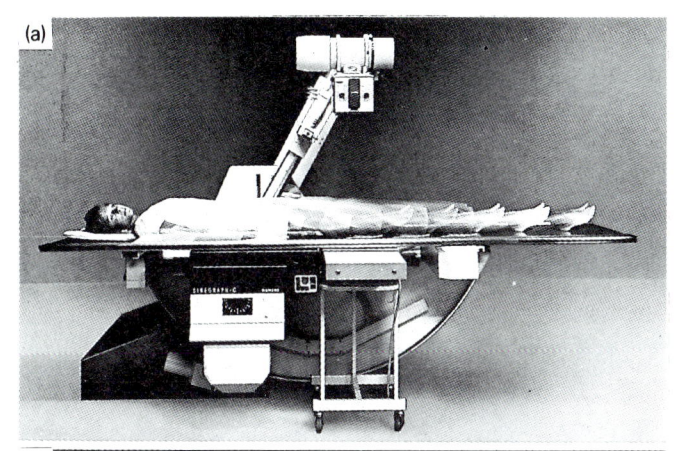

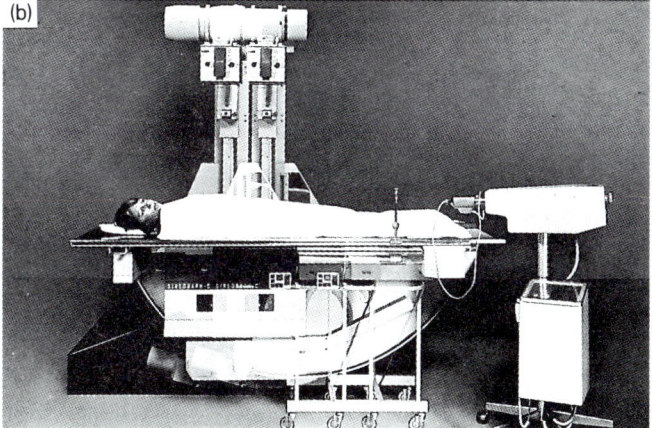

Figure 11.6 Siemens 'Siregraph-C' unit. (a) showing stepped movement of table top (b) set up for angiography

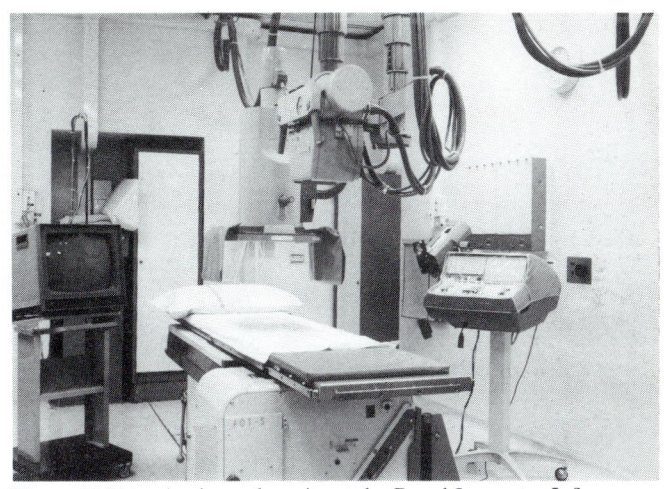

Figure 11.7(a) Angiography suite at the Royal Lancaster Infirmary

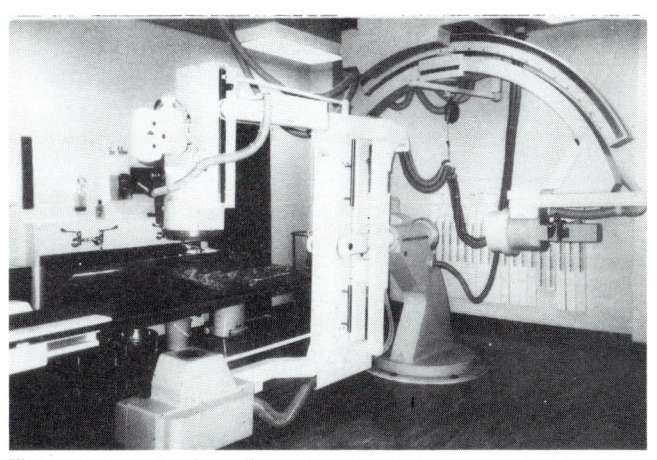

Figure 11.7(b) Angiocardiography suite at Victoria Hospital, Blackpool

MAMMOGRAPHY UNIT

As the name implies this unit is dedicated to radiography of the female breast.

The unit illustrated in Figure 11.8 is the Siemens Mammomat. It consists of a mammography X-ray tube, film

Contrast medium injectors

There are a number of injectors on the market, one example being the Medrad IV by Wolverson. The injector uses disposable syringes the contrast medium being maintained

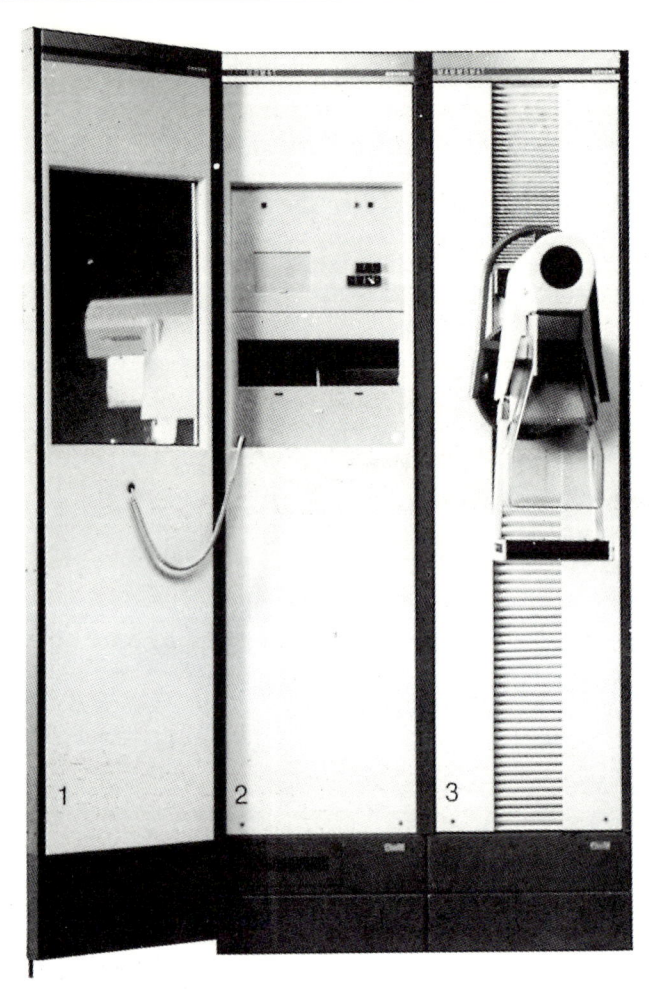

Figure 11.8 Siemens Mammomat with X-ray unit support and swivelling arm system (3) generator cabinet (2) and radiation protection screen (1)

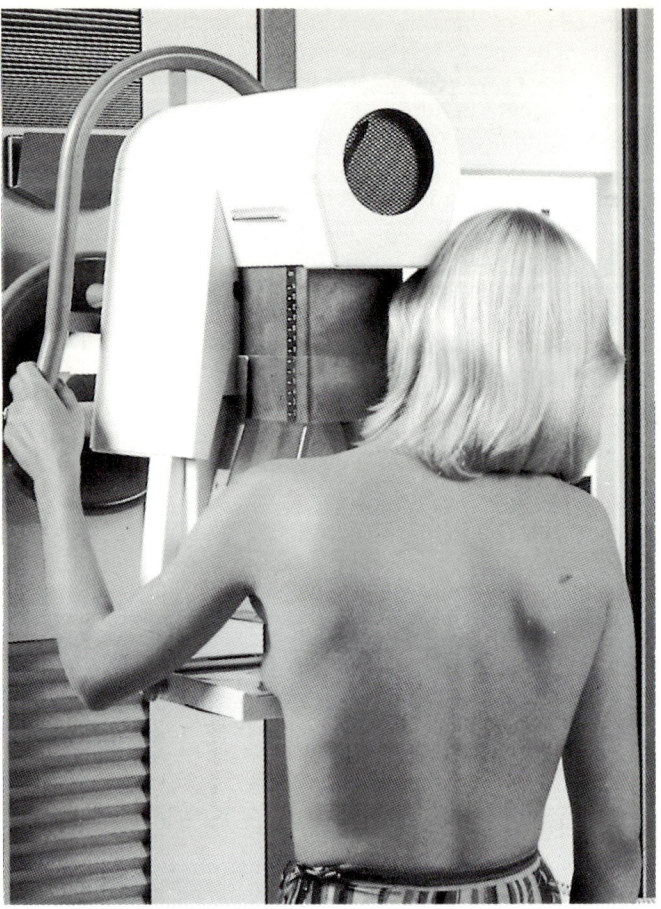

Figure 11.9 Patient positioned for radiography of the breast

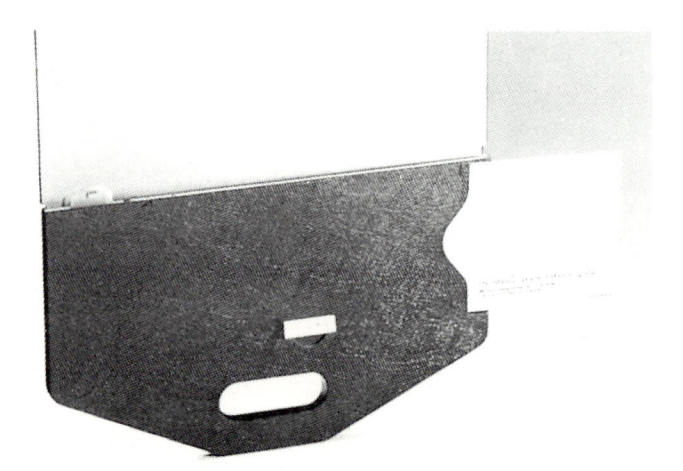

Figure 11.10 Light-tight holder for mammography film (note the patient identification system)

support and compression device which together form an integrated unit which can be raised or lowered on a vertical stand. Movement of the unit is counterbalanced and it can be angled through 270°. It indexes automatically in the vertical and horizontal projections. A transparent compression cone driven by means of a crank and controllable millimetre by millimetre reduces the volume of breast irradiated resulting in improved contrast (Figure 11.9). A series of five easily interchangeable compression devices are available to meet varying needs. Special mammography films are used in light-tight holders and an identification system enables the patient's particulars to be recorded on the film. (Figure 11.10).

The patient can be examined in the standing or sitting position. A patient chair mounted on a rail system allows the chair to be moved towards or away from the erect stand and to either side. The chair swivels on its own axis and can be moved to one side when the patient is standing.

Generator

A six-pulse generator giving 300 mA at 25 kV ensures that exposure times are short and that motional blur is minimized. Radiographic technique is programmed but free control of mA s is provided, the selector switch being concealed under a sliding cover.

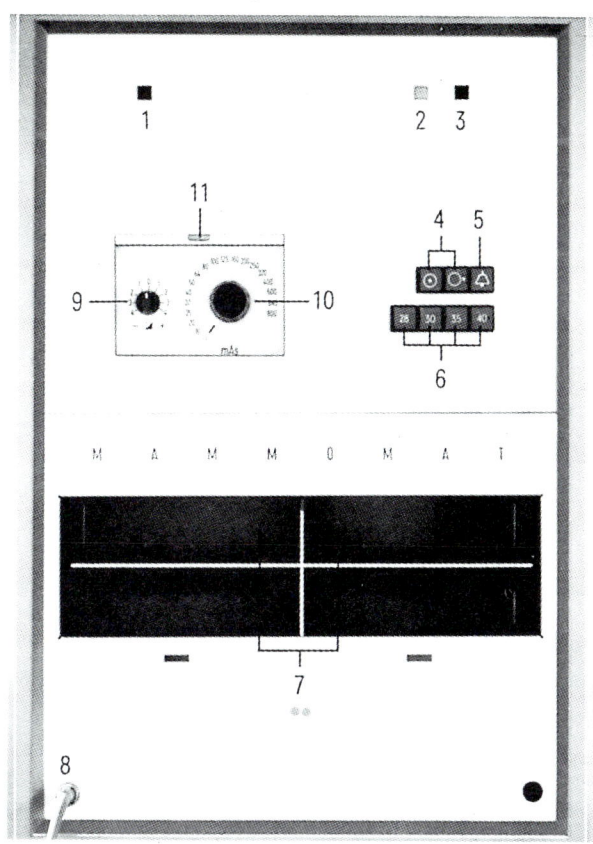

Figure 11.11 Mammomat control panel

X-ray tube

A special tube with a molybdenum anode (Chapter 5 Figure 5.23) would normally be used with this unit.

Xeroradiography

The unit can be used for xeroradiography as well as conventional film radiography, the insertion of a Xerox cassette holder automatically switching the kV to the higher values needed for that technique. The molybdenum filter is replaced by one of aluminium. If the unit is to be used solely for xeroradiography a special tube with a tungsten anode should be fitted.

Siemens Mammomat B

This unit is similar to the Mammomat just described but it has some interesting additional features.

The tube/bucky section of the unit is adjustable in height, is counterbalanced and can be swivelled through an angle of 180°. It is held in position with electro magnetic locks (Figure 11.12). It can also be inclined towards the patient up to a maximum of 12° (Figure 11.13).

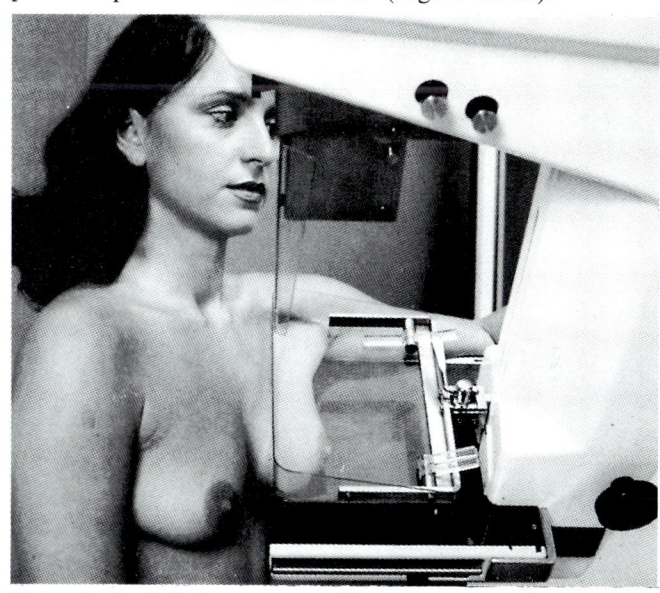

Figure 11.12 Swivel-arm system with support plate for Bucky radiographic technique

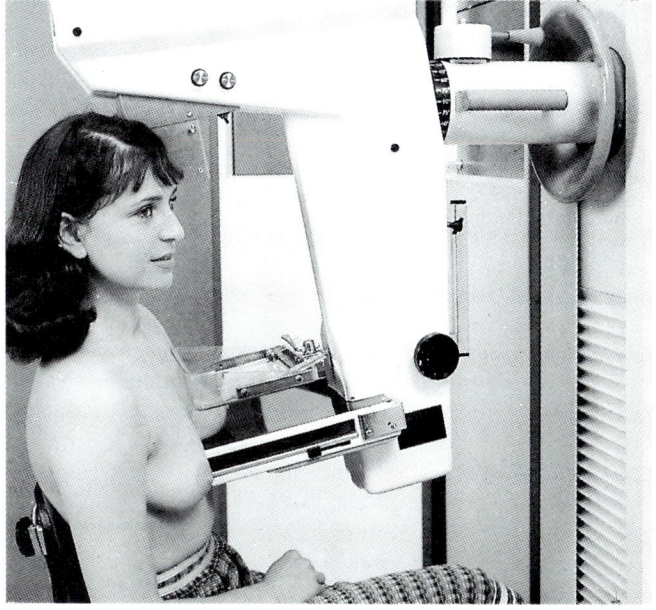

Figure 11.13 Examination of seated patient with swivel-arm system inclined forwards

It has a moving grid assembly which allows exposures down to 0.3 s to be taken without the introduction of grid lines.

The bucky support plate is made of carbon fibre to minimise X-ray absorption.

A motorised compression plate is operated by means of a foot pedal.

A light marker and special compression plate is provided for fine needle biopsy examinations. The compression plate has a rectangular opening with letters or numbers marked on the edges which are visible on the survey film. Using this device in conjunction with the light marker the entry point for the puncture can be established (Figure 11.14).

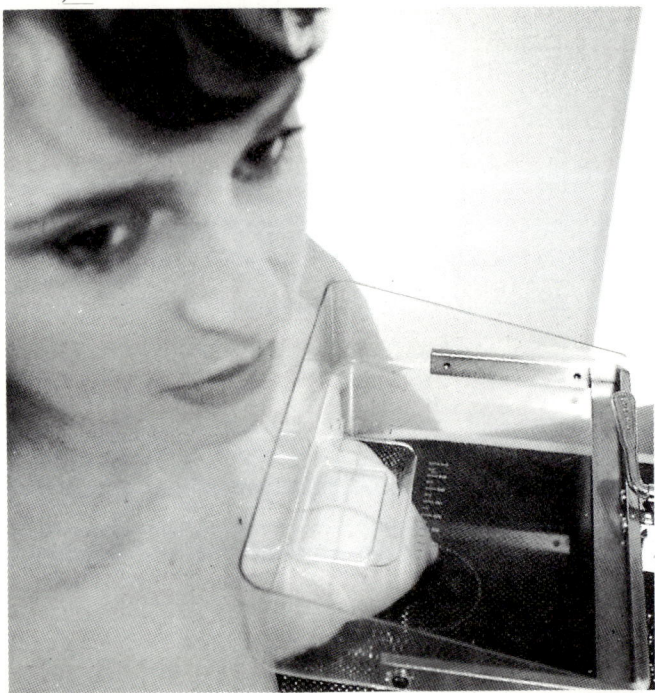

Figure 11.14 Compression plate and light market for guided fine-needle biopsy

X-ray tube	Mammography tube as previously described
Generator	6 pulse with automatic mains voltage compensation and automatic high tension stabilization during the exposure. *Output* 300 mA at 25 kV, 250 mA at 30 kV *kV range* 25 to 49 kV *Exposure time* 0.3 to 3.0 S *Automatic exposure* iontomat

Exposure techniques are programmed; voltage, current and film blackening all being selected by pressing one push button.

Quality assurance tests for mammography equipment

Quality assurance tests and various checks should be carried out on installation of the equipment, after repair and at fixed intervals thereafter.

Checks

Mechanical locks, interlocks and all moving parts should be checked to ensure they are functioning properly and fully serviceable. Tube filters should be checked to ensure they are of the correct metal and of the correct thickness. Any warning lights should be checked to ensure they are operable.

Tests

kV and radiation output measurements should be made and recorded, as described in Chapter 15, making sure that the penetrameter used for the kV measurement is able to cover the lower ranges of kV when a molybdenum anode is used.

Collimation of the beam should be checked to ensure that the beam is limited to the correct extent at the cathode end of the beam.

Resolution tests may be carried out using a tissue equivalent phantom. One such phantom is made up of 16 wax blocks in which are embedded specks, filaments and masses of various sizes. The position of the wax blocks within the container is interchangeable and a plastic half-cylinder at one end of the container simulates the anterior part of the breast (Figure 11.15).

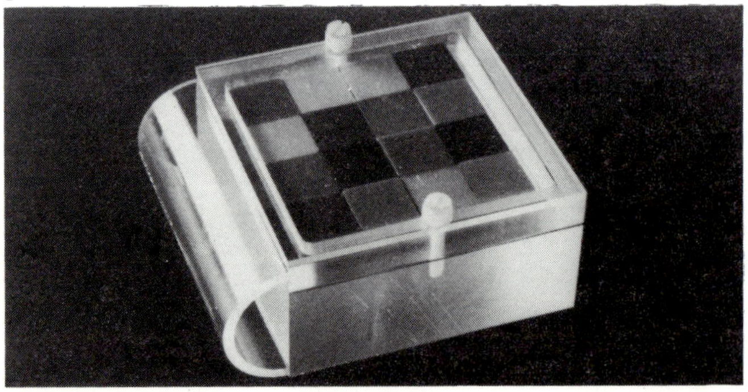

Figure 11.15 Random Phantom (SIEL)

Test films should be retained for comparison with films taken before and after so that the system may be evaluated over its lifetime.

Frequency of tests

Tests are essential at installation and after repair, thereafter every 4 months. When tube filters are interchangeable, they should be checked before each exposure to ensure that the correct filter is being used.

Equipment for paediatric radiography

Specialized equipment to meet the needs of infants and children is only justified when there is a high throughput of such patients. By its very nature such equipment is useless for adult patients. In other cases where its cost is justified however, a wide range of equipment is available from different manufacturers. One such unit is the Infantoskop by Siemens (Figure 11.16). This unit consists of a tilting table with overcouch tube, undercouch image intensifier coupled with closed circuit TV and 100 mm cut film camera. The unit can be operated from the side of the table or by remote control.

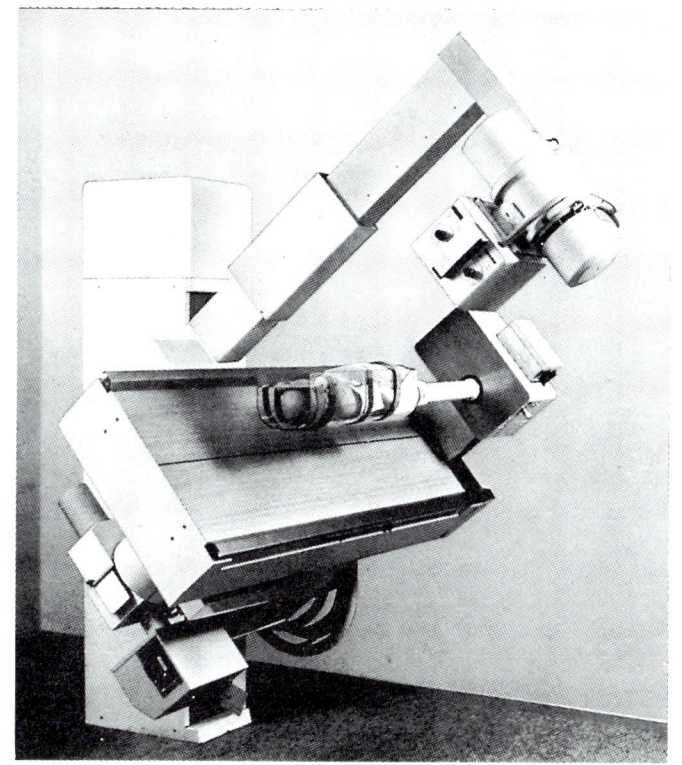

Figure 11.16 Infantoskop by Siemens

A cradle is provided into which an infant may be secured. The cradle can be rotated in either direction by a motorized drive which permits two speeds of movement. This can be done with the unit in any position. At the press of a switch the cradle may be automatically rotated into the AP position. The cradle may also be moved nearer to or away from the table top to permit enlargement techniques. Cradles of different sizes, to suit different sized infants are available (Figure 11.17). The table top can be moved longitudinally or transversely with or without the cradle. It can be tilted from vertical to 35° Trendelenburg, rotated through 90° and adjusted in height.

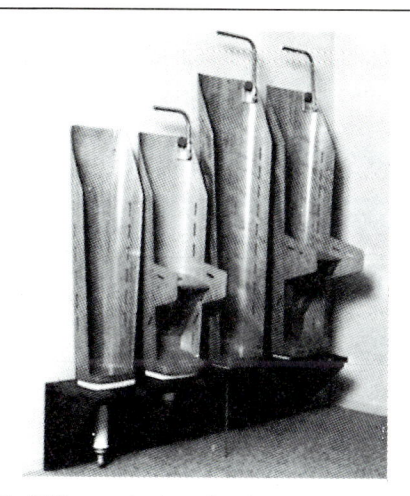

Figure 11.17 Different sized cradles for the Infantoskop

With this equipment infants and children can be examined effectively and quickly. An operating console and video monitor is provided as a single unit (Figure 11.18). It may be mounted on an overhead support, moveable in any direction, or as a stationary floor-mounted stand. Imaging is by closed circuit TV, 100 mm cut film or large sized format X-ray films.

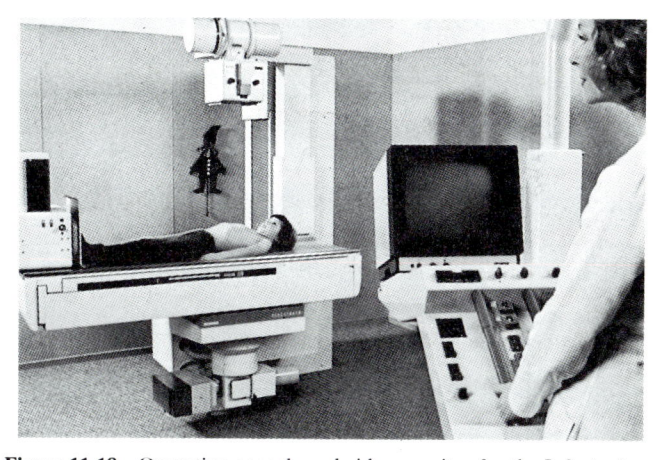

Figure 11.18 Operating console and video monitor for the Infantoskop

The *Thoracomat* is an X-ray unit by Siemens, for chest radiography of infants and children. Examinations can be carried out with the patient seated or standing (Figure 11.19) or in the case of infants in a Babix immobilizer. These immobilizers are available in five different sizes to accommodate different sized patients. The immobilizer (and infant) are positioned on a holding arm as shown in Figure 11.20; a vertically adjustable cassette holder is provided.

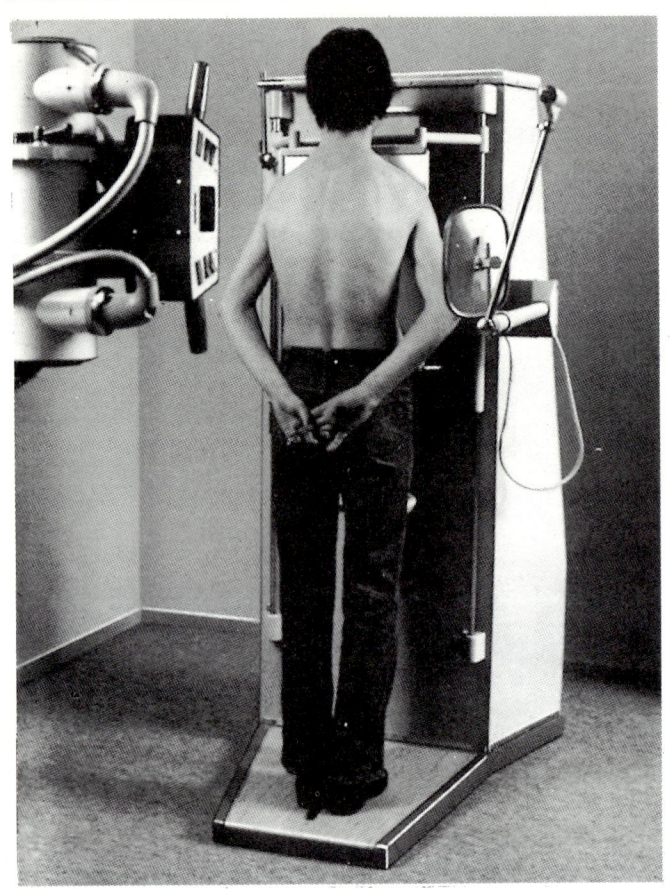

Figure 11.19 Older patient standing for examination by Siemens Thoracomat

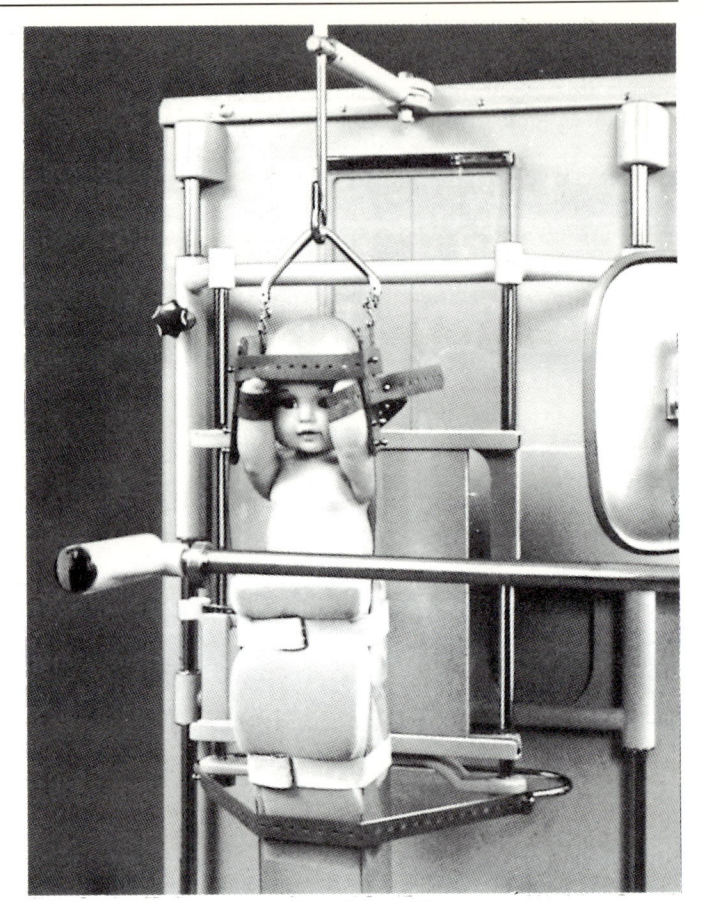

Figure 11.20 Babix immobilizer for the Thoracomat

Older children can sit on a seat which is adjustable in height and which can be rotated for lateral views (Figure 11.21). Protection is provided for the nurse who is holding a restless child, and a solid state radiation sensor provides automatic exposure control.

Respiramet X is an electronic control unit which enables radiographs to be exposed at a particular phase of respiration. A thermistor sensing device is fixed in front of the patient's mouth or nostrils. (Figure 11.22). Expired air warms the thermistor which triggers the exposure at the phase in respiration selected by the operator at the control unit.

CASSETTELESS RADIOGRAPHY

Automatic film transport systems, using magazines

To obviate the need for radiographers to carry cassettes to and from the darkroom some manufacturers provide X-ray tables which can accommodate magazines holding up to 60 X-ray films. Prior to an exposure the film is inserted automatically between screens and after exposure passed to an on-line processor or to a take-up magazine. Such a system is time saving and, when there is an on-line processor, means that the radiographer need not leave the patient to take films for processing.

Siemen's system provides supply magazines for six different film formats and gives the choice of two different speed screens (Figure 11.23). The magazines are loaded with films at the start of the working day and located under the bucky table (Figure 11.24). The patient is positioned on the table and the appropriate measuring chamber, exposure format and screen type is selected by the radiographer at a control unit located at one end of the table (Figure 11.25). The selected film and screen are transported automatically to the exposure area where the patient's name etc. are photographed onto the edge of the film from a card which is put into a slot at the beginning of each examination (Figure 11.26).

Provision is also made for L (left), R (right), AP or PA to be photographed onto the film in addition to the patient's particulars (Figure 11.25).

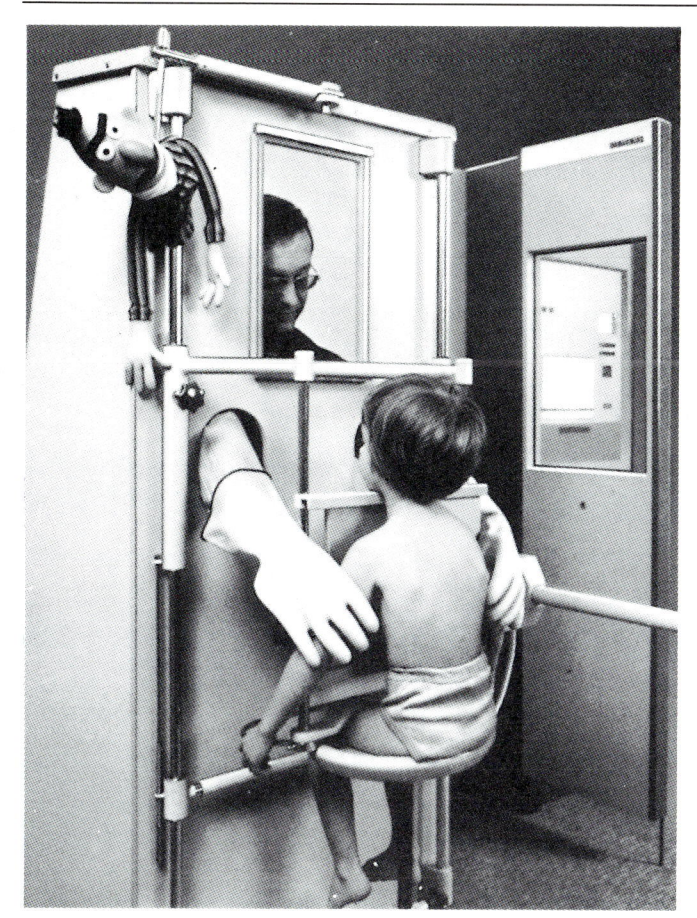

Figure 11.21 Older child on adjustable seat of Thoracomat

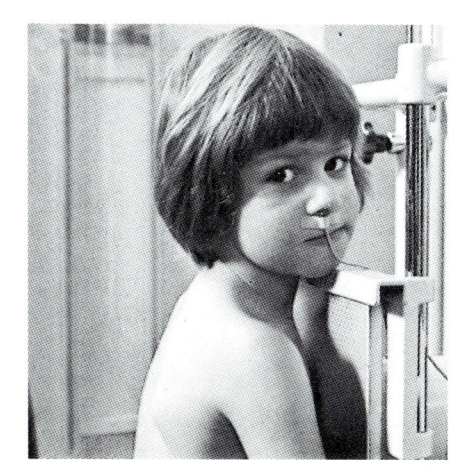

Figure 11.22 Thermistor sensing device used in the Respiramet X

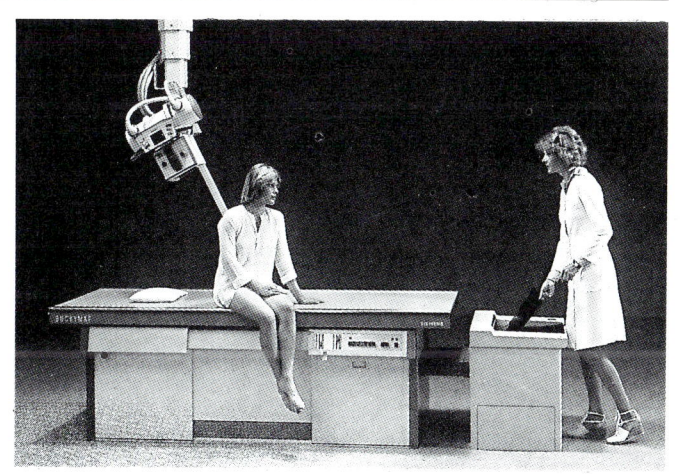

Figure 11.23 Siemens Buckymat table with on-line processor

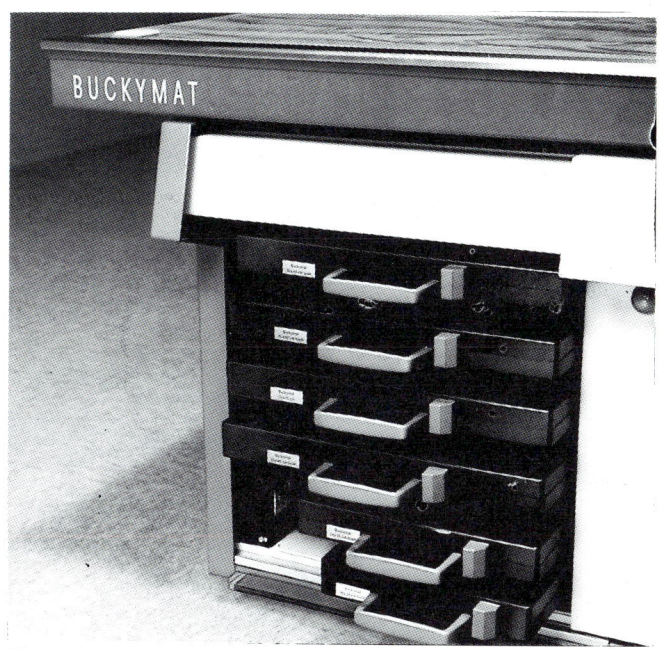

Figure 11.24 Film magazines loaded into one end of the unit

The X-ray beam is then collimated automatically to the selected film size and the exposure is made; the beam cannot over-shoot the film format but can be collimated further by the radiographer if required. The film is then transported automatically to the automatic processor or take-up box.

Such a system is cost effective when there is a large throughput of patients. It reduces patient waiting time. It increases the rate at which patients can be examined. It eliminates the need for staff to carry cassettes to and from the darkroom. It means that the radiographer need not leave the patient to process the films when 'on call'.

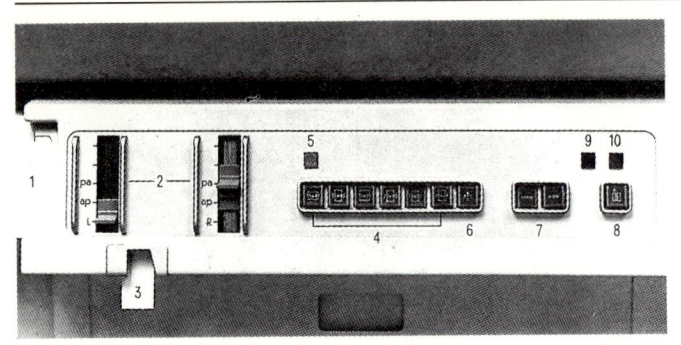

Figure 11.25 Operating panel and controls

Key:
1. Opening for EDP punch card
2. Sliders for the exposure of a.p./p.a. and L/R onto the film
3. Slot for date strip
4. Pushbuttons for film format selection
5. Warning lamp (yellow) indicating fewer than ten films in supply magazine
6. Pushbutton for free operation (e.g. radiography using cassettes)
7. Pushbuttons for intensifying screen selection
8. Pushbutton for film transport
9. Indicator light (red), film transport
10. Indicator light (green), exposure readiness

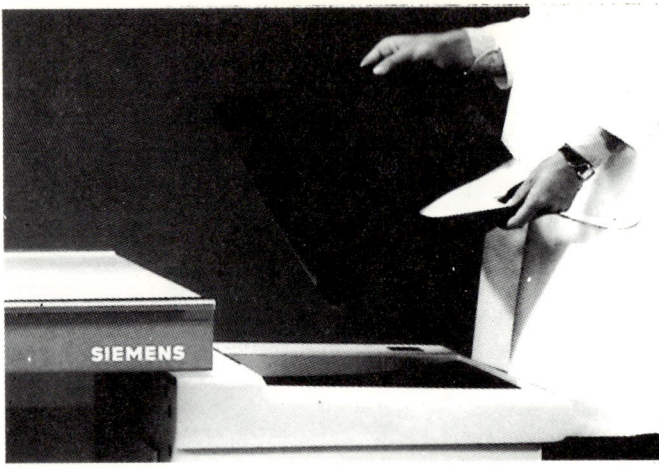

Figure 11.27 After exposure the film is passed to the processor then viewed

An automatic unit for chest radiography is only cost effective when large numbers of patients are radiographed, i.e. departments associated with chest clinics, chest hospitals, etc.

The increasing availability of daylight loading systems and daylight processors has resulted in some departments considering these in preference to the automatic chest unit, a particular advantage of the daylight loading system being the availability of different sizes of film. They are of course much slower in operation.

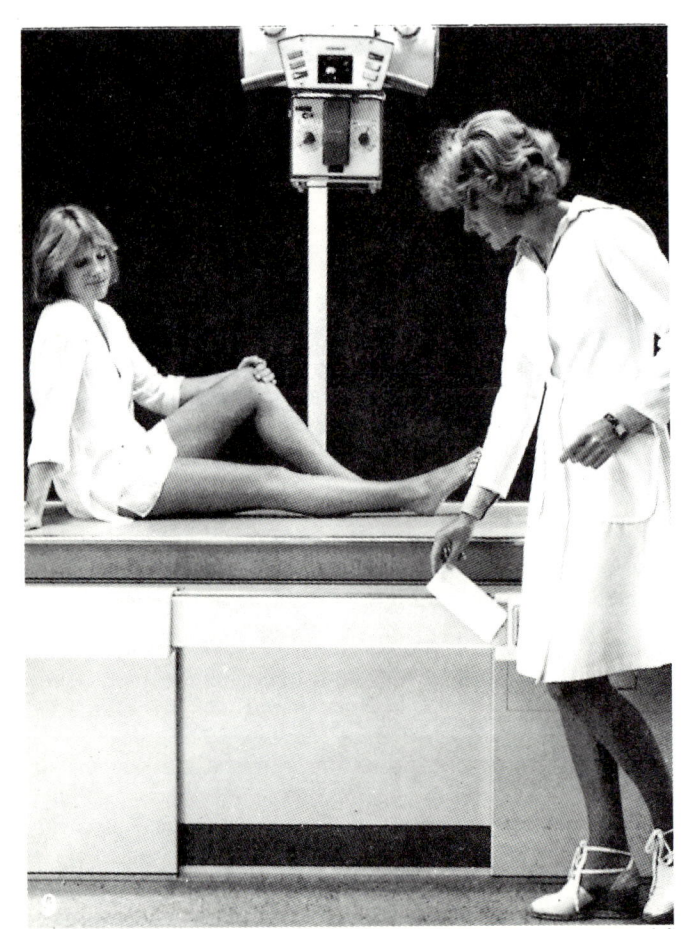

Figure 11.26 Patient's identification card is inserted for automatic film identification

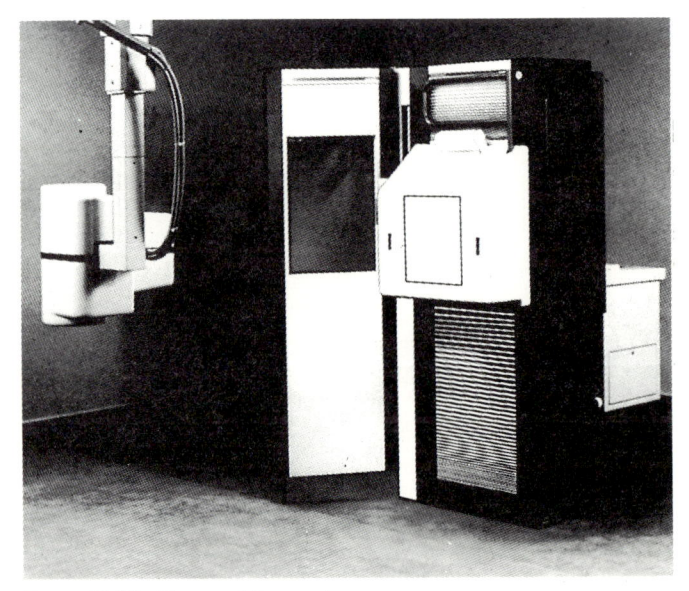

Figure 11.28 Siemens Thoramat

Chest stands using film magazines

A unit such as the Siemens Thoramat has a self-centring X-ray tube, uses magazines which accommodate up to 55 films of 40 cm × 40 cm or 35 cm × 43 cm format according to the model of choice and may be supplied with either an integrated processing unit or a receiving magazine (Figure 11.28). The patient's name, date, 'R' and 'L', etc. is projected photographically onto the film during radiography. Movement of the tube and film unit are counterbalanced or, if desired, a motor assisted drive may be fitted. The film unit has a smooth front surface for easy cleaning. A handle and a strap assist in immobilizing the patient during radiography.

12
Care, choice and installation of equipment

CARE OF EQUIPMENT	154
Servicing of equipment	154
CHOICE AND INSTALLATION OF NEW EQUIPMENT	154

CARE OF EQUIPMENT

Modern X-ray equipment is very expensive and every effort should be made to ensure that it, and its accessories, are used with care. Any faults noted by the operator should be reported immediately so as to minimize the risk of further damage to the equipment. Operators should recognize the symptoms of faulty behaviour and carry out routine checks to ensure that the equipment is performing to a satisfactory standard.

Cleanliness is essential primarily because of consideration of hygiene and secondly because dust, dirt, grease, etc. can quickly foul up a floor track etc. or possibly lead to electrical breakdown. Equipment should be *damp* dusted daily, preferably each morning and specifically with the mains switched off, noting whilst doing so any faults such as worn outer covering of high tension cables, faulty locks, etc.

This regime should be strictly adhered to and any minor faults recorded in a book kept with the equipment specifically for this purpose. The engineer can then correct such faults at the next service of the equipment. Any major faults should, of course, be reported immediately to the appropriate authority and if the operator considers it necessary, the equipment should be put out of commission until it is considered safe.

Mobile units should be subjected to a similar regime and faults recorded in a book with the major equipment. Cleanliness is, of course, of paramount importance particularly if the unit is to be used in the operating theatre. To minimize the risks of cross-infection it is common practice to keep theatre units within the environs of the theatre as the dangers of infection being carried into the theatre are obviously increased if a mobile unit is used about the hospital generally, and in consequence wheeled along many corridors before being taken into the theatre.

More detailed information regarding quality assurance tests and the frequency with which they should be carried out is given in Chapter 15.

Servicing of equipment

X-ray equipment is usually serviced by the manufacturer's engineers on a regular contract basis, the intervals between services being determined by the extent to which the equipment is used, customer's preference, etc. Servicing contracts are usually arranged on a 3-month, 6-month or annual basis.

In addition to regular servicing, equipment will need immediate attention if a major fault develops. Before purchasing equipment it is, therefore, advisable to find out how long it will take the engineer to reach the Department in the event of an emergency call out, how long it will take to get spare parts etc. as this information will determine the length of time the equipment will be out of commission (sometimes called the 'down time').

CHOICE AND INSTALLATION OF NEW EQUIPMENT

Various factors must be taken into account before any final decision is made on the purchase of new equipment. The first consideration is 'What is the new equipment needed for?' Is it to meet a new need or to replace existing equipment? Is it for special examinations such as angiography or is it to be used for general radiography? Will it be a fixed installation or mobile? and, is the money available for its purchase?

Before these questions can be answered satisfactorily futher information is needed. If it is to be a simple replacement of existing equipment we must ask whether or not the equipment presently installed meets the needs of the radiologist and radiographer. One must also ask whether or not there are to be any radical changes taking place in the hospital in the forseeable future which would alter the present requirements. Other departments must be consulted and plans coordinated so that future as well as present needs will be met.

Once we have identified the needs it is important that equipment is selected which will meet these needs as closely and as economically as possible. To do this it is necessary to obtain detailed information about the required equipment from all the major manufacturers. It is important to visit other departments which already have the desired equipment installed so that it can be seen under working conditions. Discuss with the radiographers working with the equipment any good or bad points it may have and how well it meets the needs of their department. Find out from the superintendent any difficulties he has encountered with installation, servicing and replacement of spare parts, etc.

Having decided on the equipment you feel will be most satisfactory in meeting your needs, and of course ensured that money is available for its purchase it is necessary to ensure that, if it is a fixed installation, it will fit into the space available. It is a simple matter to use scale cutouts to represent each piece of equipment i.e. table, control console etc. and to place these on a piece of graph paper on which has been drawn a scale plan of the room. Manoeuvering the pieces about on the room plan makes it easier to decide on the best location for each piece of equipment. It is necessary of course to ensure that not only is there sufficient space for the equipment but that there is enough room to give access to wheelchairs and trolleys as well as adequate space for the radiographer to work in.

It is important, in this preliminary assessment, to ensure that doors and corridors in the hospital are wide enough to get the equipment to the X-ray room and that the lift is big enough and powerful enough to accommodate mobile units etc.

Having, hopefully, obtained satisfactory answers to the questions raised in this preliminary assessment it is advisable to get the help and advice of the radiological protection advisor, an experienced hospital physicist who will advise on the necessary protection requirements. The manufacturer's engineers, because of their experience in installing equipment in other hospitals should also be consulted at an early stage. They will, in consultation with the hospital engineer decide whether or not the existing electrical cables are adequate to meet the demands of the new equipment or whether new cables will be needed. The architect, in consultation with the engineers must decide whether or not the floor is strong enough to take the weight of the new equipment and whether or not the ceiling needs to be heightened or the walls strengthened to accommodate ceiling suspended tubes, monitors etc.

When the architects' and manufacturers' provisional plans are to hand, check them over carefully so that final plans can be produced which meet the needs of the department, and the user, as closely as possible. Try to ensure that any pre-installation work is completed to schedule so as to avoid delays in the installation of the equipment and make sure that equipment delivered to the hospital prior to installation is safely stored in dry accommodation.

Accessory equipment such as cassettes, films, protective aprons etc. should be ordered in good time and safely stored until required.

After installation check all mechanical movements, scales, locks etc. Ensure that all scales are reading correctly and carry out the quality assurance tests described in Chapter 15 to provide a basis against which future performance can be judged. Finally ensure that all radiographers are familiar with the equipment and its controls *before* the first patient is examined.

13 Computers and microprocessors

COMPUTERS AND MICROPROCESSORS	156
THE BINARY SYSTEM	156
Simple binary arithmetic	157
Addition	157
Subtraction	157
Multiplication	157
Division	157
DIGITAL SWITCHING CIRCUITS	158
LOGIC GATES	158
AND gate	158
OR gate	159
NOT gate	159
NAND gate	159
NOR gate	160
The exclusive OR gate	160
CLOCKS	160
FLIP FLOPS	160
SHIFT REGISTERS	160
Information display	161
THE ANALOGUE COMPUTER	161
Operational amplifier	161
Negative feedback	161

COMPUTERS AND MICROPROCESSORS

There are two main types of computer namely the digital computer and the analogue computer. The digital computer consists essentially of an input, a processing facility, and an output. The input relates to data, the central processing unit (CPU) and its associated memory etc. to the processing facility and the output to the answer the CPU produces. If the central processing unit is a microprocessor, then the computer is called a microcomputer. Such a computer can handle only one job at a time and when many functions have to be carried out simultaneously a mainframe computer is used.

By definition the word computer means 'to calculate or estimate'. Now, how does a computer 'calculate or estimate'? Well, it cannot 'think' as we do nor has it intelligence as we know it. In fact the digital computer works entirely on the basis of deciding whether or not a value is 'high' or 'low' or whether a switch is 'on' or 'off'. How then does the computer carry out a calculation on the basis of an input voltage or signal being 'high' or 'low'? It does so by using the binary system as opposed to the decimal system for the purposes of the calculation. Let us be clear first of all as to what is meant by these two arithmetical systems. In the decimal system the numbers in each column to the left of a point increase progressively by raising ten to the power of 0 1 2 3, etc.

10^3	10^2	10^1	10^0	.
Thousands	Hundreds	Tens	Units	Point

Numbers to the right of the point decrease progressively by raising 10 to the power of -1 -2 -3, etc. giving us fractions of the whole number.

The digital computer, because it can only differentiate between input signals which are 'high' or 'low' uses the binary system to carry out its calculations. In this system no digit is higher than one and indeed all digits are either 0 or 1 which corresponds nicely to the signals 'on' or 'off', 'high' or 'low' which the computer can use. A signal which is low is called logic 0 and a signal which is high is called logic 1.

THE BINARY SYSTEM

The binary system uses the base 2 so that all numbers to the left of the point are increased progressively by raising 2 to the power of 1 2 3, etc.

2^5	2^4	2^3	2^2	2^1	2^0	.
32	16	8	4	2	1	Point

Fractions are obtained by raising the numbers to the right of the point to the power of -1 -2 -3, etc. To write, say, 162 in decimal, i.e.

Hundreds	tens	units
1	6	2

means that we have written 1 hundred, 6 tens and 2 units. In binary 162 would be written as 10100010, i.e.

2^7	2^6	2^5	2^4	2^3	2^2	2^1	2^0
128	64	32	16	8	4	2	1
1	0	1	0	0	0	1	0

meaning one 128, no 64s, one 32, no 16s, no 8s, no 4s, one 2 and no 1s which is:

```
 128
  32
   2
 ---
 162
```

How do we go about converting decimal to binary? All we need to do is divide the number continuously by 2 as shown below. The remainders reading from the bottom, gives the binary number.

Let us once again take the number 162.

```
2)162
 2)81  r 0
  2)40 r 1
   2)20 r 0
    2)10 r 0
     2)5  r 0
      2)2 r 1
       2)1 r 0
         0 r 1
```

Read the binary number from the bottom upwards, 10100010.

Each digit in the binary system is called a bit (*bi*nary dig*it*) and a group of eight such digits (commonly used by microprocessors for counting) is called a byte.

An 8 bit processor can deal with 2^7 variations in signal, i.e. it can store information in the form of 'on' 'off' signals as a binary number 11111111 which equals 255 decimal, whilst a 16 bit processor can cope with 2^{15} variations, 1111111111111111 or 65 535 in decimal. The latter is called a 64K memory.

Note: 64K in binary = 65 535 in decimal, whilst 64K in decimal = 64 000. The reason for this disparity is that 1K decimal = 10^3 whereas 1K binary = 2^{10} = 1024.

Some processors use 28 bits which can cope with up to 2^{27} variations which equals 132 217 928 bits.

The binary code is not the only way in which the digits 1 and 0 may be used to represent numbers. Another system is the grey code which is used to convert analogue quantities to digital signals. Yet another system uses binary coded decimals (BCD) where four binary digits are used to represent each digit of a decimal number and the excess three code is another system which uses the digits 1 and 0 to represent numbers. Octal (10^8) and hexdecimal (10^{16}) are other systems in use. The advantage of these is that they make more economical use of storage space in the computer, i.e. less bits are needed to store a given piece of information within the memory.

Simple binary arithmetic

Addition, subtraction, multiplication and division can all be carried out on paper in a similar way to decimal.

Addition

To add 1001101 to 0111011:

```
 111111  ← carry
 1001101
 0111011
 --------
10001000
```

Rules
0+0 = 0
0+1 = 1
1+0 = 1
1+1 = 0 carry 1
Carry 1+ 1+1 = 1 carry 1

Starting from the right, 1+1 = 0 carry 1, and so on until the last carry 1 which forms the first bit of the answer, which is 10001000

Subtraction

To subtract 010011 from 101101:

```
       101101
      -010011
borrow 1  1
       ------
       011010
```

Rules
0−0 = 0
0−1 = 1 borrow 1
1−0 = 1
1−1 = 0
1−1−borrow 1 = 1 borrow 1

Multiplication

Multiplication is carried out in the same way as for decimal but the vertical columns are, of course, added as for binary.

For example, to multiply 100110 by 101:

```
   100110
    ×101
  -------
   100110
   000000
   100110
  -------
 10111110  = answer
```

Division

Division is carried out in the same way as for decimal long division but using binary to subtract.

For example, to divide 1101001 by 101:

```
         10101
    _____
101)1101001
     101
     ___
      110
      101
      ___
       101
       101
       ___
        . . .
  answer = 10101
```

DIGITAL SWITCHING CIRCUITS

Digital switching circuits are used to switch rapidly from 'on' to 'off' or from 'off' to 'on' when a digital signal is applied to the input of the circuit. The output is always either 'on' counted as 1 or 'off' counted as 0; there are no intermediate stages. The circuit diagram in Figure 13.1 illustrates how the transistor achieves this switching function.

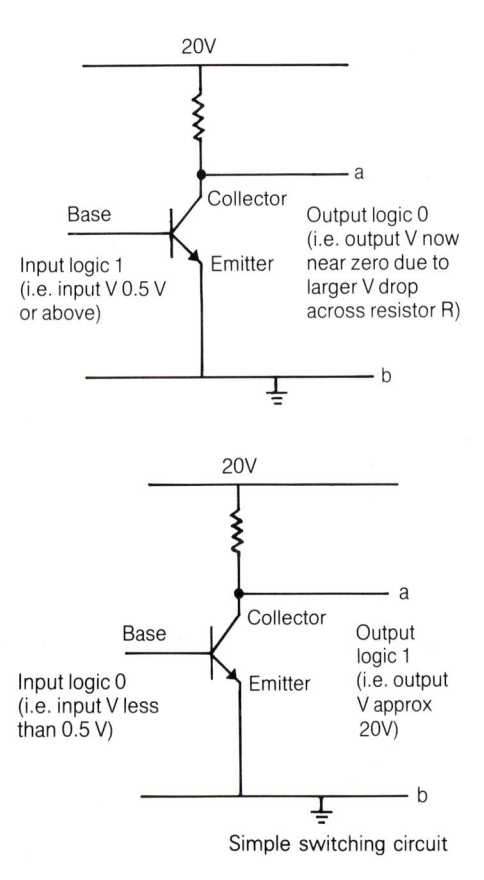

Figure 13.1 Digital switching circuit

For an input of less than 0.5 V the transistor remains cut off, i.e. any input (base) voltage between 0 and 0.5 V is insufficient to allow current flow through the transistor and the input is therefore counted as 0 and the output as 1.

When the transistor base voltage exceeds 0.5 V however, (input logic 1) the transistor switches on, a large collector current flows, the voltage across a–b drops and this output is called logic 0.

Originally, individual transistors were used to build computer circuits but the large numbers needed made them very unwieldy and the soldered joints caused a lot of trouble. These problems were overcome when integrated circuits were developed as the transistors and resistors, etc. are all incorporated on to a tiny chip of silicon. The early integrated circuits (ICs) had only a few transistors and resistors and were called small scale integrated circuits (SSIs). Nowadays large scale integrated circuits (LSIs) contain may thousands of transistors and resistors built into complex circuits, all of them contained on one tiny chip. Whilst these LSIs are quite cheap to produce they are very expensive to design.

LOGIC GATES

A logic gate uses digital signals as inputs and outputs. Logic gates are usually arranged so that a logic 1 appears at the output for some definite combination of input signals. A microprocessor is a circuit which can perform virtually any logic function. The action of the logic circuit can be described by means of a *truth table*. A truth table shows the output that will be obtained for various combinations of inputs. (Another method is to use Boolean algebra).

AND gate

A	B	X
0	0	0
0	1	0
1	0	0
1	1	1

2 input AND gate

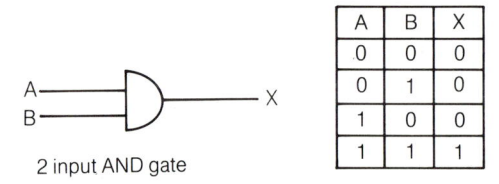

Figure 13.2 Circuit symbol for 2 input AND gate. A and B are the inputs and X is the output

Let us first of all consider the AND gate which is one of the standard logic gates. It is demonstrated by the symbol shown in Figure 13.2. Now for X to have an output logic 1, both A *and* B must also have a logic of 1. This is demonstrated on the truth table (Figure 13.2).

COMPUTERS AND MICROPROCESSORS

From the truth table it will be noted that there are four different ways in which the two input signals can be combined but that a logic 1 is obtained at the output X only for one combination, i.e. when A *and* B are logic 1. For this reason it is called an AND gate and the number of different combinations of lines in the truth table is 2^n when *n* is the number of inputs. For example, a three input AND gate (Figure 13.3) has nine different combinations or lines in the truth table ($2^n = 2^3 = 9$) shown below.

Truth table

A	B	C	X
0	0	0	0
0	0	1	0
0	1	0	0
0	1	1	0
1	0	0	0
1	0	1	0
1	1	0	0
1	1	1	1

3 input AND gate

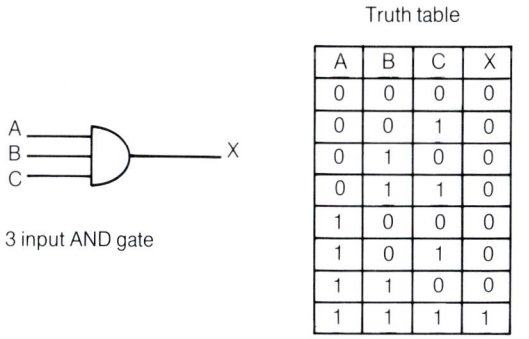

Figure 13.3 3 input AND gate

This of course corresponds to a circuit using mechanical switches as shown in Figure 13.4. As with the AND gate, current flows through X only when switches A, B and C are closed. The truth table applies equally well to this mechanically switched circuit.

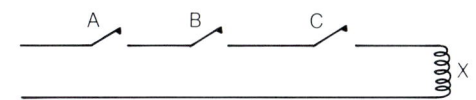

Figure 13.4 Circuit with three switches in series which corresponds to the three input AND gate

OR gate

In this circuit logic 1 at *either* A or B *or* both will give a logic 1 at X. (Figure 13.5 shows the symbol for a two input OR gate and its truth table is as follows:

Truth table

A	B	X
0	0	0
0	1	1
1	0	1
1	1	1

2 input OR gate

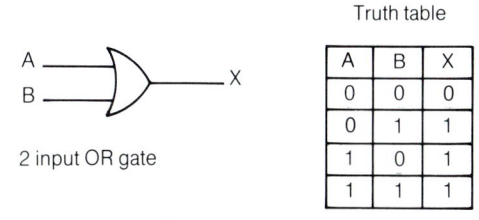

Figure 13.5 2 input OR gate

Figure 13.6 shows the symbol for a three input OR gate and its truth table is as follows:

Truth table

A	B	C	X
0	0	0	0
0	0	1	1
0	1	0	1
0	1	1	1
1	0	0	1
1	0	1	1
1	1	0	1
1	1	1	1

3 input OR gate

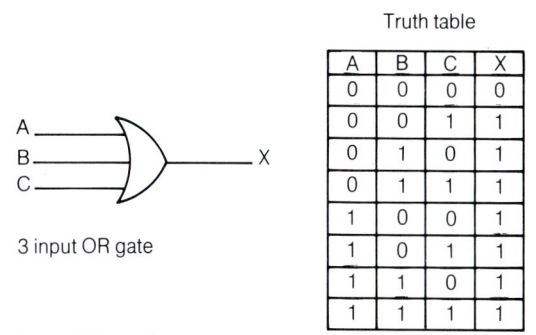

Figure 13.6 3 input OR gate

This corresponds to a mechanically switched circuit of this type which again has the same truth table as the three input OR gate (Figure 13.7).

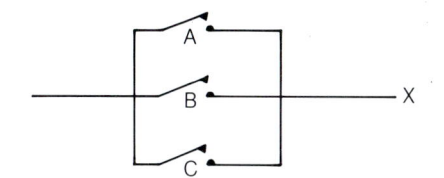

Figure 13.7 Mechanically switched circuit which corresponds to the three input OR gate

NOT gate

The logic NOT gate is an inverter circuit and therefore converts a logic 1 input to a logic 0 output and vice versa. Figure 13.8 shows the symbol and the truth table is as follows.

Truth table

A	X
0	1
1	0

NOT gate

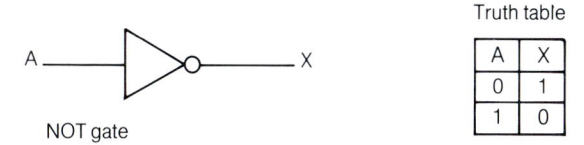

Figure 13.8 NOT gate. The small circle at the output indicates inversion

NAND gate

The combination of the NOT gate with an AND gate gives us a NAND gate (in other words a NOT AND gate). The symbol is shown in Figure 13.9 and the truth table is as follows:

Truth table

A	B	X
0	0	1
0	1	1
1	0	1
1	1	0

NAND gate

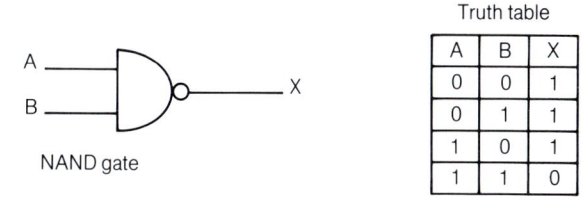

Figure 13.9 NAND gate

NOR gate

The NOR gate is shown in Figure 13.10 and its truth table is as follows:

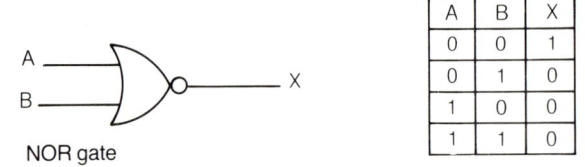

A	B	X
0	0	1
0	1	0
1	0	0
1	1	0

Figure 13.10 NOR gate

The exclusive OR gate

The OR gate gives a logic 1 at X if there is a logic 1 at either A or B or *both*. The exclusive OR gate produces logic 1 at X for a *single* logic 1 at A or B only. The symbol for the exclusive OR gate is shown in Figure 13.11 and its truth table is as follows:

Truth table

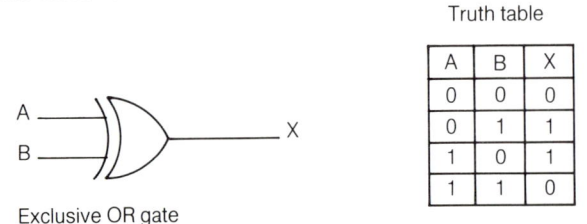

A	B	X
0	0	0
0	1	1
1	0	1
1	1	0

Figure 13.11 Exclusive OR gate

Note that in the last line of the truth table that where there are more than one logic 1 inputs the output is logic 0.

CLOCKS

To enable operations to be carried out in a proper sequence the computer makes use of clocked pulses. Thus signals arriving at a part via different paths are held up until all are received and ready to pass on to the next part of the process. The width of each clocked pulse is wide enough to allow the signal travelling by the slowest route to arrive in time for the next part of the sequence.

FLIP FLOPS

A flip flop or bistable multivibrator is stable in either the high or low output state, that is to say its output can be maintained at 1 or 0 indefinitely. For it to change it must receive an appropriate input signal such as a high or logic 1 which will make it flip or a low or logic 0 which will make it flop.

SHIFT REGISTERS

A shift register is a circuit using flip flops connected in line so that each bit of information from an output is transferred to the next flip flop at each clock pulse.

It will be recalled that a microcomputer consists of an input, a central processing unit and associated memories, and an output. The input, as we have seen, is data presented in the form of a digital signal. It may be put into the microprocessor via a keyboard similar to a typewriter, each key having an associated binary code which is fed into the computer when that particular key is pressed. The most commonly used code is called the ASCII (American Standard Code for Information Interchange). Information can be stored as numbers, letters or punctuations, etc. by pressing the appropriate keys. Other keys such as 'return' and 'shift' have functions which correspond to similar keys on a conventional typewriter. On the other hand, there may be no keyboard at all, information being fed into the computer at the same time as the kV, mA and exposure time are selected, in which case the radiographer may not even be aware that, in addition to selecting the exposure factors, he has also fed the appropriate signals to the microprocessor.

The central processing unit (CPU) processes all information put into the microprocessor and either stores it or displays it as a digital readout of kV, mA and time on the control panel. The input information relating to the exposure factors may, for example, be compared with information relating to tube rating which is stored permanently in the computer's memory and, if the selected factors were such as to cause overloading of the X-ray tube, the output signal from the computer would operate a relay preventing an exposure being made and possibly indicate 'overload' as a visual readout on the control panel. To accommodate information stored permanently in the computer, in addition to that which is stored on a temporary basis only, two memories are used, one is called ROM or read only memory and the other called RAM or random access memory.

The information stored in ROM is permanent and whilst it can be read by the microprocessor it cannot be altered by it. Because of this ROM is said to be non-volatile and the information stored within it is not lost even when the power supply is switched off. (Information can also be stored on floppy discs, magnetic tapes, etc. This stored information is also permanent, i.e. non-volatile.)

The other memory chip called RAM (random access memory) can store information written into it by the microprocessor and the stored information can also be read by the microprocessor but all information stored in RAM is lost when the power supply is switched off. Because of this it is said to be a volatile memory.

COMPUTERS AND MICROPROCESSORS

The output signal from the microprocessor can be used to control external circuits via a peripheral interface adaptor or a peripheral interface input/output chip called PIA or PIO respectively.

Information display

Information from the microprocessor may be displayed on a video screen as in the case of computerized axial tomography equipment, or on the control panel of a modern X-ray unit as a digital readout of kV, mA, etc. In the latter case a seven segment display may be used, the digit being formed by illuminating any combination of the seven segments, as shown in Figure 13.12.

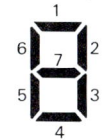

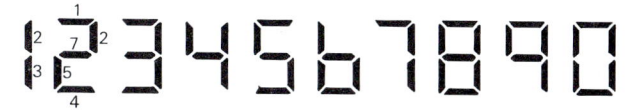

Figure 13.12 Digital readout

Digital readout of kV, mA, exposure time, mAs, etc. are commonplace on the control panels of most modern X-ray equipment and indeed modern units now use microprocessors to control and monitor many functions. They can, for instance, be used to store information relating to tube loading etc. or to block an exposure if the selected factors would overload the tube. Some units also use microprocessors to display information regarding the number of exposures still permissible when undertaking rapid sequential imaging examinations such as angiography etc. and, as we have seen, the high frequency generator uses a microprocessor to control the circuitry which produces the rapidly changing current. It will also be recalled that the microprocessor monitors the kV and mA, etc. and controls circuits which maintain these factors at preselected values.

THE ANALOGUE COMPUTER

As opposed to the two fixed states 'on' or 'off', or 1 or 0 used in the digital computer the Analogue System uses a varying voltage to represent changes analogous to those occurring in a physical system over a period of time. A control panel enables the operator to vary the voltages representative of various parts of the physical system so that a study can be made of the effects of such changes. A fundamental component of the analogue computer is the operational amplifier.

Operational amplifier

The operational amplifier is an integrated circuit used in the analogue computer to carry out mathematical operations such as addition, integration and differentiation. It will be noted from Figure 13.13(a) that the device has a negative and a positive input. If the input signal is applied to the negative input the signal will be amplified and inverted (Figure 13.13(b)). If however, the signal is applied to the positive input the signal is amplified without inversion.

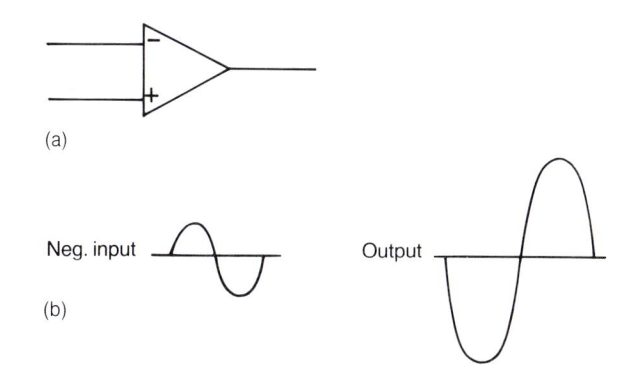

Figure 13.13 (a) Circuit symbol for operational amplifier. (b) Signal is amplified and inverted when it is connected to the negative input

Negative feedback

The operational amplifier may have a fraction of its negative output fed back to the input via a resistor (R_2 in Figure 13.14). The amplification factor is calculated by dividing resistance of R_2 by resistance of R_1.

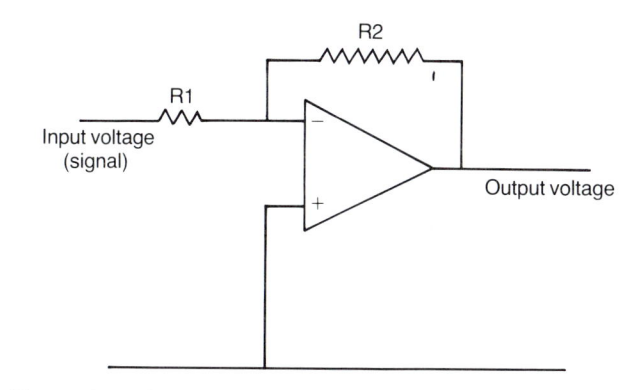

Figure 13.14 Operational amplifier with negative feedback

14
Protection and monitoring of patients and staff

THE EFFECTS OF X-RADIATION ON THE HUMAN BODY	162
PROTECTION – PRIMARY AND SECONDARY BARRIERS	163
Choice of materials for primary and secondary barriers for radiations up to 150 kVp	164
Examples of primary barriers	164
Examples of secondary barriers	164
Protection and the inverse square law	165
MEASUREMENT OF RADIATION DOSE	165
MONITORING OF STAFF	166
The film holder (film badge)	166
Assessment of radiation dose	167
MEASURING PATIENT DOSE	167

THE EFFECTS OF X-RADIATION ON THE HUMAN BODY

X-rays, in common with certain other radiations in the electromagnetic spectrum, are able to penetrate and ionize matter. This ionization of body tissues can have a number of effects such as erythema, epilation or sterility, the particular effect being determined by the dose of radiation received. Ionization may also cause structural changes in the irradiated tissue cells leading to cancer or necrosis of the cells. These effects, which may be immediate or delayed are called *somatic effects*. Another effect which may never manifest itself in any observable way in the irradiated individual is the *genetic effect*. Small doses of radiation may cause changes in the ovum of the female or the sperm of the male. On fertilization, two sets of genes, one from the male and one from the female come together. If a gene has been affected by ionizing radiation it is called a recessive gene whilst a normal gene would be called a dominant gene. On coming together the dominant gene usually overcomes a recessive and the characteristics carried on the dominant gene are passed on to the offspring. The recessive gene although dormant is, however, passed on to the next generation. Each subsequent generation will be unaffected unless two recessive genes come together. When this occurs there is a mutation; the effect of such a mutation may be quite insignificant such as a change in the colour of the baby's eyes. However, mutations are rarely beneficial to mankind and they may result in mental or physical abnormalities in the offspring. Because the genetic effects will almost certainly be increased by exposing large sections of the community to even small doses of radiation, it is important that the radiation dose received by the gonads of irradiated patients be kept to a minimum. This is achieved by shielding the patient's gonads with lead or lead rubber whenever possible.

It will be appreciated that if only a small proportion of the general public is being irradiated the chances of two recessive genes coming together at fertilization are remote. However, the workload of diagnostic X-ray departments is constantly increasing, and the number of patients X-rayed annually also increases steadily. It is apparent, therefore, that as a greater and greater proportion of the general public is irradiated the danger of mutations both now and in the future also increases. It is important, therefore, that the radiation dose to the gonads of patients of child-bearing age be kept to a minimum, consistent, of course, with meeting the needs of the clinician.

Evidence accumulated over recent years, however, has led scientific opinion to the conclusion that the hazards associated with low dose radiation are *not* entirely confined to the genetic effect and in fact it is now thought that these risks were originally overstated and they are now considered to be much lower than originally thought. Having said that, however, it is still of the utmost importance that radiation levels be kept as low as practicable, as apart from the genetic effect, which is still a hazard, there is also the somatic effect to be considered. This effect is now thought to be the most significant effect because of the risk of radiation-induced carcinomas which are thought to increase to the square of the dose after a certain threshold dose has been received. Whilst the hazards, both somatic and genetic, inherent in the use of ionizing radiations are increasingly well recognized and appreciated, the value of such radiation as a diagnostic tool is equally well recognized and appreciated. This poses the question as to whether the benefit derived outweighs the risks involved in its use. There is no simple answer to this question as the hazards, whilst better understood, do not readily lend themselves to accurate quantitative assessment. It is obvious, therefore, that radiation dose to patients generally and to certain organs specifically should be kept to the lowest possible level consistent with the need to produce a diagnostic image. It is also essential that the diagnostic use of ionizing radiations be kept under continuous review by such bodies as the International Commission on Radiological Protection (ICRP), so that particular examinations which are not felt to produce sufficient information, or which produce the information at too great a risk, may be modified or abandoned. Less hazardous imaging techniques such as medical ultrasound have recently been introduced which enable diagnostic information, in certain cases to be obtained with little or no risk to the individual under examination.

The ICRP gives guidance to the panels of experts in each country who provide the rules and regulations which govern the use of radiation in that country. In the UK we have the 'Code of Practice' for the 'Protection of Persons against Ionizing Radiations' which makes the necessary recommendations relating to the protection of patients and staff. In the Code some examinations are discouraged whilst others have been abandoned altogether. For instance, the technique of intraoral fluroscopy is prohibited whilst other examinations such as chest radiography of pregnant women by mass miniature techniques (as opposed to full-sized film radiography) and radiography of the lower abdomen during early pregnancy are strongly discouraged. In these cases it is felt that the possible hazards related to the use of radiation are not worth the information to be gained – or that the information should be obtained by using equipment which subjects the patient to less radiation dose. It is, of course, the responsibility of the radiologist and the clinician to jointly consider special cases and to determine whether or not it is worthwhile taking the risks to obtain the desired information. They may well decide to obtain the information by some other technique, such as the use of ultrasound in pregnancy etc.

When a patient is undergoing radiographic examination the tissue cells at greatest risk are those which are undergoing rapid change e.g. germ cells. These cells are to be found in the gonads, the bone marrow, the embryo and fetus, etc. The following list indicates the possible dangers due to ionization of these cells.

(1) The fetus. Radiation damage, particularly during the first 3 months *can* lead to developmental abnormalities.

(2) The bone marrow (where red blood cells are formed). Radiation damage to growing red blood cells *may* be responsible for some types of leukaemia.

(3) The gonads. Radiation damage to germ cells in the gonads *can* be responsible for genetic effects. Massive doses (not associated with diagnostic radiography) can lead to sterility.

(4) There are dangers involved in the use of very low kVp techniques such as mammography. Exposures should be kept to a minimum as cancer *may* be induced which can manifest itself in later years. Always use special equipment for this procedure, never use makeshift equipment.

(5) Damage to the lens of the eye. Where appropriate eye shields should be used if the eyes are likely to be irradiated.

Balancing the risks associated with the use of ionizing radiation for diagnostic procedures on the one hand against the advantages to be derived from its use on the other, is sometimes called 'A philosophy of risk'. It is the responsibility of the diagnostic radiographer to derive the maximum diagnostic information from the smallest radiation dose to the patient and thus reduce the dangers and possible hazards associated with its use to a minimum.

The 'Code of Practice for the Protection of Persons against Ionizing Radiation', makes recommendations which help minimize the radiation hazard to radiographers and patients. It also lays down maximum permissible doses of radiation which should not be exceeded by staff or patients. The maximum permissible dose relates to that amount of radiation which, so far as present medical knowledge is concerned, carries with it risks which are acceptable both to the individual and to the community at large. The risks are considered to be small compared with the normal hazards of life.

Maximum permissible dose (whole body) for designated persons should not exceed 13 mSv, per quarter or 50 mSv per annum and for a member of the general public 0.5 rem per annum.

Genetic and somatic effects may be stochastic or non-stochastic, *stochastic* meaning that the effects are of a random nature, i.e. we may know that 15% of the population may be affected but we cannot identify the particular individuals forming the 15%. *Non-stochastic* effects, on the other hand, mean that if an individual receives a given amount of radiation a particular effect is inevitable.

Let us now see what measures we can take to ensure that radiation dose to patients, staff and general public is kept to a minimum.

PROTECTION – PRIMARY AND SECONDARY BARRIERS

When a patient is radiographed some of the radiation is absorbed, some is scattered and some passes through the patient without change.

(Subsequent to absorption characteristic radiation is emitted. However, the body tissues are composed of atoms of low atomic number and the characteristic radiation emitted is therefore of low energy. Consequently the characteristic radiation does not have sufficient penetrating power to do much more than leave the irradiated cell.)

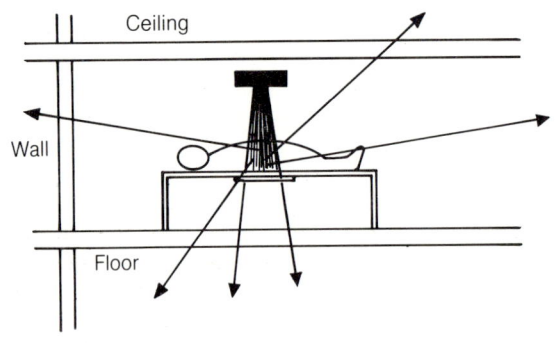

Figure 14.1 Primary and scattered radiation may pass through walls, ceiling etc.

Radiation leaves the X-ray tube by the radiolucent window (all other radiation being attenuated by the lead lining of the tube shield) and is confined to a narrow beam by the use of cones, light beam diaphragms, etc. which are fitted to the X-ray tube. It can be seen from Figure 14.1 that some radiation passes straight through the patient, table top, cassette and the X-ray room floor. In the case of the erect chest stand or erect bucky some of the radiation passes through the wall (Figure 14.2).

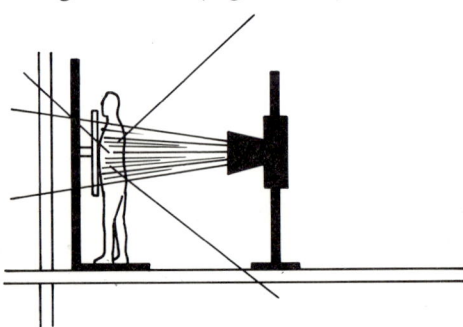

Figure 14.2 Primary and scattered radiation may pass through the wall when a chest stand is used

Staff, patients, etc. working or sitting in adjacent rooms, or the rooms above and below the X-ray room must be adequately protected against primary radiation. The appropriate sections of the floor, wall, ceilings, etc. likely to be irradiated are therefore reinforced with a material of high atomic number and density, which will attenuate the radiation sufficiently to ensure the safety of those working or sitting in the vicinity of the X-ray room. The degree of protection needed is determined by the 'occupancy factor', e.g. is the room in permanent use by, say, a typist or is it only in occasional use by any one person, e.g. patients' waiting room. The occupancy factor is high (unity) when the room is permanently in use by the same person and less than one when it has only occasional use. Materials which afford protection against primary radiation are called *primary barriers*.

So much for the primary radiation, but what about that which has been scattered by the patient, table top, cassette, floor, etc.? This scatter, whilst of longer wavelength than the primary, is nevertheless highly ionizing, and designated persons, staff and patients in adjacent rooms, etc. must be protected against it. The protective barrier need not be as thick (lesser lead equivalent) as that used to protect against primary radiation because the energy (penetrating power) of the scatter is less than that of the primary. Materials used to protect against secondary radiation are called *secondary barriers*.

Choice of materials for primary and secondary barriers for radiations up to 150 kVp

One of the most effective barriers is lead and it is used extensively for purposes of protection in the X-ray department. Because of its high atomic number (82) and high density (1.1×10^4 kg/m^3) it is particularly effective in attenuating radiation by the process of photoelectric absorption ($\propto Z^3$) and Compton scattering ($\propto$ density). Other barriers are compared to it in terms of their lead equivalence. (Lead equivalent (LE) is that thickness of lead, in mm, which affords the same protection as the barrier in question, for the same radiation quality (kVp).)

The protection afforded by a particular thickness of lead is determined by the quality of the radiation it is attenuating. As quality is a function of kVp, a given thickness of lead is said to afford protection up to a specific kVp. The lead obviously needs to be thickest when it is interacting with primary radiation and can be thinner when attenuating secondary radiation, such as scatter, which is of longer wavelength and therefore less penetrating, than the primary beam.

Examples of primary barriers

(1) The lead lining of the X-ray tube casing which attenuates all the radiation produced at the focal spot excepting that which passes through the radiolucent window and forms the useful beam.

(2) The extra protection used on floor or ceiling of the X-ray room to attenuate primary radiation and protect staff or patients, etc. who may be in rooms above or below the X-ray room, the floor or ceilings of which may be in the direct beam.

(3) The extra protection applied to a wall to safeguard those working or waiting in a room on the other side of the wall, which may be in the direct beam.

In (2) and (3) the thickness of the barrier is affected by the 'occupancy factor' as well as by kVp.

Examples of secondary barriers

(1) Radiographer's protective cubicle. As the primary beam must *never* be directed at the protective cubicle it is only necessary for it to have a lead equivalent sufficiently high to protect against scattered radiation emanating from the patient, table, etc. (Lead ply is normally used).

(2) Walls and ceiling of X-ray rooms. Barium plaster may be used instead of ordinary plaster to finish the walls and ceiling of X-ray rooms. The substitution of barium (atomic number 56) for calcium (atomic number 20) when mixing plaster increases the chances of absorption by the photoelectric process by a factor of almost 22.

(3) Lead rubber aprons, gloves, etc. These should be of such lead equivalent as to provide protection against secondary radiation. The radiographer should never be in the primary beam.

Protection and the inverse square law

The inverse square law states that the intensity of the radiation from a point source varies inversely as the square of the distance from the source providing there is no absorption or scattering in the medium. This is a case where 'distance lends enchantment' and the radiographer should stand as far back as is practicable from the primary beam during an exposure. This is particularly important when operating mobile equipment in wards etc.

MEASUREMENT OF RADIATION DOSE

The efficiency and adequacy of primary and secondary radiation barriers are checked by carrying out a radiation survey of the department. This is usually done by physicists who conduct such a survey by using ionization type survey meters, photographic film or thermoluminescent discs to measure the amount of radiation passing through the barriers or cracks in the barriers.

A typical radiation survey meter has a large ionization chamber (about 800 ml) and the exposure rate is read directly from the meter. The large sized chamber enables a full scale reading to be obtained, on its most sensitive range, of about 3 mR/h. This degree of sensitivity is needed because the barriers, if efficient, attenuate the radiation to such an extent that the amount of radiation passing through the barrier is very small. Unfortunately the electrical components of this type of meter have a response time of approximately 1 s which means they cannot be used to measure radiation produced by short diagnostic exposures. Sensitive Geiger–Meuller tubes of small volume can be used to detect radiation passing through small cracks in the barrier. (The large volume survey meter is useless for this purpose because the whole chamber must be irradiated if accurate results are to be obtained).

However, it is generally found that photographic films (personnel monitoring 'badges' for instance) are most effective for recording the integrated dose, due to many exposures occurring over a period of time, in the diagnostic X-ray department. The film 'badge' is fastened to the barrier under investigation on the side furthest from the radiation source. It is left in position for the requisite period of time, usually 4 weeks.

An ionization type survey meter, which gives an instantaneous reading, is used when information regarding radiation dose is required immediately. The disadvantages attendant on this method of dose measurement are:

(1) The instrument is sensitive to mechanical change.

(2) It may read only part of the total dose, e.g. full scale deflection of the meter may be reached before the exposure is ended.

(3) There is no permanent record.

(4) The quality of the incident radiation cannot easily be assessed.

Film 'badges' on the other hand are robust, light, and cheap, allow an assessment to be made of the incident radiation and provide a permanent record of the integrated dose received over a period of time. The greatest disadvantage associated with their use is the fact that they must be sent away to be processed and to have the dose measured. This can involve a delay of several days.

A fresh survey of the department, to check the efficiency of the radiation barriers, must be made whenever new equipment is installed, or when there is a change of position, within a room, of X-ray equipment.

In the UK a safety committee oversees the radiation protection arrangement for large hospitals or hospital groups. They are guided by a physicist called the Radiological Protection Advisor (RPA). The RPA should be informed before new equipment is purchased or when a change in position of existing equipment is contemplated so that he can ensure adequate radiation safety.

MONITORING OF STAFF

Radiographers and other designated persons are continuously monitored. Each member of staff wears a film 'badge' usually for a period of 4 weeks. At the end of this time the film 'badge' is changed, the exposed film being sent to a radiation protection laboratory where it is processed and the assessed dose recorded. Radiographers should wear their 'badges' whenever they are on duty *excepting* when they are themselves as patients undergoing radiographic examination.

In addition to film badges, ionization chambers or pen type chambers may be carried by staff when the dose received under special circunstances or for a particular examination needs to be known without delay.

Thermoluminescent powders, such as lithium fluoride, packed in a small plastic container, may also be carried by designated persons to measure radiation dose. During an exposure, radiation passes through the powder and some of the energy of the radiation is absorbed and stored by the lithium fluoride. The stored energy, which is proportional to radiation dose, is released in the form of blue-green light when the powder is heated to a temperature of approximately 300 °C. The emitted light activates a photoelectric cell and the resultant electron current is amplified by a photomultiplier tube. The amplified current then operates a meter which is calibrated in rems. The information can be read out once only. There is no permanent record. The instrument used for this purpose is called a 'reader'. (The intensity of light from the lithium fluoride is very little affected by any time interval which may occur between irradiation and heating.)

The film holder (film badge)

The film holder is made of plastic and measures approximately 5 cm × 3.5 cm when closed. It is hinged at one end to allow insertion and removal of the radiation monitoring film.

From Figure 14.3 it can be seen that the two halves of the holder are identical, each having an open window, an area of thin plastic, one of thick plastic and three metal filters. One of the metal filters consists of a slice of lead and a slice of tin, another is made up of slices of lead and cadmium, whilst the third is made of dural which is an aluminium and copper alloy.

The lead and cadmium form a compensating filter which enables the dose associated with slow moving neutrons to be assessed, whilst the lead and tin filter allows measurement of dose due to radiations in the therapy range 200 kV–2 MV.

The open window allows measurement of dose due to alpha and beta particles, whilst the thick and thin plastic

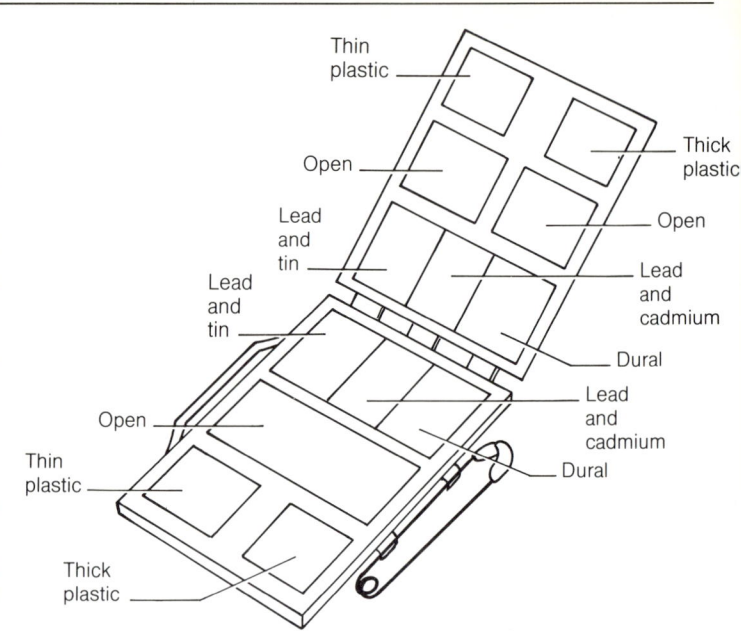

Figure 14.3 Radiation monitoring film holder

filters and the dural filter enable an assessment to be made of the dosage due to radiations in the diagnostic range.

The type of film holder supplied for routine use by radiographers and radiologists is secured to the clothing by means of a safety pin which forms an integral part of the holder. Other types of fastening are available, however, for those occasions when the use of a safety pin would not be appropriate. For example, a holder with two projections allows a linen strap to be passed through securing the holder to the user's forehead, forearm, ankle, etc. (Figure 14.4).

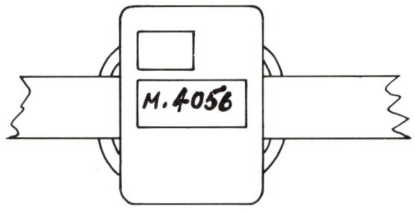

Figure 14.4 Badge specially adapted to accept linen strap. Used to secure badge to user's forehead, arm, wrist etc.

Another type of film holder, rather different in construction, is used to determine the location of an unknown source of radiation. The holder is similar to the conventional 'badge' but there is a metal pin projecting from the centre of the holder (Figure 14.5). When the film is processed the direction of the emitted radiation can be ascertained by studying the outline of the pin on this film. It may be necessary to use more than one to locate with accuracy the source of the radiation.

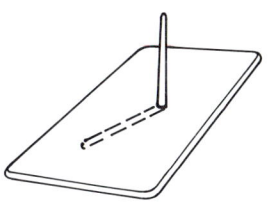

PROTECTION AND MONITORING OF PATIENTS AND STAFF

Figure 14.5 Radiation localizing badge. Dotted lines indicate 'shadow' cast by vertical pin. Outline of pin recorded on film as lesser density

Radiation monitoring film within the badge is similar in appearance to dental film. However, it differs from dental film in a number of important respects and the latter must never be used in a film holder as a substitute for monitoring film. Like dental film, monitoring film is enclosed in a light-tight paper envelope. Unlike dental film, however, it has no lead foil backing and is unique in having a fast emulsion on one side of the base and a slow one on the other. The absence of a lead foil backing ensures that radiation can reach the film from either side and that there is no secondary electron emission from the foil which would lead to increased film density and a false estimation of radiation dose.

The fast and slow emulsions enable a wide range of doses to be recorded on one film (1:10 000). Small doses of radiation are recorded by the fast emulsion whilst larger doses, (usually attributable to accidental exposure) are recorded on the slow emulsion.

When the densitometer indicates maximum density for a monitoring film, the fast emulsion is removed to enable the density of the slow emulsion to be measured.

Assessment of radiation dose

The radiation dose received by a radiographer over a period of time is assessed by measuring the density of the monitoring film from the 'badge' worn over that particular period. Equating film density to radiation dose is achieved in the following way.

Radiation monitoring films in their holders are positioned in a circle around a source of radiation of known output, such as caesium 137, and left for varying lengths of time (Figure 14.6). Alternatively films may be placed at different distances from the source and left a fixed period of time.

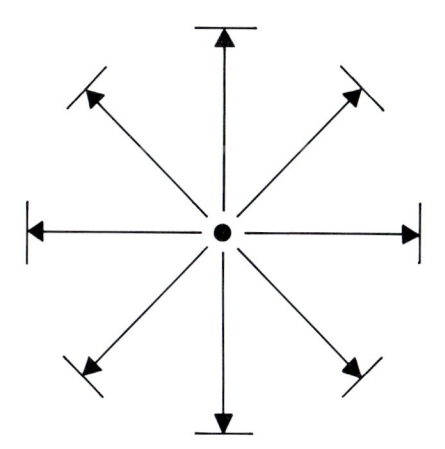

Figure 14.6 'Badges' arranged in a circle around caesium 137 source of radiation

Physicists then construct calibrated curves which enable them to relate the density recorded on the film in the badge worn by the operator to a specific dose of radiation.

MEASURING PATIENT DOSE

Patient dose can be measured using either the Diamentor (previously described) or, as an alternative, thermoluminescent discs may be used for this purpose. The latter are very simple to use and probably give a more accurate measurement of dose. They can, of course, also be placed in natural body cavities to measure absorbed dose.

15
Quality assurance of diagnostic X-ray equipment

R. PRICE

INTRODUCTION	168
ASSESSMENT PARAMETERS	168
Mechanical assessment	169
Equipment stability	169
Accuracy of scales	169
Light beam diaphragm alignment	169
Grid alignment	170
Radiation safety	170
Electrical safety	171
Earth continuity and condition of insulating material	171
Tube overload protection circuit	171
X-ray beam parameters	171
Assessment of focal spot size	171
Resolution methods	174
Radiation quality	175
Exposure time	177
Tube output	178
CONCLUSION	178

INTRODUCTION

Quality assurance is an organized process to establish and monitor the performance of the diagnostic imaging system. The justification for introducing a programme of quality assurance testing is to enable the production of radiographs of a consistently high quality but with minimal radiation doses and without incurring unnecessary costs.

Therefore, if the role of quality assurance is concerned with control of system efficiency, the process should commence before any equipment is released for use. The first step is to make sure that selected equipment is the most appropriate for the situation in which it is to be used. There is little point monitoring equipment and expressing dissatisfaction with its performance when the user has not clearly communicated the requirements to the manufacturer. This approach to quality assurance is recommended by Hendee and Rossi[1] whose quality assurance chain is shown in Figure 15.1.

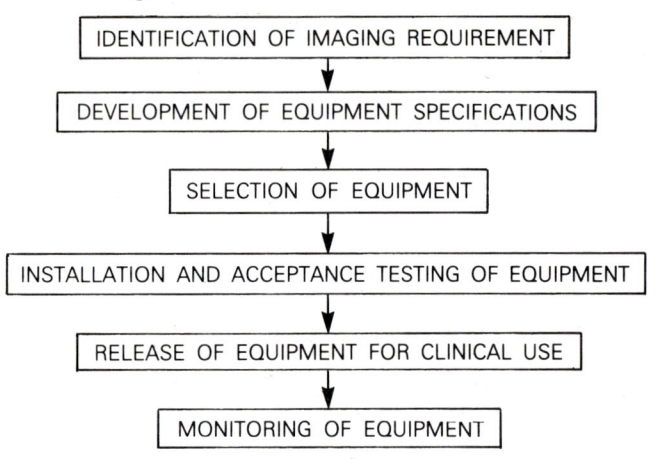

Figure 15.1 Quality assurance chain[1]

The first three links in the chain are discussed elsewhere in this book; this chapter will be concerned with the procedure following installation. Acceptance testing is a crucial element in the process. Without monitoring it is impossible to verify whether or not the manufacturer's specifications are met or if the unit meets the user's requirements. Test results at this stage provide a base line to which subsequent measurements may be compared.

Following the release of equipment for clinical use, routine monitoring would be undertaken during the unit's life so that any deviation from the established performance can be identified and corrected where necessary.

ASSESSMENT PARAMETERS

The assessment routine described is that which would be applicable to a unit used for general radiography. The tests carried out during both the acceptance and the routine monitoring phases are described. The protocols adopted for both phases are of necessity similar; however, the frequency of individual tests during the latter phase will vary significantly.

Tests are discussed under three headings, those related with mechanical alignment, stability and safety; radiation and electrical safety; and thirdly, those relating to the X-ray beam parameters. These are shown in Table 15.1.

Table 15.1 Assessment parameters for diagnostic X-ray equipment

Mechanical	Radiation and electrical safety	X-ray beam
Equipment stability	Tube filtration	Focal spot size
Accuracy of scales	Tube leakage	Radiation quality
Light beam diaphragm alignment	Continuity of earth	Exposure time
	Condition of insulating material	
Grid alignment	Tube overload protection circuit	Tube output

Note, that the reason for grouping tests as shown in Table 15.1 above is for convenience of description. The major justifications for the test procedures were given in the opening paragraph of the chapter and it should be a relatively simple task to relate each individual parameter to one or more of the stated aims. For example, non-congruency between light and X-ray fields may cause a radiograph to be repeated because areas have been excluded; the repeat means that patient dose is increased as well as associated costs.

Mechanical assessment

Equipment stability

It is essential that there is no evidence of any mechanical fault or instability. For example, brakes and tube locks must work efficiently whilst tube movement should be smooth in each of its allowable directions. Associated equipment, X-ray table and grid mechanisms must be stable and not prone to unwanted vibrations during exposure.

Sharp or jagged edges are dangerous and could result in personal injury as could any screw not flush with the surface. The grid tray must be freely moveable and enable the operator to insert and remove a cassette with comparative ease. Following installation any instability or fault must be rectified before releasing the unit into general use.

Accuracy of scales

Calibrated scales must indicate what they are supposed to measure, whether it be focal film distance (FFD) or tube angulation.

The pointer on certain types of angular scales which indicates tube rotation can sometimes stick or move when not required. This can be a source of irritation to the radiographer and should be corrected without delay.

There is no need to remind the reader that, for all practical purposes, X-radiation obeys the inverse square law and any inaccuracy with regard to the FFD scale will influence exposure factors. Miscalibration is therefore undesirable, particularly where the aim is to standardize exposure factors for units sharing similar workloads.

A check of the FFD scale accuracy is relatively simple. The plane of the focal spot should be clearly marked on the tube housing and its height above any reference plane, e.g. table top, can be measured with a rule. Any error can readily be calculated.

Alternatively, application of geometric principles will confirm accuracy. Test equipment consisting of a sheet of lead with two small holes separated by a known distance plus a cassette with film screen combination is all that is required. It is also possible to use the Wisconsin focal spot test tool for this purpose. It has two holes on either side of the resolution phantom 3 cm apart. The height of the holes above the film is known (object film distance) and the distance between the hole images can be measured directly from the radiograph. The distance from the focal spot to the holes (focus object distance) is unknown and is calculated with reference to similar triangles. The FFD is therefore the focus object distance plus the object film distance. Arrangement of the equipment and test principle is illustrated in Figure 15.2a and b. This test need only be undertaken following installation.

Light beam diaphragm alignment

The light beam diaphragm attached to the underside of the X-ray tube has two important functions, to enable the radiographer to centre the X-ray beam and to collimate the field of radiation to the area of interest.

The test objective is, therefore, twofold, to check both the accuracy of coincidence of the central ray with the centre of the radiation field and the congruency between light beam and X-ray beam.

Both the Wisconsin beam alignment and collimator test tools may be used for this test. The former consists of a plexiglass cylinder 15.0 cm in height. Each end of the cylinder is sealed by further plexiglass end pieces. When the cylinder is standing as for the test, the metal screw inset in the top end piece is directly above the washer inset in the bottom. The collimator test tool consists of a sheet of plastic inset with a rectangle formed from copper wire. The rectangle is divided into four equal areas by two other lengths of wire which are marked and numbered at 0.5 cm intervals. The collimator test tool is placed upon an

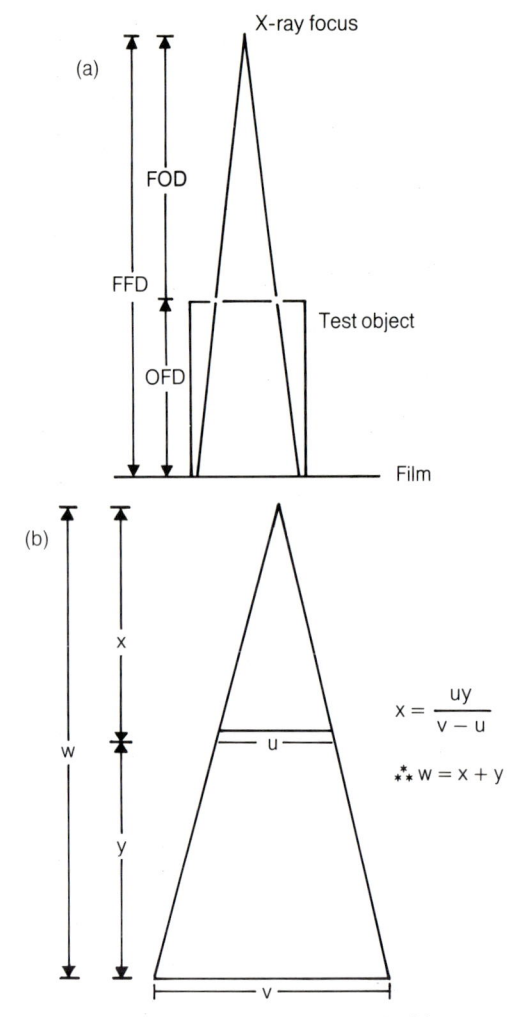

Figure 15.2 Test equipment (a) and test principle (b)

$$x = \frac{uy}{v - u}$$

$$\therefore w = x + y$$

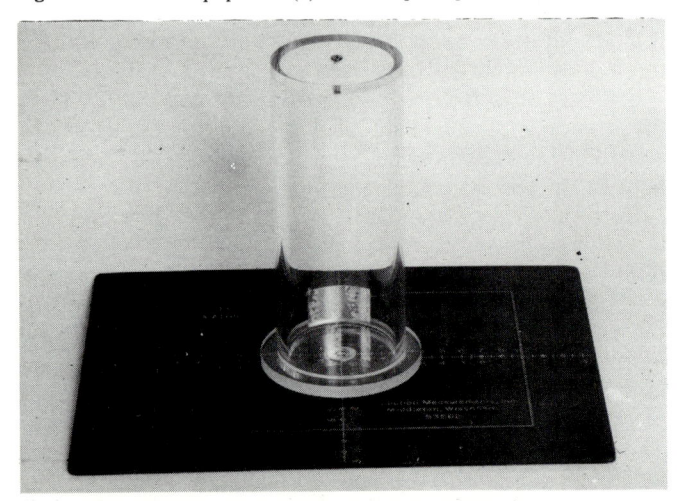

Figure 15.3 Beam alignment and collimator test tools

18×24 cm cassette. The focal film distance should be 100 cm. The light beam is collimated to the rectangular frame. The beam alignment test tool is placed in the centre of the light field. This arrangement is shown in Figure 15.3. An exposure is made, typically 60 kVp and 5 mAs for a medium speed film and screen combination.

In the absence of any British or European standards it is recommended that the limit of the radiation field be within ±1% or 1 cm of the rectangular inset in all directions at 100 cm focal film distance.

If the image of the screw is not visible outside of the washer the beam is less than 1.5° from the perpendicular. An acceptable test radiograph is shown in Figure 15.4.

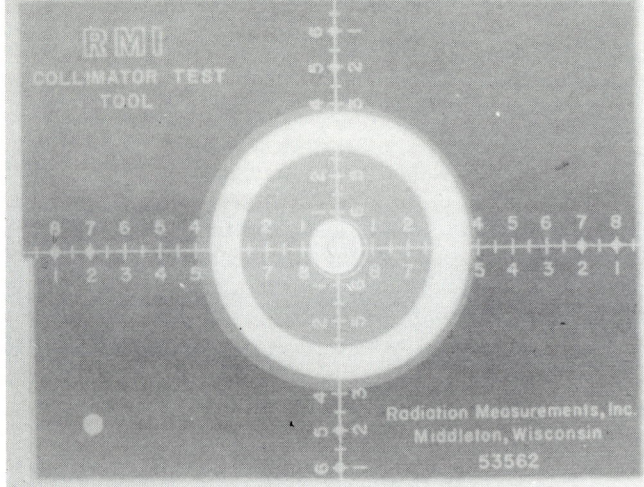

Figure 15.4 Radiograph of test objects. Following installation the test should be repeated at 2-monthly intervals and following any procedure where the light beam diaphragm has been dismantled and reassembled

Grid alignment

A secondary radiation grid either incorporated within the X-ray table or an upright stand, must be correctly centred and perpendicular to the X-ray beam. Misalignment, non-uniformity due to a constructional error, or damage, will result in a variation of transmitted radiation intensity across its width.

A test radiograph of the grid should not show any appreciable density difference across the film. The test exposure should be such as to produce an optical density of between 0.5 and 1.0 for a visual assessment.

A grid incorporated into X-ray equipment is usually well protected and there is little need to repeat this test less than at 6-monthly intervals.

Radiation safety

Both the total tube filtration and radiation leakage would be measured as part of a radiation survey which will be conducted on all new equipment, modified equipment or where techniques have changed. Radiation surveys will be carried out under the auspices of the Radiological Protection Adviser.

Recommendations for total filtration and allowable leakage are given in the *Code of Practice for the Protection of Persons against Ionizing Radiation arising from Medical and Dental Use* (HMSO, 1972).

Inadequate filtration results in greater patient dose whilst excessive filtration serves no useful purpose and will directly result in an increase in tube and generator loading.

Total filtration is composed of inherent tube filtration, added aluminium filtration and light beam diaphragm. It is assessed by measuring the half-value layer of aluminium at a known kV. Needed for the assessment are suitable aluminium filters and an ionization chamber. The X-ray beam is centred and collimated to the chamber which should be at 100 cm from the focus. The kV is selected and an exposure made without an aluminium filter in the beam. The mA s should be such that a dose of some 100 mR is recorded. Exposures are repeated after supporting each thickness of aluminium midway between tube and chamber.

The kV used for the procedure is estimated by the penetrameter method. A suitable ionization chamber and dosemeter is that described in a later section. Total filtration may then be determined from published data.

The Code of Practice, referred to earlier, recommends that 'Leakage radiation at a focal film distance of 1 metre does not exceed 100 mR in 1 hour', but also implies that this figure could be realistically reduced to 10 mR. Measurements may be undertaken with ionization chamber and dose rate meter.

Electrical safety

Earth continuity and condition of insulating material

It is essential that those metal parts of the equipment that the operator may come into contact with are either insulated or at earth potential. The latter is achieved by providing a continuous path of very low resistance to the earthing electrodes which are set into the ground.

The radiographer is protected from current-carrying cables by insulating material and where possible cables should run in metal trunking or conduits which are themselves earthed.

Both the continuity of earth and condition of cables will be checked following installation and as necessary by an electrician. When in use the radiographer must be ever vigilant in looking for signs of damage to insulating material and, particularly in older units where earthing strips run across the floor, any cracking, thinning or corrosion should be reported immediately and entered in the equipment log book. In addition the radiographer under health and safety regulations can request the Health and Safety Executive to make an inspection where any safety hazard, electrical or otherwise, is suspected.

The radiographer will contribute to overall safety standards, minimize damage, and thereby costly repairs by avoiding maltreatment of electrical equipment. Under no circumstances should equipment be moved by pulling cables.

Tube overload protection circuit

To check this circuitry the procedure is quite simple and should be undertaken following installation and at least at 6-monthly periods. In order to undertake the check the tube rating chart is required.

For each mA station the maximum allowable kVp and exposure time, ascertained from the rating chart, should be selected. The tube overload warning system should not operate and the exposure combination is recorded. The kVp should then be increased until the warning indicator operates and a note of the value is made. Reduce the kVp and repeat with the time selection noting the value that triggers the warning indicator. No exposure should be possible unless the combinations are within the allowed ratings. Should the protection circuit not operate at any combination disallowed by the rating chart, under no circumstances should an exposure be attempted. The manufacturer must be informed immediately and a warning placed on the control panel to indicate the danger.

X-ray beam parameters

The radiographer requires that for given similar situations and techniques the performance of the X-ray tube and generator will be consistent. Without such a guarantee it would be impossible to make any prediction of radiographic quality, this in turn would result in an unacceptable level of reject films with associated increase in radiation dose and costs.

It is a relatively straightforward procedure to establish the performance of a unit at installation and then to monitor its performance throughout its working life. There are a number of test tools commercially available which are designed to provide information relating to the output beam parameters. Some of the tests are now described.

Assessment of focal spot size

The smaller the finite source of the X-ray beam the less geometric blurring within a radiograph. Unfortunately, as foci become smaller the choice of exposure factors is limited. This is particularly so, when for a given kVp and mAs the selection of a short exposure time may be precluded as, at the increased mA, the overload circuit may prohibit an exposure. In practice a compromise is reached between power handling and geometric characteristics by the application of the well-known line focus principle. Fortunately, however, excluding macroradiography, large changes in focal spot size are not detectable in the image and the prime need for measurement lies in the focal spot's role in power handling capability. A focal spot smaller than its quoted size will very likely result in a shortened tube life whilst a focus which is larger than the recommended tolerances results in underutilization of the generator.

To measure the focal spot size in relation to its power handling characteristics, reference will be made to the British Standards Institution publication BS 5269, Part 1, 1975, *Measurement of the Dimensions of Focal Spots of Diagnostic X-ray Tubes using a Pinhole Method* to whom acknowledgement is given for permission to reproduce information contained within that publication.

The test tool consists of a pin-hole camera, shown in Figure 15.5. Note the relative size of the test object in comparison to the centimetre scale.

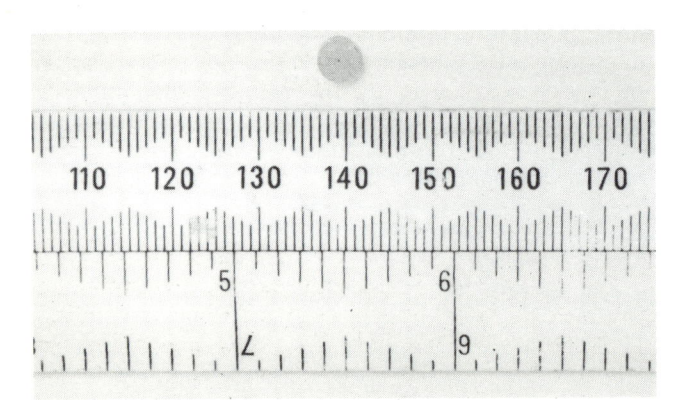

Figure 15.5 Pin-hole camera

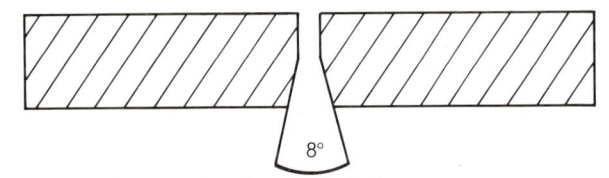

Figure 15.6 Cross section through pin-hole camera

Note that the hole shown is on the side of the camera remote from the focus during the test. Indeed, the size of the pin-hole, quoted as being 0.03 mm in diameter, is too small for the eye to resolve. A cross-section through the camera is shown in Figure 15.6. The visible hole in Figure 15.5 is the fluted diameter which allows for divergence of the X-ray beam and avoids an effect known as tunnelling which would result in a distorted image of the focus. The pin-hole camera shown is made from a 90% gold and 10% platinum alloy. A lead pin-hole camera may suffice to demonstrate the focus shape for interest but should not be used for any measurement as lead is subject to 'creeping' and it is impossible to guarantee that the pin-hole remains of a given size.

The arrangement of the camera for the test is shown in Figure 15.7.

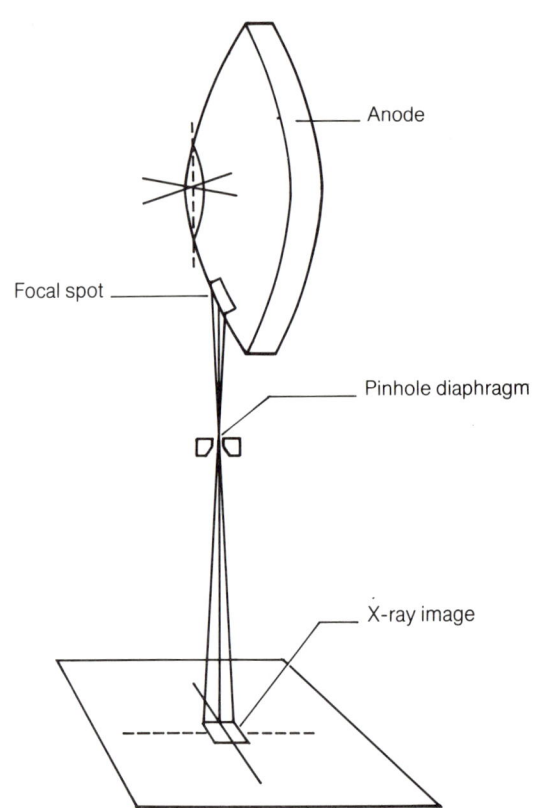

Figure 15.7 Pin-hole camera test

It is the effective focal spot that is measured, and is defined as:

'the projection of the focal spot on the plane which is perpendicular to the central perpendicular line of the window of the tube shield'.

It should not be confused with the actual focal spot which is a rectangle 3–4 times the length of the effective size. The actual focal spot is defined as:

'the section at which the anode of an X-ray tube intercepts the electron beam'.

It should be obvious to the reader that the appearance and therefore size will vary in accordance with the relationship between the pinhole camera and central perpendicular line of the tube shield. The changing focus size is illustrated in Figure 15.8 which shows images produced with a multi-pin-hole diaphragm.

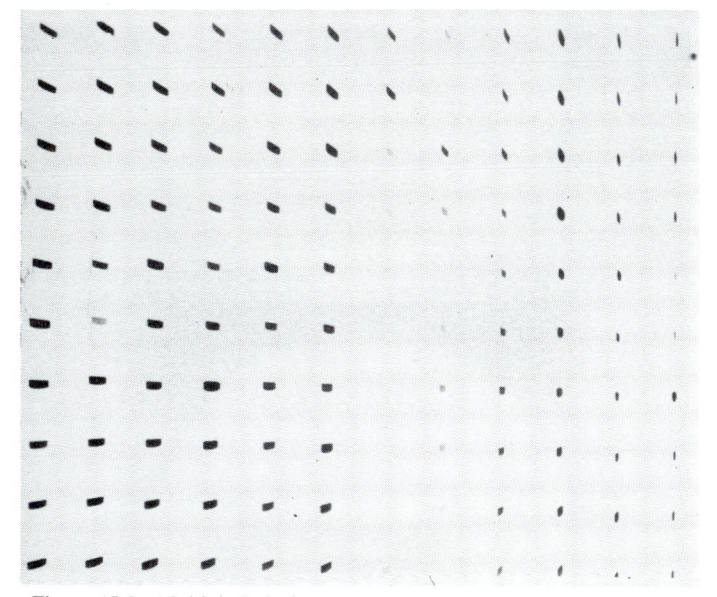

Figure 15.8 Multipin-hole images

However, the alignment should have been checked previously with the aid of the Wisconsin Beam alignment tool and any gross errors rectified by the engineer before measuring the focus. Where the alignment is satisfactory, the pin-hole, supported in a brass holder, is held by a suitable stand and placed in line with the centre of the light beam diaphragm. The distance from the pin-hole to the focus should be equal to or greater than 100 mm. This presents no problems in practice as the light beam diaphragm window is in excess of this distance from the tube. To assist in measurement an enlargement factor of ×3 is recommended for a nominal focal spot of 0.3–1.2 mm, ×2 for 1.2–2.5 focus and ×1 for a focus of 2.5 or greater.

The enlargement factor is expressed by the ratio:

$$\text{Enlargement factor} = \frac{\text{Pin-hole-to-film distance}}{\text{Focal spot-to-pin-hole distance}}$$

The exposure conditions for the test are shown in Table 15.2.

The British Standard does recommend the use of non-screen film but the mA s required to provide sufficient density tends to be rather excessive. Use of a high resolution film/screen combination is quite satisfactory. A common error is to overexpose and one may get the impression that the focus is a uniformly emitting homogenous spot rather than the split intensity distribution demonstrated by the pin-hole image shown in Figure 15.9 which is typical.

Table 15.2 Exposure conditions for pin-hole test

Maximum rated voltage U (kV)	Test voltage	Test current
$U \leq 75$	Maximum rated voltage	50% of maximum current permissible for 0.1 s at the test voltage
$75 < U \leq 150$	75 kV	
$U \geq 150$	50% of maximum rated voltage	

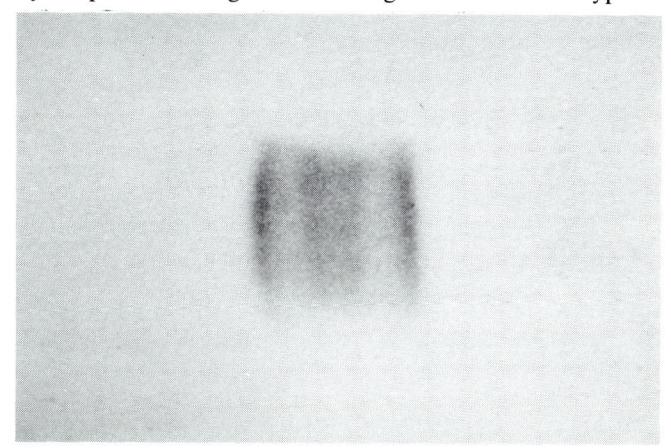

Figure 15.9 Pin-hole image showing split intensity distribution

The size of the image is measured with the aid of a magnifying glass with a built-in graticule with 0.1 mm divisions and with a ×5–10 magnification. Measurements need to be made in two directions, parallel and perpendicular to the anode cathode axis. Focal spot dimensions are calculated by dividing the dimensions of the image by the enlargement factor. In addition, it is recommended that a correction factor of 0.7 is applied to the longest dimension but there are conflicting ideas on this point and values of 0.8 and 0.9 have been suggested. However, the effective focal spot dimension is expressed as $(FL \times FW)^{\frac{1}{2}}$ where FL is the focal length and FW the width.

The allowed manufacturing tolerances of focal spot dimensions are given in Table 15.3.

Table 15.3 Manufacturing tolerances of focal spot dimensions

Focal spot	Nominal Dimensions	Tolerances %
Fine	0.8	−0 − +50
Small	0.8–1.5	−0 − +40
Large	1.5	−0 − +30

Resolution methods

A disadvantage of the size measurement obtained with the pin-hole method is that limitation in resolution produced by any focus is not only a function of size but also of the shape and intensity distribution.

There are, in existence, a number of resolution phantoms available for focus measurement. Three are shown in Figure 15.10.

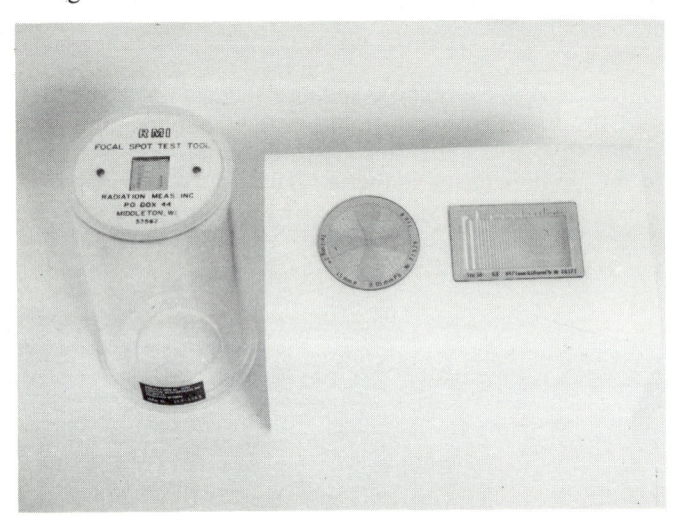

Figure 15.10 Resolution phantoms. Wisconsin focal spot test tool, star phantom, bar phantom

Whichever phantom is used, it is imaged at a stated magnification factor. It is possible to calculate the focal spot size by the degree of blurring present in the image. Both the Wisconsin and bar phantom consist of discrete line pair spacings and the calculated result is subject to error. In addition using the bar phantom will require two images, because the line pairs are aligned in one direction only. The star phantom overcomes both these problems and is the method described.

As with the pin-hole camera the star phantom must be correctly aligned with the central axis of the X-ray beam. The phantom is supported parallel to the X-ray tube central horizontal axis with an alignment such that equal pairs of opposite quadrants lie parallel and perpendicular to the anode–cathode axis. There must be at least 30 cm between phantom and focal spot and the distance from focus to film such that there is a magnification factor of ×5 for a nominal focus of 0.6 mm or less, ×3 for a focus greater than 0.6 mm and up to 1.0 mm, ×2 greater than 1.0 mm and up to 2.0 mm and a ×1.5 magnification for a nominal focus of 2.0 mm or more. In any case the blurring diameter shown on the images in Figure 15.11 should be greater than 30 mm. Note the greater blurring diameter with the broad focus.

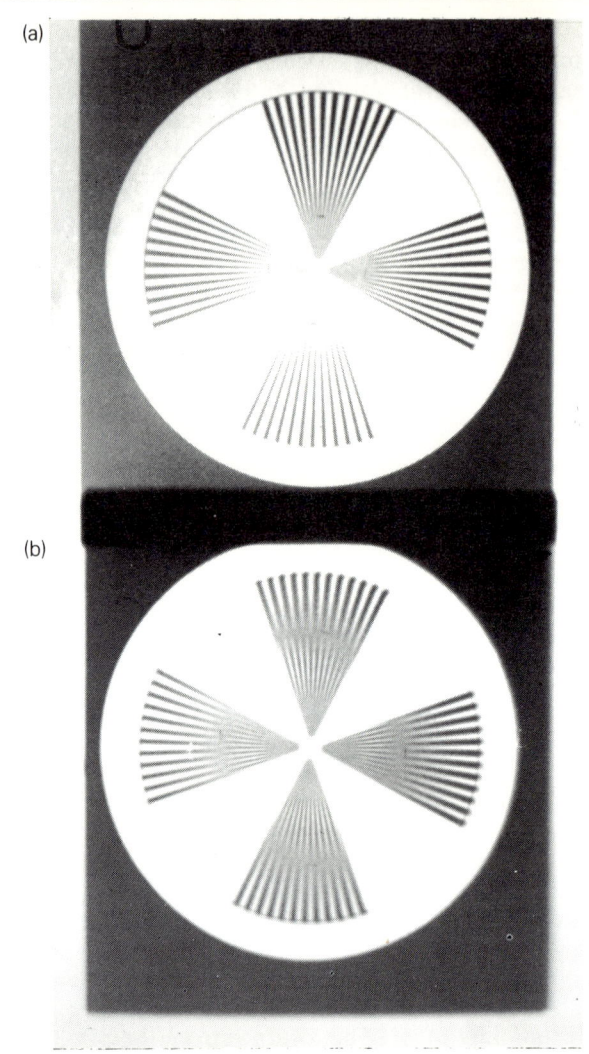

Figure 15.11 Star phantom image. (a) fine focus (b) broad focus

As an exposure guide, kVp and mA values may be chosen in accordance with the pin-hole recommendations. However, the great saving is that an mA s of only approximately 5 is required to produce an average density of 1.0 with a high resolution film/screen combination. There is therefore no danger of damaging the target.

For a star phantom with a 2° spoke angle the dimensions of the focal spot size may be expressed thus:

$$FL(W) = \frac{2\pi D}{180(M-1)}$$

where FL and FW are the focal lengths and widths, respectively, D the blurring diameter and M the geometrical magnification.

The equivalent size is then expressed as $(FL \times FW)^{\frac{1}{2}}$

where the equivalent size is defined as: 'the size of a theoretical homogenous focal spot which would produce a similar failure of resolution'.

The typical split intensity distribution of a focus is due largely to the electron optics of focusing and, therefore, such a focus consists of two separate emitting areas. The resolution of such a focus is going to be less than if it were to have a uniformly emitting surface. The equivalent size, therefore, states the dimensions of a focal spot as if it were an homogenous focus. The equivalent size for such a split intensity distribution focus will be greater than that of the effective size of the same focus determined by the pin-hole method. In the case of a uniformly emitting, biased focus, as commonly used in macroradiography, the equivalent size will equal the effective size.

Some comparisons are presented in Table 15.4.

Table 15.4 Comparison of pin-hole and star phantom focal spot sizes. Measurement of focal spot sizes are only indicated following installation

Nominal size (mm)	Pinhole (mm)	$(FL \times FW)^{\frac{1}{2}}$ (mm)	Star phantom (mm)	$(FL \times FW)^{\frac{1}{2}}$ (mm)
0.6×0.6	0.80×0.65	0.72	0.92×0.88	0.91
1.2×1.2	1.75×1.25	1.48	2.12×1.60	1.84

Measurements may be made as required but experience has shown that none or little change in size occurs following installation.

Radiation quality

Of the factors influencing image contrast, the selection of kilovoltage is made by the radiographer. To ensure consistency of contrast it is important that the kilovoltage is as selected and does not change with time.

Historically, radiographers have selected beam quality in terms of kVp; this, however, is not the only factor affecting quality. Filtration, generator waveform and target material are additional factors. It is well reported that radiographers have to select different values of kVp in one room compared to another when conducting similar investigations. This latter point could also be due to incorrect calibration in that the same quality X-rays are not produced by different units for the same selected kVp.

One method used to measure beam quality is to determine the half-value thickness by placing aluminium filters in the beam. The disadvantage of this in terms of image quality is that radiographic results cannot be predicted. It is possible for different kVp values and filtration to produce beams with the same half-value layers but with the radiographic quality being dissimilar.

To overcome the above disadvantage penetrameter cassettes have been developed which give an indication of the 'effective kilovoltage'. The better known of these are the Ardran and Crooks penetrameter, the Wisconsin X-ray test cassette and the Sussex cassette.

This effective kilovoltage is sometimes referred to as constant potential equivalent and is defined as:

'that quality of radiation filtered to near homogeneity, such that it is of similar quality to the known reference beam.'

The test objective is to determine the calibration and consistency of kilovoltage calibration at selected mA stations. The cassette to be described here is an Ardran and Crookes GEC penetrameter. The cassette is based upon a modified X-ray film cassette and is shown in Figure 15.12(a) and (b). Its dimensions are 25 cm × 20 cm.

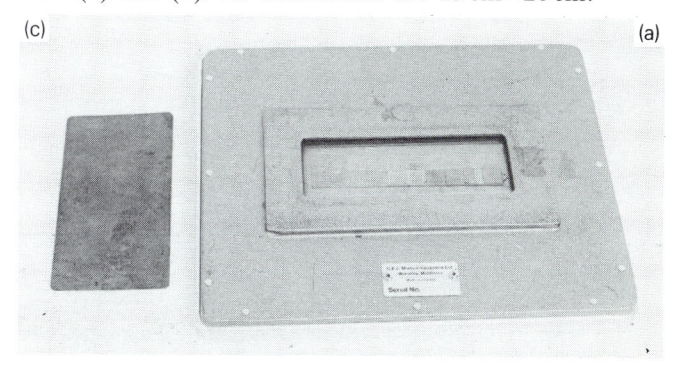

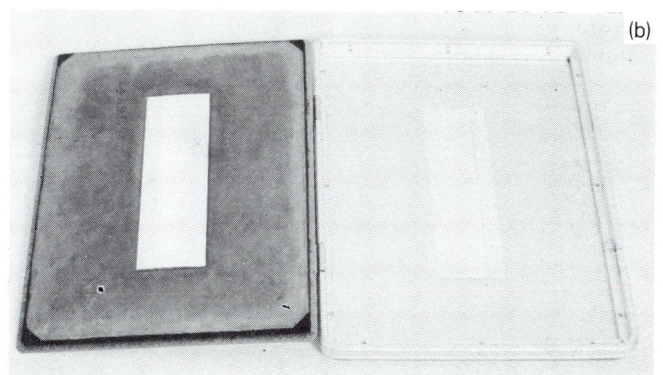

Figure 15.12 Ardran and Crookes GEC penetrameter. (a) closed (b) open (c) copper filter

The inner aspect of the tube side of the cassette is masked with a sheet of lead with four rows of adjacent parallel holes 5 mm in diameter and 10 mm apart. Below the two outer rows of holes are placed strips of high definition (slow) intensifying screens and beneath the two middle rows there are two strips of a fast intensifying screen. Above the two middle rows is the copper penetrameter. A cross-sectional diagram through the cassette demonstrates this arrangement (Figure 15.13).

When a film in the cassette is exposed to X-radiation the attenuation in the copper will reduce the densities

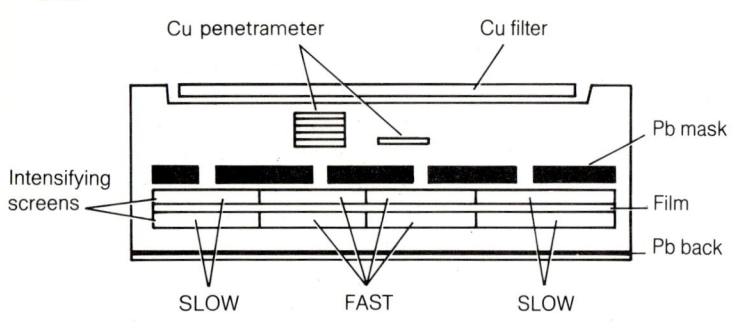

Figure 15.13 Cross-sectional diagram of Ardran and Crookes penetrameter

which decrease with increasing copper thickness. The image of the outer holes will be of similar density and provide a reference value. There should be a certain thickness of copper (copper reference number, CRN) that matches the outer reference densities and if the penetration of the beam (by increasing kVp) is increased then it follows that a greater thickness of copper is required to match the reference. By calibrating the cassette to beams of known kVp it is possible by densitometric analysis to establish the selected kVp's of other units.

The calibration procedure which may be undertaken at the National Physical Laboratory requires a series of exposures at known kVs and waveform type. The calibration curve is a graph of matching copper thickness (CRN) against kV (Figure 15.14).

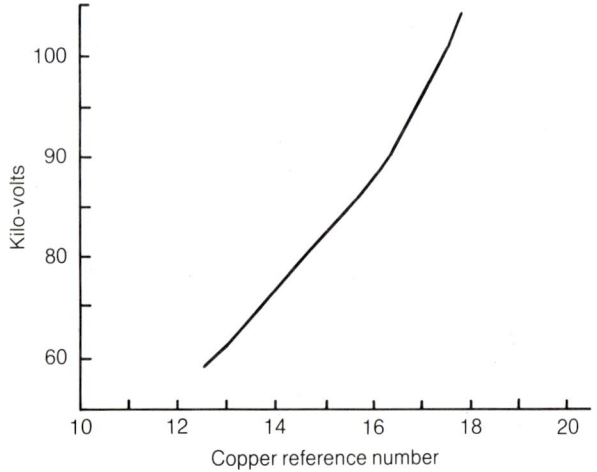

Figure 15.14 Calibration curve

The response of the penetrameter, i.e. the CRN for a given beam quality, is dependent upon the speed ratio of the intensifying screens, e.g. 4:1. The thickness of copper needed to reduce the radiation to $\frac{1}{4}$ of its original intensity is approximately the fourth value layer of copper and will be equivalent to the CRN, in which, alternatively, the cassette may be calibrated.

Screen speeds are not critically controlled and will vary with time; it is therefore recommended that cassettes are intermittently calibrated, say 2-yearly, for the first 4 years of their life. After this time experience has shown little change to occur.

When assessing kV values above 50 the 1.45 mm copper filter, as shown in Figure 15.12, is used. Its purpose is to filter low and medium energy parts of the X-ray beam making the penetrameter relatively insensitive to changes in voltage waveform.

The cassette, loaded with a conventional film is placed on the X-ray table with the long axis perpendicular to the anode–cathode axis. The light beam is collimated to the penetrameter. If the beam is set at 50 kV or more the copper filter is used.

An exposure is made at the selected kVp with sufficient mA s to produce an optical density on the reference steps between 0.5 and 1.0. The film is then processed in an automatic processor. The procedure is repeated for each kV setting to be assessed. A particular disadvantage of this cassette is that each exposure requires a different film and unavoidably takes time. Other cassettes enable a series of exposures to be made upon the same film. A typical radiograph is shown in Figure 15.15.

Note: The outer reference densities are similar whilst the densities under the penetrameter vary. The inner dot having the same density as the outer reference dot is the CRN whose value in terms of kV can be determined from the calibration curve.

Densitometric analysis is necessary for the exact match and it is very likely that reference and CRN densities will be dissimilar. The following example illustrates how the exact match is determined.

Example

CRN (step no.)	Optical density	Optical density of reference dot
14	1.32	1.10
15	1.06	1.10

The density of step 15 is subtracted from step 15. The difference between these steps is divided into the difference between step 14 and the reference density. The quotient plus the step number will give the exact match.

$$\therefore \text{CRN} = 14 + \left(\frac{1.32 - 1.10}{1:32 - 1.06}\right) = 14.8$$

There are no British or European specifications of performance. However, the following guidelines have been suggested[3].

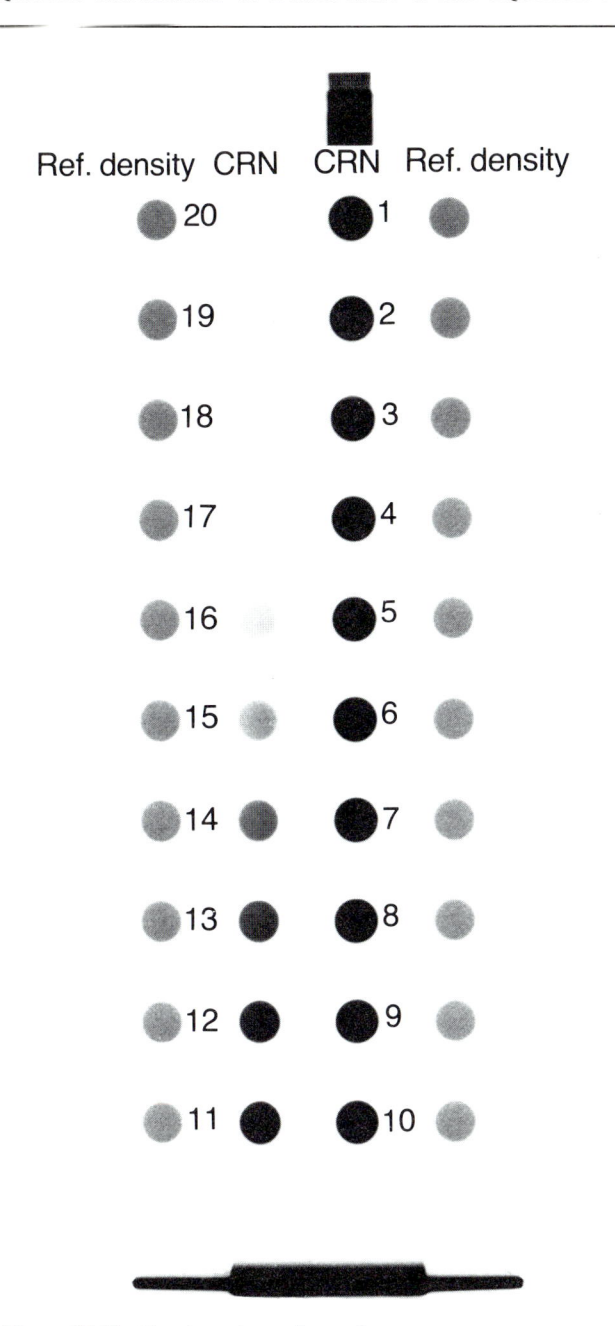

QUALITY ASSURANCE OF DIAGNOSTIC X-RAY EQUIPMENT

Figure 15.15 Penetrameter radiograph

(1) In the diagnostic range ±5 kV between penetrameter measurement and nominal (dial) kV is acceptable.
(2) A discrepancy of between 5 and 10 kV should be brought to the attention of the manufacturer.
(3) A discrepancy of 10 kV or more should be thoroughly investigated.

The reader should be aware that these tolerances are quite large. Consider two generators in adjacent rooms sharing a similar workload. Both are set at 60 kVp – one has a measured value of 65 kV, the other 55 kVp. Such a discrepancy is unacceptable and would require attention.

The American guidelines are more stringent where it is stated that a ±4 kV difference requires manufacturer's investigation[1].

Frequency of testing, following installation, should be at 3-monthly intervals, or following repair or servicing.

Exposure time

For a given tube voltage and current the quantity of radiation and hence the film blackening is controlled by altering the exposure time. Whilst a consistent percentage error throughout the time scale may be of little immediate worry, any inconsistency in the reproducibility of selected times can be disastrous. The consequence of such a situation is an increased probability in the reject film rate. The test objective, therefore, is not only to determine the accuracy of the set exposure but also its consistency.

The traditional method of checking exposure time has been with a 'free wheeling' spinning top. The top, in its simplest form, consists of a metal disc with a hole drilled near the circumference. This disc is mounted upon a pointed stem upon which it can be made to rotate.

In use the top is placed upon a cassette and rotated. A suitable kVp and mA are set plus the nominal exposure time, e.g. 0.1 s. During the exposure each pulse of radiation produces blackening upon the film according to the position of the hole. With a 50 Hz supply for 0.1 s there should be ten dots upon the film, whilst with half-wave rectification only five dots should appear.

When used with three-phase equipment, falling load or capacitor discharge units, a continuous band of blackening is produced. As the speed of rotation is unknown no attempt should be made to assess exposure time. This method is now for all practical purposes obsolete as other methods are much quicker and, in addition, suitable for use with three-phase units.

The problem pointed out above is overcome by using a motor-driven spinning top. In this device the spinning top is driven by a synchronous motor. The test tool should be fitted with a motor that produces one revolution of the disc in 1.0 s when used with a 50 Hz supply, otherwise a correction factor will need to be applied to measured exposure time. In use the test tool which is shown in Figure 15.16 is placed upon an X-ray cassette, switched on, and an exposure is made at the selected time.

Included within the test tool construction is a stepwedge, which allows any differences in film blackening at a given mAs and kVp to be noted. This allows not only the

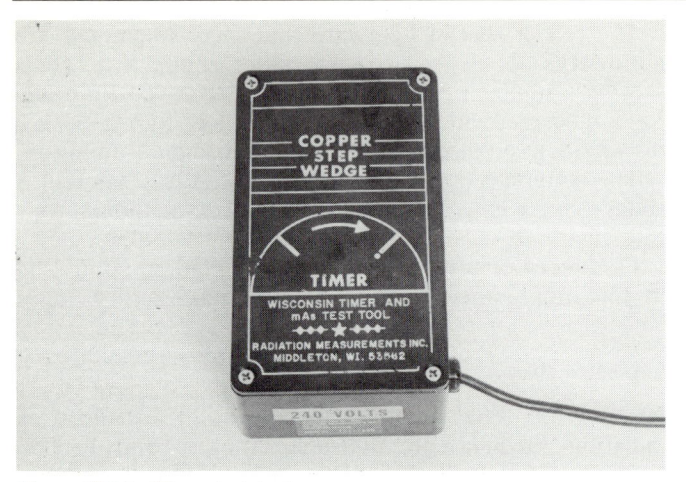

Figure 15.16 Timer test tool

consistency of factors to be checked but also the reciprocity between time and mA. Any discrepancy in film blackening may not just be due to an exposure time error, but may be due to discrepancies in kVp and/or mA values. Should this be the situation then further specific tests are indicated. However, in practice, because of the small number of steps and limited thickness this test is of limited value as it is very easy to overexpose and produce high optical densities when comparison becomes difficult. Typical radiographs are shown in Figure 15.17(a) and (b). Note the different appearance between a three-phase and single-phase unit.

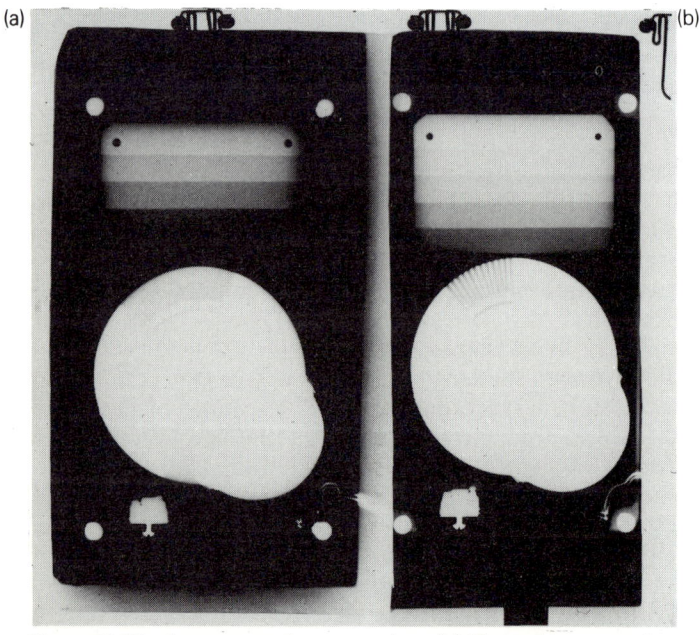

Figure 15.17 Assessment of exposure time. (a) Three-phase generator; (b) single phase generator

The exposure time is calculated from the following:

$$\text{Exposure time} = \left(\frac{\text{angle subtended by exposure arc}}{360°}\right) - 2°$$

360° is the number of degrees in one revolution or 1.0 s and 2° is equivalent to the width of the slit. Certain models are unsuitable for measuring exposure times greater than 1.0 s or for multisecond exposures where, for the latter amount, measurement of arc width is extremely difficult.

By far the most convenient method of assessing exposure time is to use a digital X-ray timer, of which there are a number commercially available. Typically, such units consist of a semi-conductor detector probe which is placed in the centre of the X-ray field. An exposure is made and the exposure duration may be read immediately in digital form. A wide range of exposure times may be checked quickly, both for accuracy and reproducibility. However, one word of warning is to avoid a too rapid rate of exposure or the tube may overheat and be permanently damaged.

In conjunction with a digital timer, a storage oscilloscope is a useful addition where the radiation output waveform with time may be displayed or inspected.

Once again there are no British performance specifications and the guidelines given below are those quoted in the American publication.[1]

(1) A given exposure time station should be reproducible within 5% or better.
(2) The accuracy of the indicated exposure time should be 5% or better for timer settings of 10 ms or greater.
(3) For times less than 10 ms, an accuracy of 20% is acceptable with the digital X-ray timer method.
(4) For single-phase units the actual number of exposure pulses must be equal to the expected number of pulses for times less than 0.1 s.
(5) For times greater than 0.1 s, an accuracy of ±1 pulse is acceptable.

It is suggested that frequency of testing be at 3-monthly periods following installation.

Tube output

The radiographer requires that, for given similar situations and techniques, the output of the X-ray tube and generator will remain consistent.

X-ray output in relation to nominal selected exposure factors may be measured with the aid of an ionization chamber and suitable dosemeter. A suitable combination is shown in Figure 15.18.

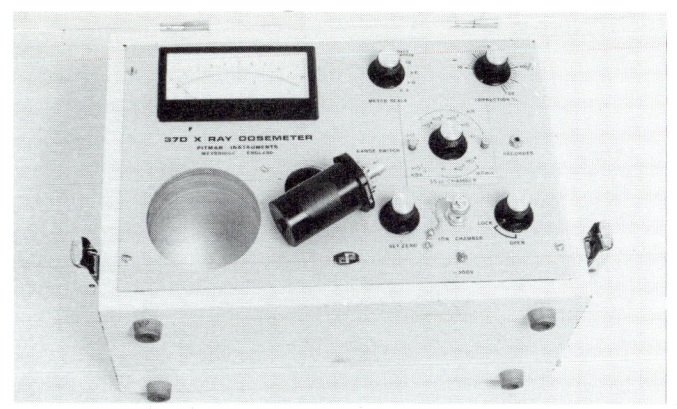

Figure 15.18 Dosemeter and ionization chamber

The relationship of exposure (mR) or tube output in mR/mA s can be measured for a range of selected factors. For example, a convenient method is to keep the mA and time constant but vary the kVp throughout the range. The mR/mA s plotted against kVp should produce a linear relationship.

For a given kVp, the above procedure should be repeated but, in the first instance, time is kept constant and mA is varied. Secondly, for a given kVp and mA, the exposure time is varied. There should be a linear increase in mR for both the mA and time variations, and the mR/mA s should remain constant.

Consistency of a single exposure can be checked by making four separate measurements with given factors. For example, 70 kVp, 0.1 s and excluding falling load operation, the mA value should be that which is commonly used, one with fine focus, the other with broad focus. A note of caution, once again, is to avoid overheating the tube with a rapid series of exposures. For all measurements the ionization chamber is placed at 100 cm from the tube focus.

There are no British standards for the performance specifications and at present measurements are used to ensure a unit's self-consistency.

Exposure measurements are extremely useful in practice and, provided that kVp and timer calibration have been confirmed by tests described earlier, non-linearity in exposure due to mA differences may be identified.

Indeed, following acceptance testing where a full assessment is undertaken, exposure measurements repeated after intervals of 5000 exposures can form the basis of routine monitoring where kVp and timer tests need not necessarily be undertaken unless a ±10% change in output is demonstrated.

CONCLUSION

In the preceding section, a protocol that may be adopted to monitor the performance of general X-ray equipment has been discussed. However, it must be noted that quality assurance is rather more than monitoring X-ray equipment performance.

A radiograph is produced after the radiographer has selected and manipulated components of an interdependent and integrated imaging system. A complete quality assurance programme must therefore take into account all facets of the imaging system. It is just not good enough to monitor X-ray equipment only and ignore other elements, e.g. processing conditions, darkroom lighting conditions and film screen content. Whilst faulty equipment may well be manifest as poor radiographs, so may other elements of the imaging chain and indeed may well produce similar effects as result from poor tube and generator performance. In practice, and in conjunction with assurance tests, a weekly reject film analysis should be undertaken from which it will be possible to categorize the causes of reject radiographs under headings such as exposure, technique, processing, etc. In the case of a suspected variation in performance of the X-ray tube and generator, further specific tests as outlined previously are then indicated.

The radiographer must have the key role in the equipment monitoring process. It is the radiographer who produces the radiograph and decides whether or not to accept or reject the film. The radiologist demands a high quality of radiographic performance, the radiographer must demand that the imaging system performs to its optimum. The only way to be assured of this is to monitor system performance on a regular basis. Costs and radiation dose are both reduced when the reject film rate is reduced.

Unfortunately, whilst there has been a great deal of interest shown in quality control there are not, as yet, any British or European regulations relating to performance characteristics. Without such regulations it is difficult to ensure that the performance of individual units is standardized. At best, all that can be achieved is that a single unit maintains a degree of self-consistency. Furthermore, without enforceable regulations, there are not any standard test methods and tools, and a certain degree of caution must be recommended when comparing test results of the same parameter, assessed by different test methods. There has, fortunately, been some movement in this direction and penetrameters, as previously indicated, can be calibrated at the National Physical Laboratory.

References
1. Hendee, W. R. and Rossi, R. P. (1979). *Quality Assurance for Radiographic X-ray Units and Associated Equipment.* US Dept. of Health Education and Welfare Publication (FPA) 79-80041
2. Henshaw, E. T. (ed.) (1976). *The Physics of Radiodiagnosis.* Scientific Report Series, 6. The Hospital Physicists Association. Revised Edn. ISBN 0 904 181 049
3. Topic Group Report 32 (1980). *Measurement of the Performance Characteristics of Diagnostic X-ray Systems Used in Medicine.* Part 1. X-Ray Tubes and Generators. The Hospital Physicists Association. ISBN 0 904 181 170

16
Ultrasound

V. CHALLEN

SOUND WAVES	180
LONGITUDINAL AND TRANSVERSE WAVES	180
RELATIONSHIP BETWEEN VELOCITY, WAVELENGTH AND FREQUENCY	181
Amplitude	181
Velocity	181
Wavelength and frequency	182
DISPLAYING THE RETURNING ECHOES	182
Types of real-time scanners	183
Mechanical method	183
Electrical method	183
ULTRASOUND PRODUCTION	184
PULSE–ECHO TECHNIQUE	184
RESOLUTION AND TRANSDUCERS	184
Axial resolution	184
Lateral resolution	184
TRANSDUCERS FOR SPECIAL PROCEDURES	185
IMAGING SEQUENCE	185
MEASUREMENTS IN THE POSTPROCESSING PHASE	186
DOPPLER	187
SAFETY OF ULTRASOUND	187

SOUND WAVES

Ultrasound is now well established as a valuable diagnostic tool. It has advantages in that it is a non-invasive technique, is free of X-radiation hazard and, as far as is known at the present, atraumatic.

What is meant by the term ultrasound? We all know what sound is, guitar strings, vocal cords, tuning forks, etc. emit sound when they vibrate. The vibrations of these objects produce vibrations of the molecules of the air that is then passed on from one molecule to the next and so on. The disturbance of the air causes the ear drum, the ossicles and the endolymph to vibrate on nerve endings which change these mechanical vibrations into electrical vibrations, which are then transmitted to the brain for interpretation.

The number of vibrations per second that a source of sound undergoes is termed its frequency, and is measured in hertz (Hz). Audible sound ranges in frequency from 30 Hz to 20 kHz. The prefix ultra in ultrasound means beyond or on the other side of, therefore ultrasound means sound beyond the audible range, i.e. any frequency above 20 kHz, although the majority of diagnostic ultrasound equipment will be found to operate in the 1–10 MHz range.

Using ultrasound to produce an image, i.e. seeing with sound, seems like a contradiction in terms. However, if we consider, as above, how the ear manages to convert mechanical vibrations into electrical vibrations, all we need is a piece of apparatus, the scanner, which does the same; one which converts ultrasound waves into electrical impulses which can be displayed in a number of different ways on a screen.

Ultrasonography is based on the principle of a pulse–echo technique. At a very basic level, a short pulse of ultrasound is directed through the skin of a patient and travels through the tissues until it reaches a reflecting surface, a so-called interface. Part of the beam will continue on through that surface, and part will be reflected as an echo back to the scanner. The scanner is then able to convert that reflected mechanical vibration into an electrical signal which can be shown either as a dot or a spike on an oscilloscope or video screen. The time taken for the echo to return can be estimated and, if we know the speed of the echo, the distance of the reflecting surface from the skin may be calculated too.

LONGITUDINAL AND TRANSVERSE WAVES

In radiography we are used to thinking in terms of electromagnetic waves which are *transverse* waves, i.e. the electromagnetic vibrations are at right angles to the direction of motion of the wave (Figure 16.1).

In ultrasound the waves are *longitudinal* (for the most part). Each molecule vibrates to and fro along the same line as the direction of motion of the wave (Figure 16.2).

ULTRASOUND

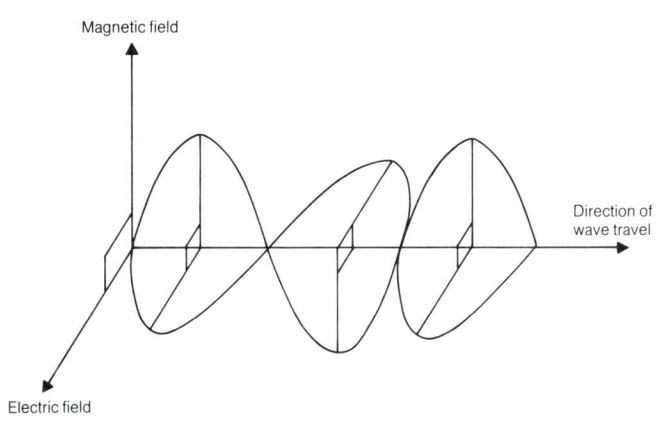

Figure 16.1 Electric and magnetic fields at right angles to each other and to the direction of wave travel

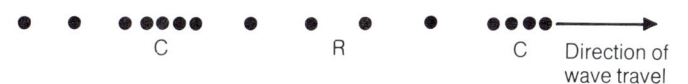

Figure 16.2 Molecules in air subject to regions of compression and rarefaction along the direction of wave travel

Motion of the molecules gives rise to regions of compressions (C) and rarefactions (R) and a longitudinal wave may be represented as a transverse wave in terms of a pressure difference at any moment in time (Figure 16.3).

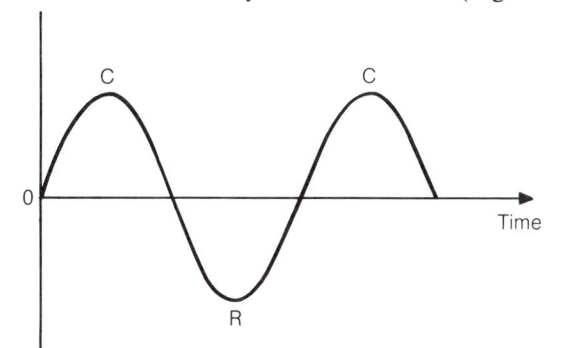

Figure 16.3 Waveform indicating compressions (C) and rarefactions (R)

RELATIONSHIP BETWEEN VELOCITY, WAVELENGTH AND FREQUENCY

In common with other types of waveform, the following features can be noted (Figure 16.4).

A – amplitude, i.e. the maximum change in the pressure from the average value (measured in decibels (dB))

V – velocity, i.e. the speed of the wave in the direction of travel (measured in metres/second (m/s))

λ – wavelength, i.e. the distance between similar points on the waveform (measured in millimetres (mm))

f – frequency, i.e. the number of vibrations per second (measured in megahertz (MHz))

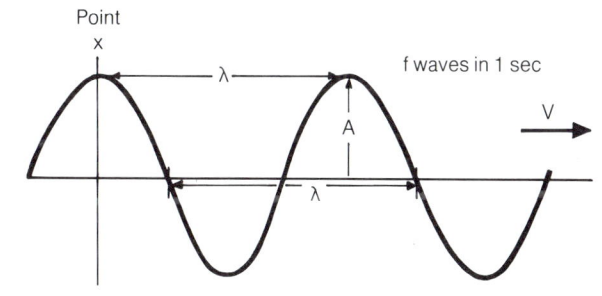

Figure 16.4 Features of a wave form

Velocity, wavelength and frequency are related by a simple expression. Consider from Figure 16.4 a point X past which sound waves are travelling. In one second f waves will pass X each with a wavelength of λ. The distance which the first wave past X will have travelled in one second will be $f \times \lambda$.

Therefore $V = f \times \lambda$

Amplitude

Amplitude or power of an ultrasound beam is synonymous with loudness of an audible sound. For convenience the amplitude of ultrasound echoes are measured in decibels. However, it must be realized that the decibel is not an absolute measure, merely a ratio between the amplitudes of two different sound waves.

Velocity

All electromagnetic waves, whatever their source, travel at the same velocity, i.e. the velocity of light which is approximately 3×10^8 m/s in a vacuum. The velocity of sound waves is variable and depends on the *density of material* through which the sound travels and the *temperature* of that material.

As the conduction of sound depends on the direct mechanical transmission of vibrations of molecules, sound cannot travel through a vacuum. Gases are poor conductors of sound as their density is low, i.e. the molecules are too far apart. Sound travels through air at 331 m/s.

Bone is also a poor conductor of sound as it is of high density; the molecules are unable to vibrate freely and therefore cannot transmit the vibrations efficiently. Sound travels through bone at approximately 4000 m/s.

Soft tissue structures of the body are of similar density, so the velocity is assumed to be constant for all soft tissue at normal body temperature. Sound travels through soft tissue at approx 1500 m/s.

The relationship between tissue density and velocity of sound is termed the acoustic impedance – which will be referred to again later.

Wavelength and frequency

On returning to the equation, $V = f \times \lambda$, we can deduce that the higher the frequency, the shorter the wavelength.

i.e. $$\lambda = \frac{V}{f}$$

e.g. if $V = 1500$ m/s, $f = 10$ MHz

$$\lambda = \frac{1500}{10 \times 10^6}$$

$$\lambda = 1.5 \times 10^{-4} \text{ m}$$

$$\lambda = 0.15 \text{ mm}$$

If $V = 1500$ m/s, $f = 3$ MHz, $\lambda = 0.5$ mm

As with light, the resolution that is obtained is dependent upon wavelength, so that better resolution can be obtained by employing higher frequencies. However, tissue attenuation increases with frequency and this limits the depth of tissue to be imaged. There must, therefore, in any examination be a compromise between the highest frequency for optimum resolution, and one which is low enough for adequate tissue penetration. Different frequency transducers are therefore available for differing parts of the body.

DISPLAYING THE RETURNING ECHOES

As previously mentioned, the returning echoes generate electrical impulses which may be displayed on screen in a variety of ways. The three different modes of display are referred to as A, B and M.

The size of the echo can be registered in terms of the amplitude of the deflection of a spike from a horizontal baseline – the so-called A-mode (Amplitude) mode. Here no attempt is made to produce an image. The echoes received, on being converted into an electrical signal, are amplified and then displayed on a cathode ray tube. The spot which forms the trace on the screen moves across to the right-hand side at a steady speed. The echoes produce a vertical spike on the trace corresponding to the returning echoes.

The *horizontal axis* represents the time taken for the echo to return – therefore the distance from the transducer to the reflecting surface (Figure 16.5).

The *vertical axis* corresponds to the strength of the echo.

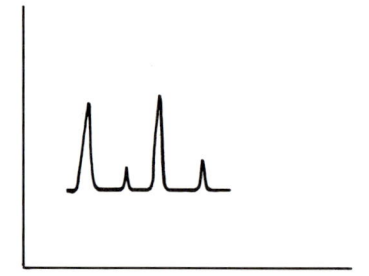

Figure 16.5 A-mode

A-scans are predominantly used to measure the distances between structures, e.g. midline structures of the brain.

Time position scans or M-mode (Motion) is a variation on the A-mode in that each spike is replaced on the baseline by a single bright dot, the degree of brightness indicating the strength of the echo (Figure 16.6).

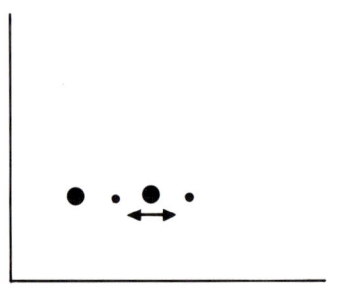

Figure 16.6 Bright spot replaces spike on A-mode. If a structure moves along the base line (◄─►) it will alter the position of the spot

If one of the returning echoes is from a moving structure, the position of the dot will move along the horizontal time base. If we also cause the horizontal time base with its line of dots to move from bottom to top of the screen, the result will be a display of straight lines indicating stationary structures and wavy lines indicating moving structures. The wavy lines show the position of the structures at any one moment in time.

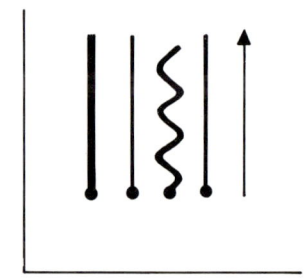

Figure 16.7 TP or M-mode

TP or M-scans are predominantly used to detect and demonstrate fetal heartbeat and the movement of heart valves (Figure 16.7).

B-mode (Brightness) forms the basis of a system which demonstrates pictorial images of two-dimensional cross-sections through the body. As with the M-scan the spikes of the A-mode are replaced by dots of varying brightness but instead of orientating the spots on a horizontal axis, the line of dots are orientated in the same direction as the transducer is positioned. When the transducer is moved along or across the patient's body an integrated image of all the stored signals is displayed, demonstrating a slice of the patient (Figure 16.8). The thickness of the slice will be related to the ultrasound beam width.

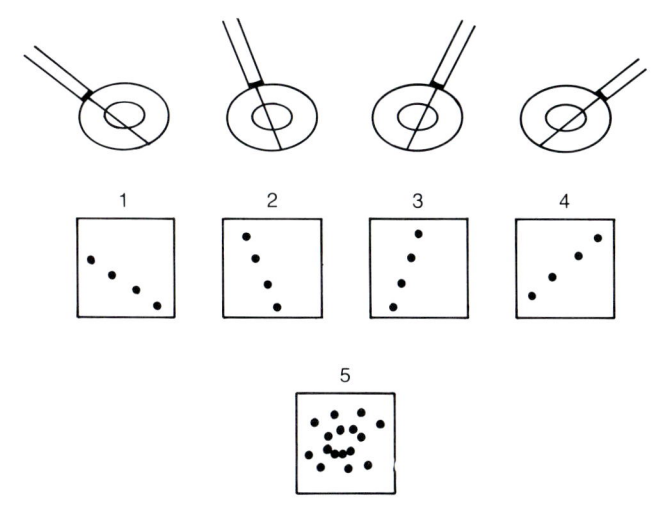

Figure 16.8 B-mode

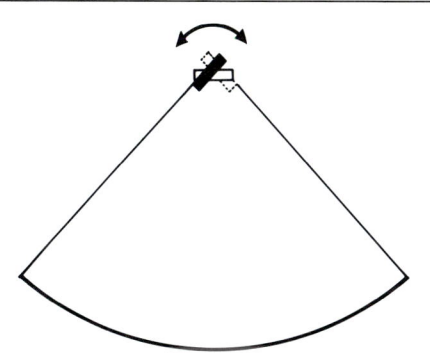

Figure 16.9 Oscillating transducer

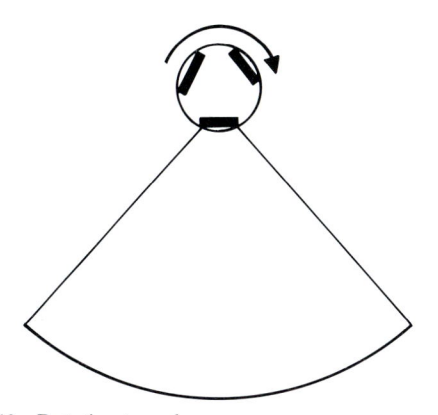

Figure 16.10 Rotating transducer

B-scans are predominantly used to demonstrate the abdominal and pelvic contents in the pregnant and non-pregnant patient.

Real-time is a term from the computer world and involves the processing of data as it arises and the provision of a current picture of events as they occur. Real-time scanners are essentially B-scanners with automated and speeded up transducer movement so that any movements within the field of scanning may be observed as and when they occur.

Types of real-time scanners

Mechanical method

(1) Oscillation of one transducer to produce a sector (Figure 16.9).
(2) Rotation of two or more transducers – also to produce a sector (Figure 16.10).

Manufacturers provide a fixed angle, e.g. 90° or 105°.

Electrical method

(1) Linear phased array consists of a row of up to as many as 400 thin transducer chips which are activated in sequence in groups of about five, in such a way as to create an electronic lens. The image produced will be rectangular rather than sector shaped (Figure 16.11).

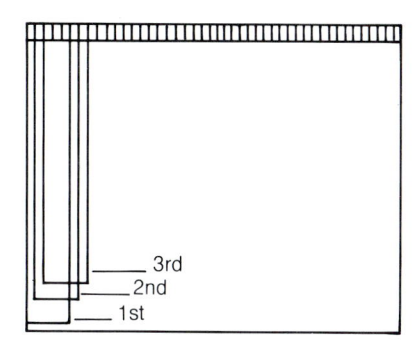

Figure 16.11 Linear array transducer. First pulse produced from activation of first five transducer chips, second pulse produced from activation of chips 2–6 and third from 3–7 and so on until all have been activated to produce a rectangular-shaped field

(2) Sector phased array consists of a row of about 20 small transducers. The activation of groups of transducer chips may be delayed in such a way as to cause an angled beam to be emitted and thus produce a sector-shaped image. Depending on the delay in activation sectors of differing angles are possible.

(3) Annual phased array consists of concentrically arranged rings of transducer elements rather like the annual rings on a tree trunk. Activation of the transducer elements creates an electronic lens and produces a very thin beam width.

ULTRASOUND PRODUCTION

Ultrasound is produced by an *electroacoustic transducer* employing the *piezo-electric effect*. The word transducer is derived from trans – meaning across, and duce – to lead. It therefore means a device which can lead across electric and sound fields; it is a two-way device which can convert an electrical signal into ultrasound and then ultrasound back into an electrical signal.

Piezo, from the Greek, means to press. Therefore, piezo-electric means pressure-electric effect. Some naturally occurring crystalline substances, e.g. quartz, exhibit this effect. When they are squeezed or pressure is applied they produce a small electrical potential. The returning echoes from the body squeeze or deform the crystal and in doing so generate minute alternating voltages which can be amplified and recorded and displayed in a variety of formats, e.g. as a spike in A-mode or as a bright dot in B-mode.

Conversely, when a potential difference is applied to the crystal it becomes squeezed or deformed and in doing so generates a small pressure wave – the ultrasound pulse.

Ultrasound transducers make use of an artificially produced ceramic called lead zinronate titanate (PZT) which if heated may lose its properties. It is important, therefore, that transducers, if required to be sterilized, should be made so by means other than heat sterilization, e.g. gas sterilization. Care should also be taken not to drop or in any other way cause mechanical damage to the transducer as the ceramic crystals are very sensitive to shocks.

PULSE–ECHO TECHNIQUE

An ulstrasound wave on reaching an interface with a medium of different acoustic properties may be reflected or refracted in the same manner as the behaviour of light at the junction of materials having different refractive indices.

The degree of reflection and refraction is determined by the incident angle at which the sound wave reaches the interface and by the difference in the *acoustic impedance* between the two media involved.

The acoustic impedance (Z) of a particular tissue is a product of the velocity of sound in that tissue (C) and the density of the medium (ϱ).

$$Z = C \times \varrho$$

When a sound wave crosses an interface between soft tissue structures, only a small proportion of the sound is reflected, the remainder carries on through the tissue until it reaches another interface. As the velocity of sound in most soft tissue is nearly constant, the only factor altering the acoustic impedance is the density of the tissue. If the difference in both speed of sound and density of the material is great, most of the sound will be reflected – thus effectively acting as a barrier to the sound. Bone has a high acoustic impedance in comparison with soft tissue, and therefore most of the wave is reflected, and structures beyond cannot be imaged; air has a low acoustic impedance in comparison with soft tissue, thus also causing most of the incident sound beam to be reflected. This latter feature illuminates the need for the use of a coupling medium between the transducer and skin surface to avoid the trapping of air between the two. It also emphasizes the problems that may arise in imaging an abdomen which is full of bowel gas.

RESOLUTION AND TRANSDUCERS

The ability of an ultrasound scanner to separate two structures which are very close together is called resolving power or simply resolution. The two types of resolution in ultrasound are axial and lateral.

Axial resolution

This is the ability to separate two structures or interfaces which lie in the path of the beam and this ability is dependent mainly on the wavelength of the ultrasound pulse. Pulse length may be controlled at the transducer by either physical damping of the crystal (by the use of a backing block composed of tungsten embedded in plastic) or by electronic damping of the crystal (by reversal of the polarity of the crystal to arrest vibration) in order to produce a single wavelength of sound.

Lateral resolution

This is the ability to separate two structures which lie across the beam and is dependent on the width of the beam. If two structures are closer together than the width of the beam only a single echo will be produced and two separate structures will not be resolved. The ideal is therefore to produce a very narrow beam width.

Because ultrasound is a wave, the waves spread out when passing through an opening; the effect is termed diffraction. In general the spread increases as the width of the opening decreases, thus decreasing the width of a transducer in order to produce a narrow beam would have the reverse effect from that desired (Figure 16.12).

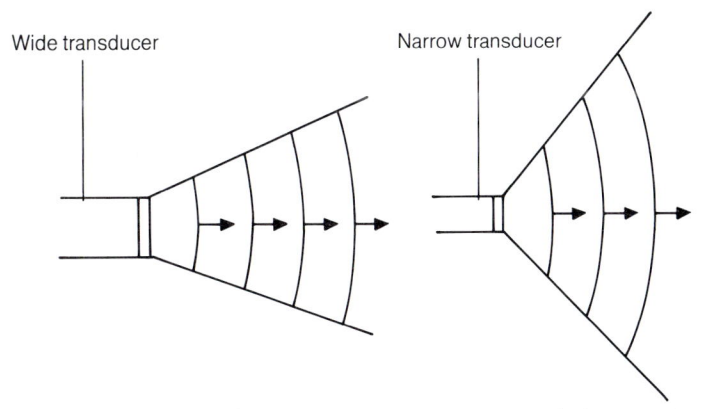

Figure 16.12 Diffraction of a sound beam. In general the spread increases as the width of the opening decreases

This problem may be overcome by focusing the beam either by the use of an acoustic lens or by the use of a concave transducer (Figure 16.13).

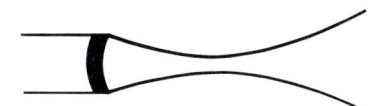

Figure 16.13 Use of concave transducer to narrow the beam

Spreading of the beam will still occur due to diffraction but the focusing effect reduces the beam width to an acceptable level at an appropriate distance from the transducer producing a particular focal zone for that transducer.

Note: It is not possible to focus the beam very close to the transducer head.

In linear array scanners focusing of the beam is accomplished by the creation of an 'electronic lens'. This is achieved by varying the time at which individual chips are activated. It allows for a variation in the focal zone to be made, so that focusing can be achieved in the near, middle or far field through electronic manipulation.

A further dynamic focusing is also possible. Here focusing is continuous in that the focal zone automatically follows the sound pulse as it travels through the body so that the transducer is always focused at the depth from which the echo is being received – thus optimizing the resolution at all depths within the image.

TRANSDUCERS FOR SPECIAL PROCEDURES

A wide variety of transducers are available, in addition to standard transducers, in all shapes, sizes and frequencies, depending on their particular application.

(1) *Minute* transducers which can be attached to probes or needles;
(2) *Rotating* transducers for insertion into body orifices;
(3) *High resolution* transducers for imaging structures of small dimension which may be near the surface of body;
(4) *Biopsy* transducers which are essentially the same as standard transducers with the addition of a central channel through which a biopsy needle can be passed.

IMAGING SEQUENCE (Figure 16.14)

(1) *Pulse–echo*. The pulse generator produces a focused beam from the selected transducers. Meanwhile, returning echoes from the patient are received by the transducer.

(2) *Preprocessing*. These returning echoes are small and need to be amplified. Because of the differential attenuation of the beam at different tissue depths, differential amplification of the echoes is required and provided for by a function referred to as TGC (time gain compensation). Gain is measured in decibels (dB).

   Near gain determines the gain of echoes returning from interfaces nearest the transducer.

   Slope determines the depth where near gain ends and the TGC ramp commences.

   Sloped rate controls the slope of the TGC ramp – the rate at which gain is added to the returning echoes dependent on their depth.

(3) The operator will have selected the display mode (A, B, M) and, once processed, the returning echo information is converted from analogue to digital form via the A/D (analogue-to-digital) converter.

(4) *Processing*. Once in digital form the echo information may be processed by computer and manipulated in a variety of ways.

(5) *Postprocessing*. Postprocessing is carried out in the image store but the effects are seen once the image is on the display system.

   The operator has several controls at his/her command – a few of which are referred to in Figure 18.14.

(6) In order to produce an image the digital signal is converted back into analogue form via the D/A converter.

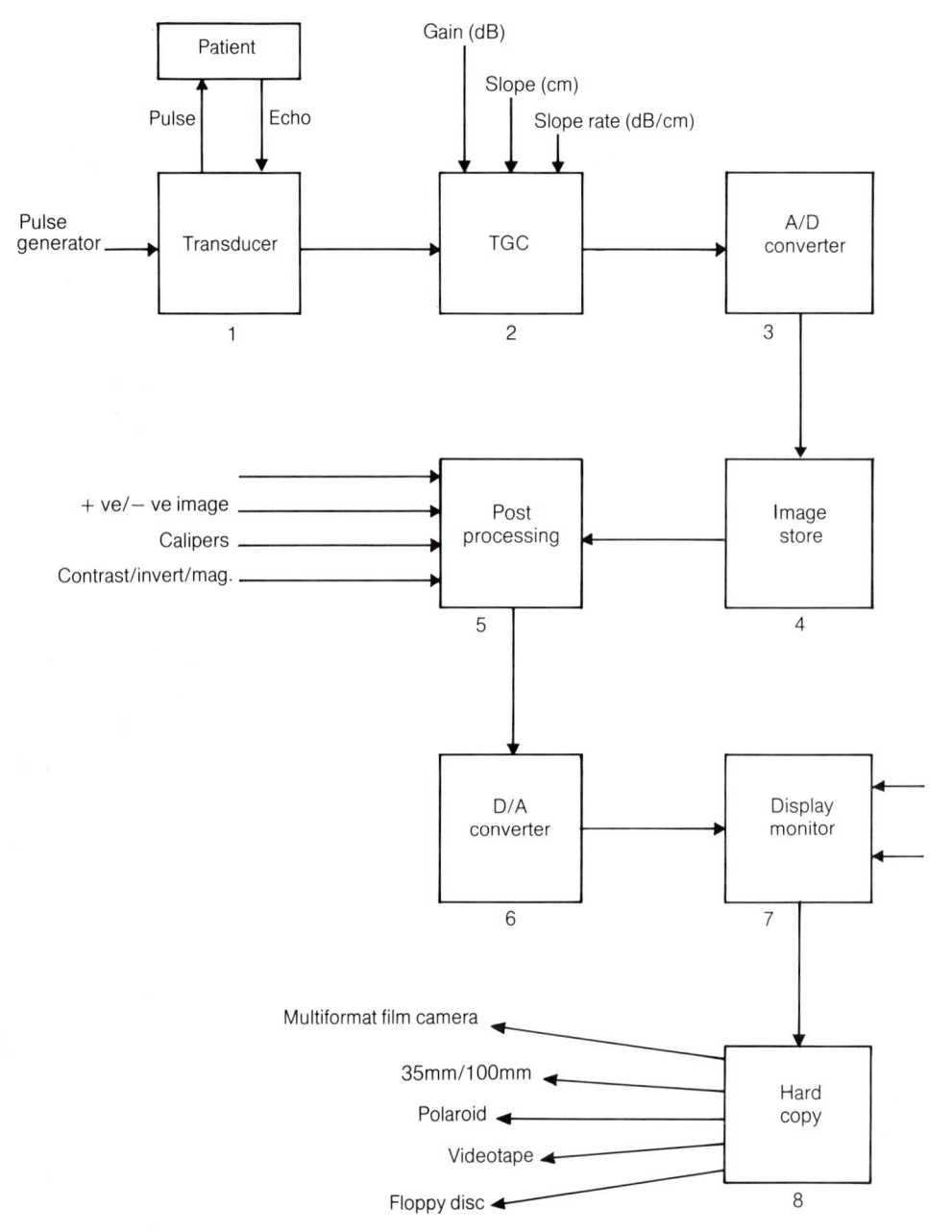

Figure 16.14 Imaging sequence

(7) The image is displayed on the screen of a video monitor. A freeze-frame facility is available in order for the operator to view and to take measurements from the still frame of a real-time scan.

(8) In order to obtain a permanent copy of the image displayed on the monitor, there is a wide choice of so-called hard copy available.

MEASUREMENTS IN THE POSTPROCESSING PHASE

The measurement of certain parameters within the image is important in both obstetric and non-obstetric applications of ultrasound. Measurements may be achieved by the use of electronic calipers. Here the operator places two dots on the image and the processor calculates the distance between the two; also by the use of a joy stick facility several dots may be placed, for example, around the fetal abdominal circumference and circumference area may be calculated by the processor.

A more accurate method of measurement is the use of a light pen caliper. Here the operator points the pen at the screen, a dot is generated indicating the starting point of the measurement and the pen is moved over the image tracing out the desired measurement. Many manufacturers provide, with this facility, not only a simultaneous read out of the desired measurement but also correspondingly related tables sometimes indicating upper and lower standard deviations of the particular measurement.

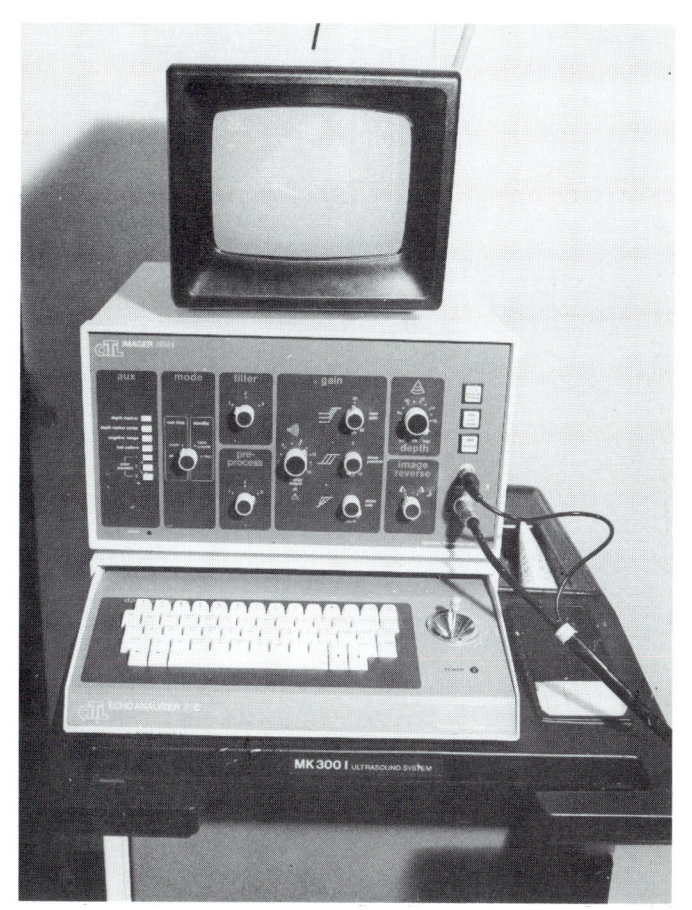

Figure 16.15 The aTL real time scanner

DOPPLER

The apparent change in frequency involved when there is relative motion between a source of sound and an observer along a line joining them is called the Doppler effect. We are all familiar with the drop in pitch of a police car siren as it sweeps past. A similar effect occurs in ultrasound where, if a structure in the body is subject to continuous sound, the returning signals will have an increased or decreased frequency depending on whether they are moving towards or away from the transducer.

A transducer for Doppler will differ from the pulse–echo technique transducer – as it will require a separate transmitter and receiving transducer since it will be transmitting continuously.

An example where this technique is used is in the detection of blood flow within veins and arteries.

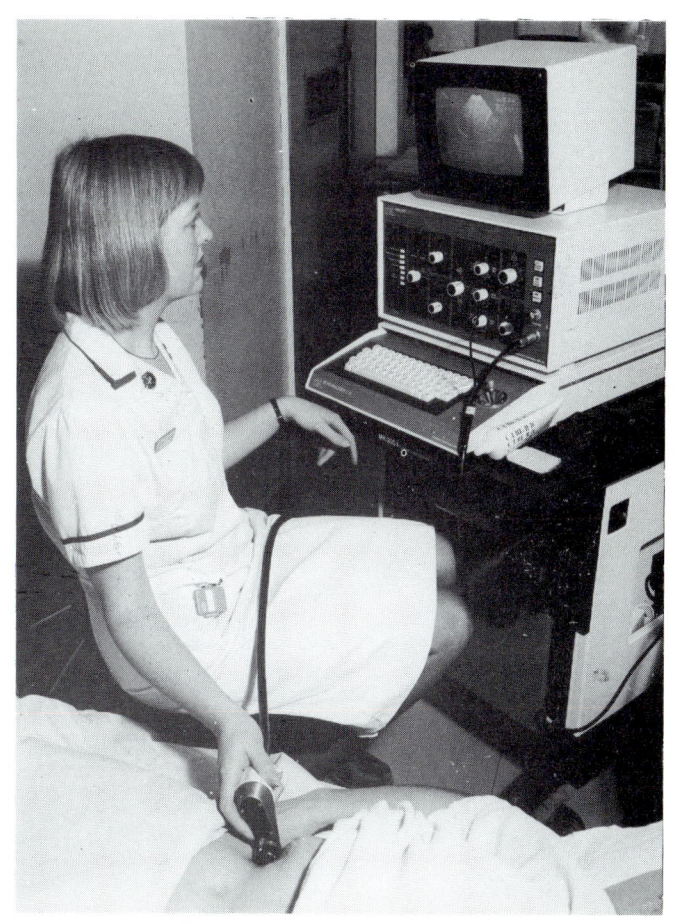

Figure 16.16 Radiographer scanning an abdomen

SAFETY OF ULTRASOUND

Very high intensity ultrasound has been found to produce physical effects within tissue through which it passes, i.e. cavitation (bubble) formation, temperature rise, mechanical stress. However, all these effects have only been found when power levels are several times greater than those used in medical diagnosis.

The power output (intensity level) of an ultrasound beam is measured in mW/cm² and according to the AIUM 1976 no adverse effects have ever been demonstrated in mammalian tissue at intensities less than 100 mW/cm². All commercially available ultrasound equipment has power outputs (acoustic intensity) at levels well below this figure.

One of the major safety factors for the pulse–echo technique of imaging is that the transducer is only emitting for about one thousandth of the time and listening for the remainder of the time for the returning echo.

Figure 16.17 Hand held transducer

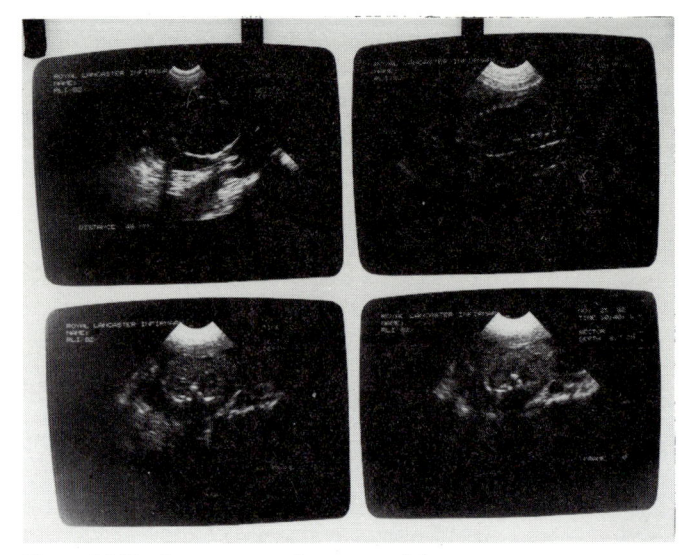

Figure 16.18 Sector scans of pregnant abdomen

17
Nuclear medicine
D. MANNING

INTRODUCTION	189
THE SCOPE OF NUCLEAR MEDICINE	189
Therapeutic nuclear medicine	189
Organ uptake measurements	189
Measurements on specimens	190
'In vitro' tests	190
Organ imaging	190
RADIONUCLIDES AND RADIOPHARMACEUTICALS	190
DETECTION DEVICES	191
Gas counters	191
Ionization chambers	191
Geiger-Müller counters	192
Scintillation detectors	192
Applications	193
GAMMA CAMERAS	193
Efficiency of gamma ray detection	193
Spatial resolution	194
The collimator	194
The photomulitplier array and positioning electronics	194
Temporal resolution	195
Energy resolution	195
Field uniformity	195
GAMMA CAMERAS FOR SPECIAL FUNCTIONS	196
Scanning gamma cameras	196
Tomographic cameras	196
APPLICATIONS OF NUCLEAR IMAGES	196
RADIATION HAZARDS	197
Dealing with spills	197

INTRODUCTION

Nuclear medicine is a general term that is used to describe a wide range of diagnostic and therapeutic techniques. The common cord that links these techniques is the use of radioactive materials. Furthermore, these radioactive materials that are used are in an unsealed state and can therefore be administered to patients or used to study body fluids in laboratory conditions.

In the late 1940s radioactive materials first became readily available and it was quickly seen that many of these could be incorporated into molecules for use in the biological sciences. The potential for studying organs and physiological systems as well as the treatment of some diseases was apparent and a whole new field of radiation medicine was opened. The speciality has continued to grow and diversify to the extent that there are specialities within nuclear medicine that attract the expert knowledge of physicists, biochemists, pharmacists, physiologists, haematologists and oncologists as well as radiologists and radiographers.

THE SCOPE OF NUCLEAR MEDICINE

As already indicated nuclear medicine is a very broad based speciality and it is beyond the scope of this book to cover its entire range in any detail. There are natural divisions to the subject that we may summarize, however (Table 17.1).

Table 17.1 Divisions within nuclear medicine

(1) Therapy
(2) Organ uptake measurements
(3) Measurements on specimens
(4) 'In vitro' tests
(5) Imaging

Therapeutic nuclear medicine

This has a limited but important role to play in the treatment of disease processes. The techniques involve the administration of a large radiation dose to a specific organ or site within the body by means of an unsealed radioactive source. The route taken by the radiopharmaceutical may be through a simple injection into a body cavity. This is the case in yttrium-90 colloid treatment of malignant effusions of the pleura. On the other hand, the biological pathway may be more complex as in the treatment of thyrotoxicosis or some carcinomas of the thyroid gland with oral iodine-131. In either event accurate radiation dosimetry is essential if the treatment is to be effective.

Organ uptake measurements

These tests involve the accurate, quantitative measurement of organ function by means of radiopharmaceuticals.

The range of this aspect of nuclear medicine is very wide and there is considerable overlap into the imaging division (Table 17.1). In fact, modern equipment allows for the simultaneous acquisition of both organ images and the quantitative measurement of their uptake in most cases. Examples range from quite simple functional studies of thyroid activity using radioiodine to the highly complex analysis of regional metabolic activity in the brain using a number of radio tracers including the positron-emitting radionuclides carbon-11 and oxygen-15.

Measurements on specimens

For the most part, measurements on specimens involve techniques more familiar to the medical laboratory scientist than to the radiographer. They all involve the administration of a known quantity of radioactive material to a patient and the subsequent collection of specimens of body fluids, tissues, blood, urine or faeces to study a physiological system. An example is the estimation of red cell survival time after labelling some of the patient's erythrocytes with chromium-51.

'In vitro' tests

These tests are unique in that no radioactivity is given to the patient. Instead the tests are carried out on body fluids – usually serum or plasma – which are taken from the patient and mixed with radionuclides 'in vitro' or 'in the test tube'. The field known as radioimmunoassay falls into this category and allows for the accurate measurement (assay) of tiny amounts of body hormones. It is a rapidly expanding field of nuclear medicine and has already realized much of its enormous potential in providing cheap, accurate and non-invasive diagnostic testing for a wide range of conditions.

Organ imaging

It is this aspect of nuclear medicine that most closely concerns the radiologist and radiographer. The principle behind all nuclear organ imaging techniques is that a quantity of radioactive material administered to a patient localizes in specific areas of the body. The specified areas of concentration are determined by the pharmaceutical form of the radionuclide and its route of administration. So, in the normal subject every radiopharmaceutical has a known biological pathway, distribution pattern and excretion route or routes which can be studied externally. The means of external study is firstly by detection of the radiation emitted from within the patient and then the conversion of this information into a visible image.

In the next section we shall consider some of the radioactive materials that can be administered to patients in order to study diseases by this method.

RADIONUCLIDES AND RADIOPHARMACEUTICALS

There is no doubt that a great number of the elements in the periodic table have isotopes that are radioactive. What is more, many of these materials can be produced artificially in nuclear reactors or particle accelerators. But only a very few are suitable for diagnostic use in nuclear medicine and especially in organ imaging techniques. The suitability of a radionuclide depends on a number of features which we could consider as being 'ideal' for diagnostic purposes. These are:

(1) Short half-life. By this, we mean the physical half-life of the radionuclide. It should be about twice the time required to complete the test, as a rough guide.

(2) Low energy gamma ray emission. Gamma rays in the energy range 100–250 keV are most suitable for external detection and present few problems in shielding and handling.

(3) No particle emissions. Alpha and beta particles are difficult to detect externally and give a very high local radiation absorbed dose to both handler and recipient.

(4) Low toxicity.

(5) Ready availability. Because of the preferred short half-life the material must be easily accessible, otherwise very large activities would have to be kept 'in stock'.

(6) Cheap.

A radionuclide which comes closest to fulfilling these requirements is technetium-99m ($^{99}Tc^m$) which is the daughter of the fission product molybdenum-99.

It has the following features:

Half-life – 6 hours,
Emission – pure gamma (140 keV), no particles, Generator produced from a molybdenum-99 source.

Technetium is a metal and would have limited use if it were not made into a variety of different compounds for organ localization. Any radionuclide which is compounded into a suitable form for patient administration is known as a radiopharmaceutical and Table 17.2 lists some of the common forms in which technetium is so made. Most of these radiopharmaceuticals are made up within the hospital by adding sterile $^{99}Tc^m$ pertechnetate to freeze-dried kits available commercially.

NUCLEAR MEDICINE

Table 17.2 Common pharmaceutical forms of technetium-99m

Radiopharmaceutical	Administered dose	Investigations
$^{99}Tc^m$ Sulphur colloid	90–400 MBq	Liver, spleen, bone marrow
$^{99}Tc^m$ Methylene diphosphorate	400–800 MBq	Bone
$^{99}Tc^m$ Albumen or red cells	400–800 MBq	Vascular flow
$^{99}Tc^m$ DTPA (Diethylenetriaminepentaacetic acid)	200–400 MBq	Renal function
$^{99}Tc^m$ Microspheres	90–180 MBq	Lung perfusion
$^{99}Tc^m$ Pertechnetate	90–580 MBq	Brain, thyroid, gastric mucosa

With its near ideal characteristics $^{99}Tc^m$ would appear to be the nuclide of choice for all imaging techniques. Unfortunately, there are times when radionuclides with less attractive features must be used because they are the only ones that will localize in the area of interest, or they are the only ones that will combine with an essential molecule in the pharmaceutical. Examples of these radiopharmaceuticals are:

Selenium-75 methionine	pancreas localization
Selenium-75 cholesterol	suprarenal cortex localization
Iodine-131 or Iodine-123	thyroid tissue
Gallium-67	tumour localization
Krypton-81m gas	pulmonary ventilation

Each of these materials has features which may not be ideal, but are entirely suitable for the task mentioned. Before leaving the topic of radionuclides and radiopharmaceuticals we should consider the factors involved in calculating the radiation dose to the patient and that the optimum (or best compromise) activity that can be administered for a given examination. Already mentioned are gamma ray energy, physical half-life, and particle emmissions as implicating factors. But when the radiopharmaceutical is injected, inhaled or swallowed it resides in the patient for a time that depends on the biological pathway into which it is incorporated. This time duration is described in terms of a *biological half-life* because of the exponential way in which excretion always occurs. The radiation absorbed dose to the patient will depend not only on the physical half-life of the radionuclide but also on the biological half-life of the pharmaceutical. In short, the radiation dose is calculated from the *effective* half-life of the radiopharmaceutical and is given by

$$\frac{1}{\text{Effective half-life}} = \frac{1}{\text{Biological half-life}} + \frac{1}{\text{Physical half-life}}$$

DETECTION DEVICES

It is the gamma rays emitted from radiopharmaceuticals that are most easily and efficiently detected by counting and imaging devices external to the patient. Detection of beta-particles is sometimes necessary in sample counting but equipment using the same principles is usually employed. There are two physical processes that lend themselves to this detection task: scintillation events and gas ionization.

Gas counters

When gases are irradiated they will ionize provided that the energy deposited in them is sufficiently high. For most gases, the energy necessary to produce an ion pair is about 30 eV; so for gamma rays in the range of energies used in nuclear medicine absorption results in an abundant supply of ions.

If the irradiated gas is subjected to an electric field the ions produced will be separated and collected, providing a means of both detecting and measuring the radiation. (Figure 17.1 illustrates the general principle behind gas detection of radiation.) The two main types of gas counters used in nuclear medicine are ionization chambers and Geiger–Müller counters.

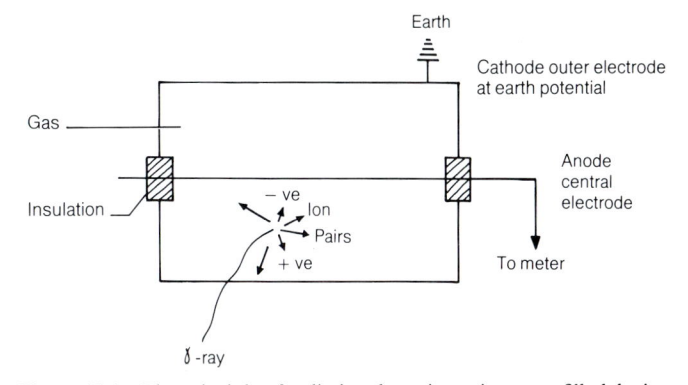

Figure 17.1 The principle of radiation detection using a gas-filled device

Ionization chambers

These generally use air as the gas producing ion pairs and can be used to measure exposure in roentgens (R). This makes them very suitable for use as radiation protection instruments. They also find application in the measurement of relatively high activity sources such as radiopharmaceuticals that have been drawn into syringes or vials before injection. When used for this purpose, it is more efficient for the chamber to be shaped in a similar way to the 'well-counter' type of scintillation device (Figure 17.4). These are then called re-entrant ionization chambers.

Geiger–Müller counters

These are very similar to ionization chambers in that they detect radiation by the ionization of gas and the collection of the ion pairs produced. However, the voltage between the collecting electrode and the 'cathode' wall is much higher. It is usually set at between 300 and 1500 v depending on the size of the tube and results in a multiplication in the number of ions collected. The multiplication comes about from collisions between the ion pairs produced initially and the atoms of the gas. Geiger–Müller tubes are used mostly for simple detection tasks rather than accurate measurements of quantity or energy. They find application as small hand-held contamination monitors in most nuclear medicine departments (Figure 17.2).

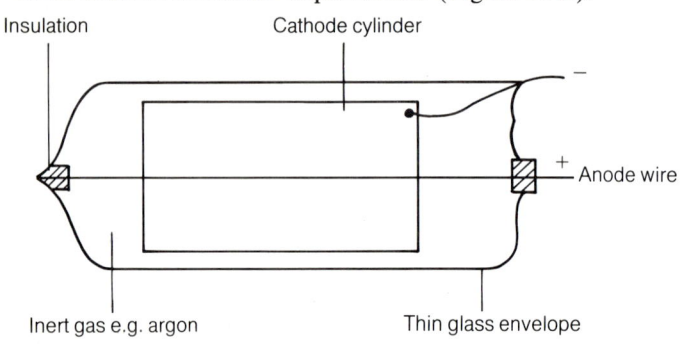

Figure 17.2 Basic construction of a simple Geiger–Müller tube. Note the use of inert gas at low pressure

Scintillation detectors

A number of materials emit a weak flash of visible light when they absorb energy from ionizing radiation. This is well known in the radiographic world where 'scintillators' in the form of fluoroscopic or intensifying screens are in common use. However, if the emitted light is converted into an electronic pulse the detection system becomes more flexible and quantitative. In fact, as the intensity of the light emitted is proportional to the energy absorbed in many scintillators, precise statements can be made about the energy of gamma rays detected from an analysis of the resulting light pulses. This is known as gamma ray spectroscopy.

The construction details of a simple scintillation detector are shown in Figure 17.3. The scintillator material most commonly used is NaI(Tl). This is crystalline sodium iodide which has added to it a small amount (about 0.1%) of thallium (Tl) as an impurity. The impurity 'doping' is found to increase the efficiency of light output from such crystals.

The instrument works by the emission of a flash of light from the NaI(Tl) crystal when a gamma ray photon undergoes attenuation. This light is converted into a num-

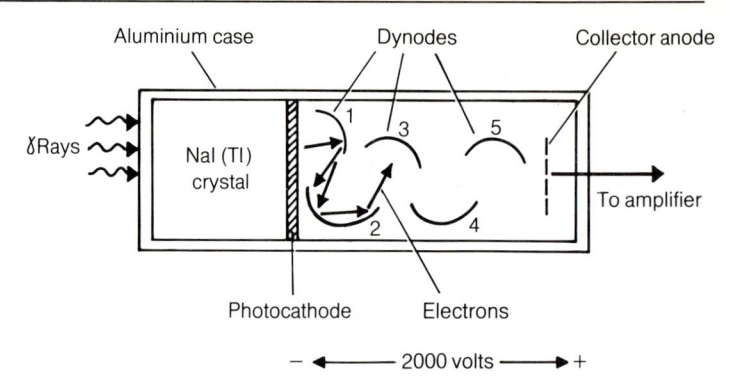

Figure 17.3 A simple scintillation counter and photomultiplier. Not all the dynodes hve been shown

ber of low energy electrons at the photocathode end of the photomultiplier. The photocathode is made of a bialkali material such as caesium–antimony and similar materials coat the dynodes (up to 13 in number) which are at progressively greater positive potential. Electrons from the photocathode are then accelerated from one dynode to the next along the photomultiplier chain dropping through a total potential difference of about 2000 V. Each dynode will emit two or three electrons for every one that strikes its surface and the accumulated 'gain' through the 13 stages can therefore be as high as 10^6.

The output from the photomultiplier can be fed to an amplifying circuit for use in powering rate meters, scalers or display units.

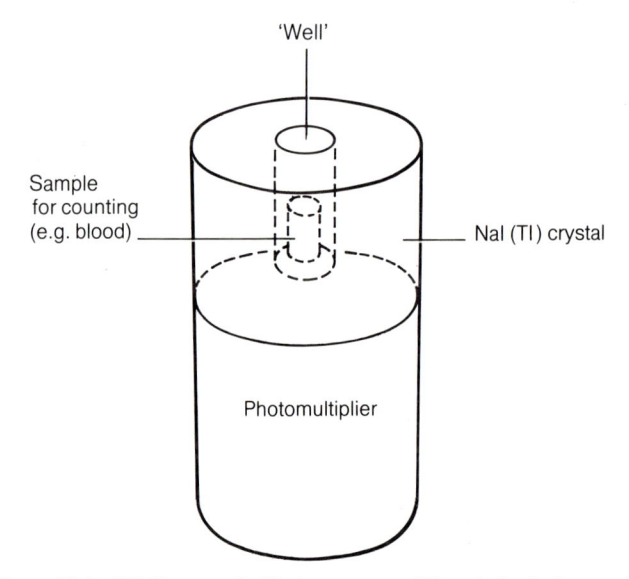

Figure 17.4 'Well'-type scintillation counter. The whole device would be enclosed in a lead-shielded compartment in actual use

NUCLEAR MEDICINE

Applications

Scintillation detectors are in widespread use in nuclear medicine. The shape and size of the detector crystal can be varied to suit the task in hand. For example a 'well-type' scintillator as shown in Figure 17.4 would be very efficient at counting the activity of small samples of blood plasma, CSF, urine, etc.

The detector can also be made very small, light and portable for use as a contamination monitor and dose-rate meter.

Alternatively, very large scintillation detectors can be made which provide the user with an image of the regional distribution of radioactivity in the field of view. These are known as gamma cameras and will be discussed in the next section.

GAMMA CAMERAS

Since its development in the 1950s, the gamma camera has evolved to become the principle method by which radionuclide images are formed. An analysis of the task of producing these images provides a clear indication of the operating requirements of a gamma camera.

(1) Radioactive concentrations within the patient emit gamma rays.

(2) These gamma rays must be detected efficiently.

(3) The origin (source) of the gamma radiation must be accurately determined (spatial resolution).

(4) The time at which the source was detected must also be accurately determined (temporal resolution).

(5) All other radiations must be excluded from the detection events (energy resolution).

(6) The gamma camera detection field must be uniformly sensitive.

Modern devices which are required to perform static, dynamic and even tomographic examinations take account of all these factors in their operating process (Figure 17.5).

Efficiency of gamma ray detection

Although other detection materials have been used in gamma cameras, thallium activated NaI crystals are the detectors in all commercially available models. From the point of view of spatial resolution the crystal should be as thin as reasonably possible to avoid geometric losses between the crystal and photomultiplier tubes. At the same time if the crystal is too thin, it will be a poor absorber of gamma ray photons. The usual thickness is 1–1.5 cm which is a reasonable compromise for photon energies up to 200 keV. The efficiency of detection for any gamma camera is a parameter easily checked in a quality control programme. The usual method of performing this checking is to place a radioactive source of accurately known activity a fixed distance from the detector face and to count over a specified period – say 100 s. The sensitivity is then measured as the counts per second per megabecquerel of activity.

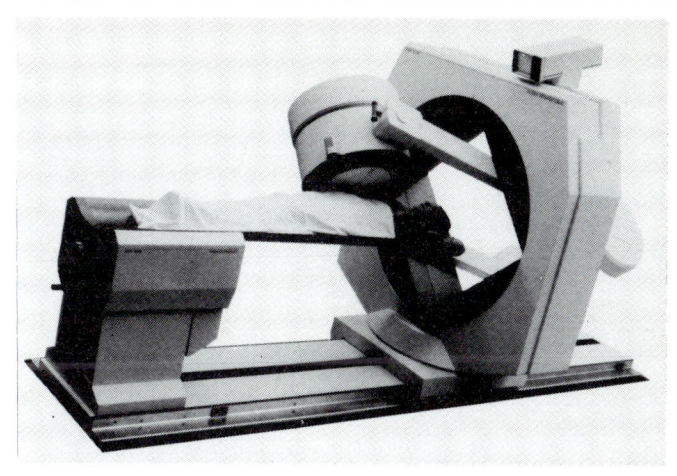

Figure 17.5(a) A gamma camera detector assembly with both scanning and rotating, single photon emission tomography (SPECT) facility
Photograph by kind permission of Picker International Ltd.

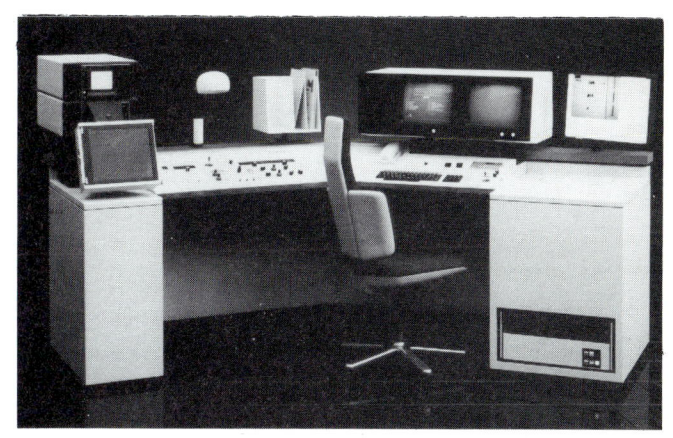

Figure 17.5(b) Gamma camera control console. Note that a computer display screen on the right hand side enables digitised information from the gamma camera to be displayed. The oscilloscope on the left has a persistent image for operator viewing and below it a 10"×8" compact recording camera produces permanent copies for a second, rapid fade oscilloscope.
Photograph by kind permission of Picker International Ltd.

194   EQUIPMENT FOR DIAGNOSTIC RADIOGRAPHY

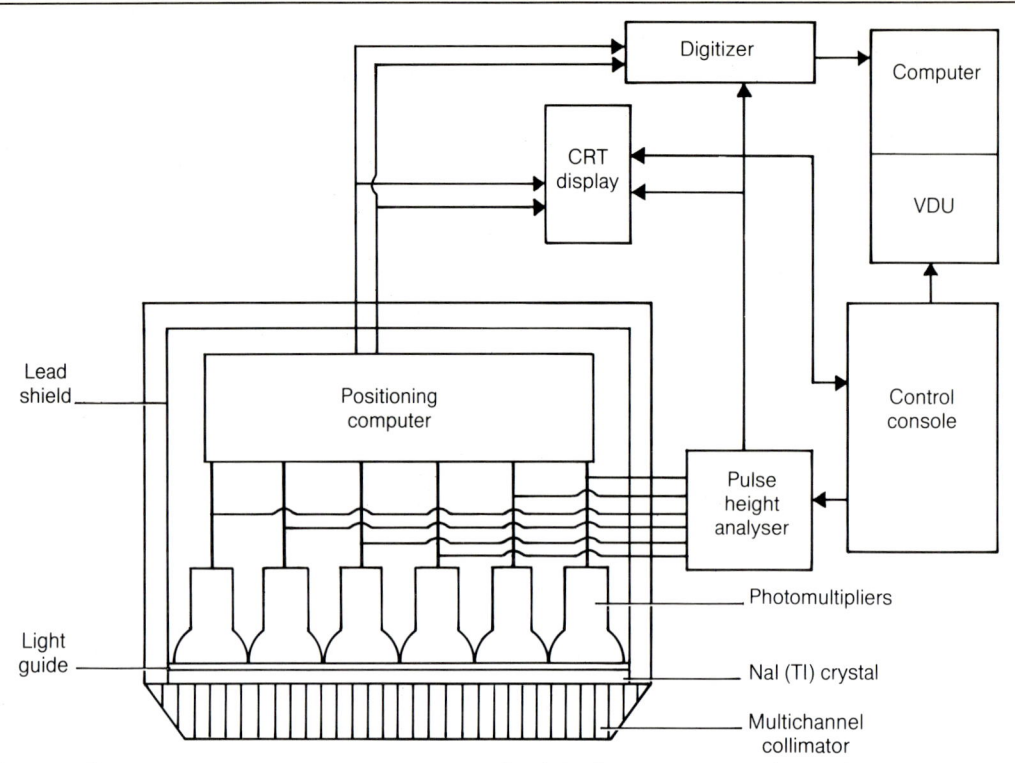

Figure 17.6 Block diagram of gamma camera head, display components and control systems

Spatial resolution

This is the ability of a gamma camera to determine with accuracy the position of a point source of radioactivity. It depends upon two major components of the gamma camera head shown in Figure 17.6.

The collimator

This is a multichannel device made, usually, of lead and often with parallel holes. Collimators for special functions have been developed with the holes divergent to cover a wider field of view, or conversely, to magnify images of small objects by convergence of the holes (Figure 17.7). In any event the function of a collimator is to provide an accurate correlation between the emission of a photon from the object source and the position of that photon striking the detector crystal. Only those photons that travel parallel to the collimator holes are allowed unattenuated passage to the crystal. In some respects the collimator uses the same methods as secondary radiation grids in diagnostic radiography.

The photomultiplier array and positioning electronics

Modern gamma cameras pack between 37 and 91 photomultiplier tubes, often circular but sometimes hexagonal, into

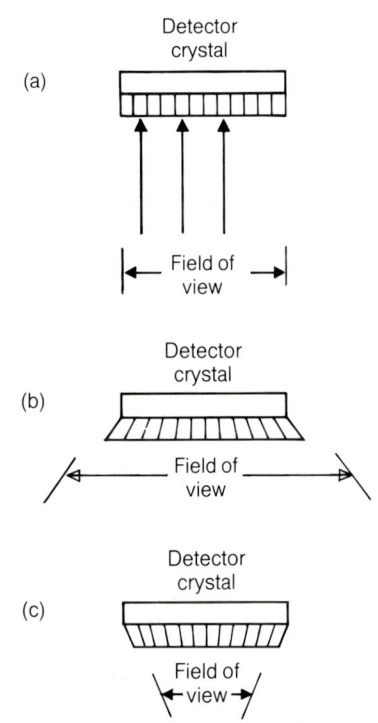

Figure 17.7 Gamma camera collimators: (a) parallel hole, (b) diverging, (c) converging

an array that covers the whole crystal detector surface. When a gamma ray photon is absorbed in the crystal the scintillation light is emitted isotropically. The light is detected by several nearby photomultipliers but the fraction seen by any one of them will be proportional to its distance from the event. Consequently, each tube will emit an electronic pulse in proportion to its proximity to the flash. These pulses are fed to a positional computer which calculates the scintillation position in terms of X and Y co-ordinates and also its brightness in terms of a Z or amplitude coordinate.

Good collimator design and digital computation of scintillation position have provided the user with high resolution gamma camera systems capable of detecting lesions as small as 5 mm diameter. Under routine use, the resolution of any gamma camera can vary from time to time and weekly resolution checks with a phantom are to be recommended (Figure 17.8). These checks could form part of a complete quality assurance programme for imaging departments as outlined in chapter 15. Quantitative measurements of spatial resolution should be carried out on acceptance of the equipment and require line spread function measurements using a multichannel analyser. Details of this and other tests are laid out in the DHSS Document *Performance Assessment of Gamma Cameras*, Part I, 1980.

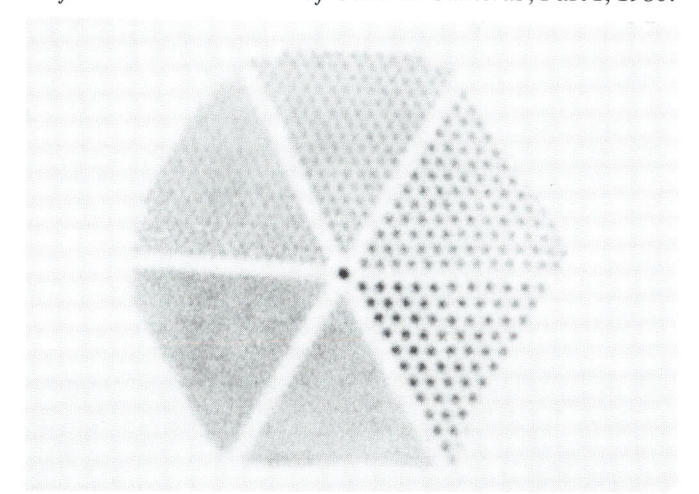

Figure 17.8 Image of a gamma camera resolution test object. This one is made of a lead sheet drilled with holes of varying spacing and is called a 'pie' phantom

Temporal resolution

The ability of a gamma camera to separate in time two scintillation events that occur in the crystal is called its temporal resolution. It is variable between different makes of instrument but is measured in terms of the number of counts per second that a camera can handle before a count-loss of 10% is experienced. A typical figure might be 30 000 counts per second and is derived from a plotted graph of counts/activity as in Figure 17.9. This is an important parameter in estimating how a gamma camera will perform in studies involving the fast movement of high activities of radionuclides in blood vessels (dynamic studies). These examinations have become a major part of radioisotope imaging.

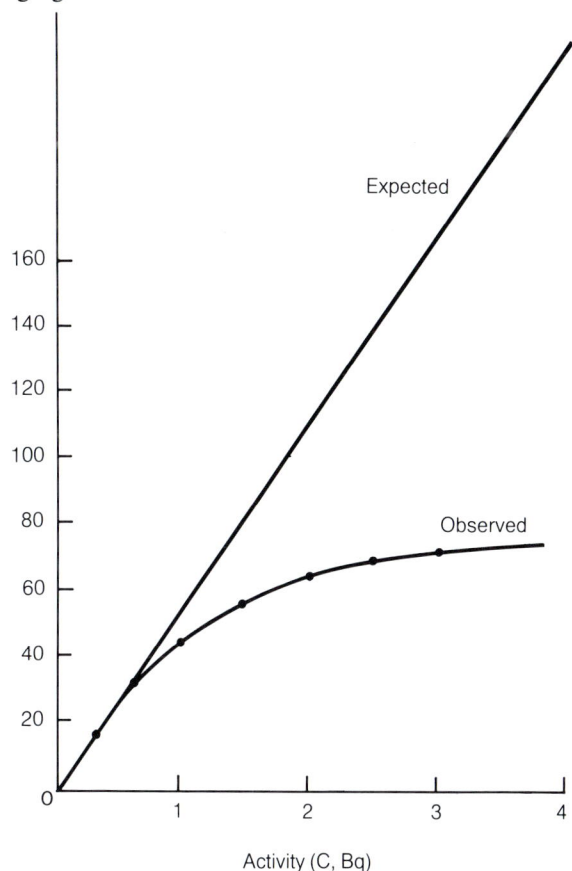

Figure 17.9 Temporal resolution. Typical curve of count-rate against activity in assessing count-rate performace of a gamma camera

Energy resolution

This feature of gamma cameras means that they can be used to detect any selected gamma ray energy at the exclusion of others. It is performed by the pulse height analyser (Figure 17.6) and functions by excluding background radiation from detection and in dual isotope imaging where two radionuclides of different energies might be injected in close succession.

Field uniformity

When all the photomultipliers in the detector array work at equal sensitivity, then the uniformity of the field of view of a gamma camera is at its maximum. Checks on this parameter should be daily routine and can be carried out with a uniform source of radioactivity large enough to cover the gamma camera field of view. Failure of field uniformity would provide images showing inaccurate representations of the spread of activity within an organ or system.

GAMMA CAMERAS FOR SPECIAL FUNCTIONS

Although we have considered only the basic instrument, gamma cameras can be constructed or modified in a number of ways to fulfil special requirements. The two most important ones are scanning gamma cameras and tomographic gamma cameras.

Scanning gamma cameras

Scanning versions of gamma cameras have evolved to meet the needs of certain examinations where large areas of the body are imaged. Typically, whole skeleton bone imaging is a technique that benefits from this type of device in reducing the examination time by a substantial amount. This is an important factor when one considers that many of the patients presenting for bone imaging are distressed by painful skeletal metastases.

Tomographic cameras

These special devices perform computerized tomography by detecting the emissions of radioactivity within the patient. The technique is therefore known as Emission Computerized Tomography (ECT) and is divided into two subtypes of imaging method.

The first method does not, strictly speaking, use a gamma camera in the way described. It uses two rotational detection devices to detect annihilation radiation emitted from a patient after the injection of a positron-emitting radionuclide. The technique is known as positron emission tomography (PET) and uses image reconstruction techniques similar to the methods of MRI and X-ray CT scanners.

The second method uses a rotating gamma camera in a circular or elliptical orbit around a patient injected with a gamma ray-emitting radionuclide. This technique is known as single photon emission tomography (SPECT) and produces sectional images of radioactive distributions.

APPLICATIONS OF NUCLEAR IMAGES

It is outside the scope of this book to provide a detailed breakdown of all the techniques of radionuclide imaging and how they are performed. But, it is useful to consider how nuclear medicine imaging compares with the other imaging methods available. It is a more difficult task than it might appear because when comparisons are made it becomes apparent that in most cases we are not comparing like with like. Generally, radiographic, X-ray CT, ultrasound and some MRI methods display anatomical details where nuclear scintigrams show physiological information. Furthermore, gamma camera devices are usually linked with microprocessors or minicomputers that will analyse the image data to produce functional information in graph form. In this context MRI and digital vascular imaging are aiming at similar goals to nuclear medicine in quantifying some features of the images they produce.

From the point of view of the patient's comfort, a radionuclide examination is less invasive, quicker (generally) and involves less risk than its radiographic equivalent. Radiation dose to the patient is usually at a level equivalent to or less than the radiographic examination of the same area (Tables 17.3 and 17.4) but there are two important differences. One is that the 'target organ' receiving the greatest dose is always the skin in radiography whereas in

Table 17.3 Representative values of radiation dose from diagnostic X-ray procedures

Examination	Absorbed dose per examination (grays)			
	Skin	Bone marrow (Mean)	Gonad (F = female)	Other organ (centre)
Skull (radiography)	14 mGy	0.4 mGy	0.01 mGy	Brain 2 mGy
Chest (radiography)	0.25 mGy	0.05 mGy	0.02 mGy	Lung 0.1 mGy
Abdomen (radiography)	14 mGy	1 mGy	2 mGy (F)	
Cholecystography (cholangiography)	30 mGy	1.5 mGy	1.5 mGy (F)	Liver 3 mGy

Table 17.4 Absorbed doses for various diagnostic nuclear medicine procedures

Nuclide	Form	Typical activity administered	Absorbed dose (gray per procedure)			
			Gonads	Marrow	Total body	Other
^{67}Ga	Gallium citrate	74 MBq	6 mGy	12 mGy	5 mGy	liver: 9 mGy
^{99}Tc^m	Pertechnetate	370 MBq	2 mGy	2 mGy	2 mGy	stomach wall: 25 mGy thyroid: 13 mGy
^{99}Tc^m	Sulphur colloid	74 MBq	0.2 mGy	0.6 mGy	0.2 mGy	liver: 7 mGy spleen: 4 mGy
^{131}I	Sodium iodide	7.4 kBq	0.1 mGy	0.1 mGy	0.1 mGy	thyroid: 260 mGy stomach wall: 0.3 mGy

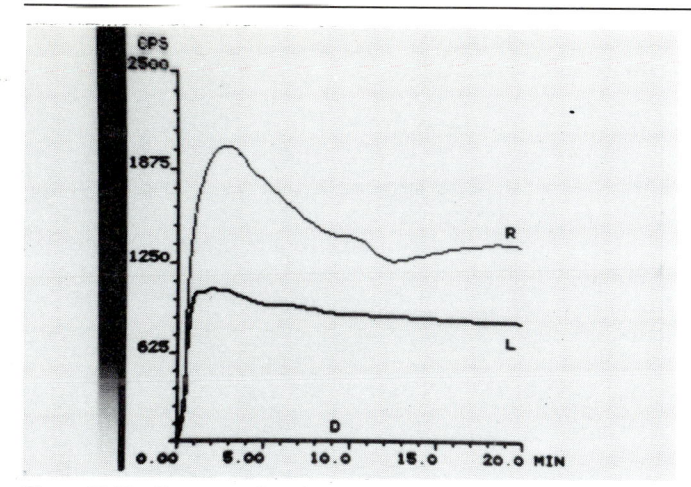

Figure 17.10 Renogram function curves for right and left kidneys. Note how activity is plotted against time by the gamma camera computer. The kidney is poorly functioning

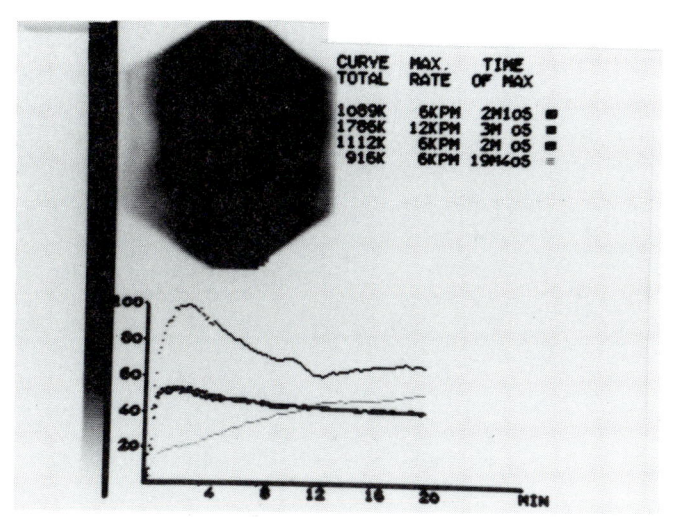

Figure 17.11 Gamma camera image and function curve of kidneys in a radioisotope renogram examination

nuclear medicine the 'target organ' varies with excretion route. The second difference is that in nuclear medicine the patient is himself a radiation source and should be regarded as such from the point of view of radiation protection.

The applications of radionuclide imaging seem to be ever widening but a great deal of attention is presently being paid to cardiovascular investigations. The use of PET and, more recently, SPECT techniques for looking at the heart wall and its dynamics is particularly topical. The full potential too of imaging with radionuclide labelled antibodies has not yet been realized and holds great promise in almost all disease investigations, but particularly in tumour detection. So the future for nuclear medicine looks very strong and we can expect it to play an increasingly powerful role in diagnostic organ imaging departments in the coming years.

RADIATION HAZARDS

Radiation problems and hazards in nuclear medicine are of a different nature to those encountered in dealings with X-radiation. Radiation from an X-ray tube can be turned off, it is directed at a target (the patient), and it is enclosed in a lead-lined container. Futhermore, radiation exposures are usually only performed when the personnel involved are behind a safety shield. None of these features applies to radionuclide radiation. The major hazard concerning radionuclides used in nuclear medicine is in the unsealed way in which they are handled.

Radioactive liquids and gases require careful intelligent handling if they are to be used safely, and as the prime risk is in contamination of personnel or the environment some simple rules are required:

(1) All drawing up into syringes must be carried out over a drip tray behind a protective barrier.

(2) Rubber gloves must always be worn when handling sources.

(3) Face masks reduce the risk of inhaled aerosol droplets or volatolized radioactive liquids.

(4) No eating, drinking or applications of cosmetics (especially lipstick) is allowed in a radionuclide laboratory or imaging room.

(5) Benchtops must be monitored at frequent intervals throughout the working day.

(6) Hands must be monitored after any handling procedure and washed thoroughly.

(7) Patients for imaging represent a 'leaking source' of radioactivity. Their urine, faeces, saliva and sweat is often a contamination hazard and should be treated as such.

With these points in mind, the risk of contamination and ingestion by personnel and other patients is minimized. This leaves only the problem of protection against primary radiation source. The source can be the radioactive sample before injection, within the syringe or after injection within the patient. In the case of the radiopharmaceutical before injection then lead shielding in pots before drawing up into lead-shielded syringes is a very efficient means of protection. But when the activity is within the patient a most effective reduction in personnel exposure can be

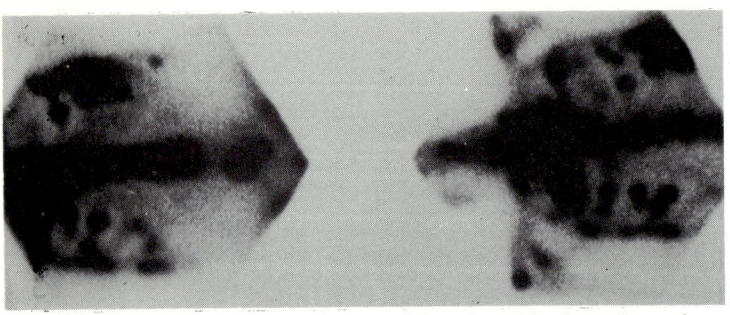

Figure 17.12 Gamma camera images of thoracic and lumbar spine and ribs after the injection of technetium-99 m labelled methylene diphosphonate. The patient is suffering from metastatic carcinoma of the prostate. Note the areas of increased radioactivity in the spine and ribs

achieved with a time and distance technique. Spending as little time as possible close to the patient will keep staff exposure (and that of other patients) to a very low level.

Dealing with spills

Finally, we should consider the procedures to adopt in the event of a spill of radioactivity within the hospital. For the most part, diagnostic doses of radioactivity do not constitute so great a risk as to be considered a 'major spill' in the event of an accident. The distinction between 'major spill' and 'minor spill' is not a clear-cut measurement of the activity involved, however, and a look at the Code of Practice for the Protection of Persons against Ionizing Radiations arising from Medical and Dental use will reveal that it depends also on the radionuclide involved and its physical state, i.e. liquid, solid or gas. A general figure to use is that if more then 3.7 GBq (wet) or one-tenth of this activity (dry) is spilled then an incident requiring implementation of prearranged procedures has occurred. In this event the Radiological Protection Adviser must be informed. Spills of lesser activity do not warrant any drastic emergency action but require only simple remedial action involving local staff and decontamination procedures. These procedures simply mean the cleaning and monitoring of the area concerned to prevent widespread radioactive contamination. In these circumstances many of the points listed in the simple rules for handling radionuclides will be the guide to action. As with all contaminated articles in nuclear medicine disposable items can be sealed in a paper bag appropriately marked and incinerated directly or held until their activity is below 1.1 MBq. Other items such as mops and buckets should be washed, monitored, labelled as contaminated and stored separately.

To put the radiation hazards into context, nuclear medicine procedures clearly involve a higher radiation dose to personnel than similar examinations using X-rays. But the risks are small indeed and with proper care it is possible to keep exposure down to a small fraction of the maximum permissible levels.

18
Computerized tomography

N. M. SPENCER

BACKGROUND	199
PLANNING A CT INSTALLATION	199
TYPES OF SCANNER	201
Comparison of third and fourth generation scanners	202
X-RAY TUBE	202
FILTRATION	203
PATIENT DOSE FROM CT SCANNING	203
VARIABLE GEOMETRY	203
SCANOGRAM	203
THE CT IMAGE	203
IMAGE COMPUTATION	204
RESOLUTION	204
WINDOW WIDTH AND LEVEL	204
IMAGE RECONSTRUCTIONS	205
STORAGE OF CT SCAN DATA	205
QUALITY ASSURANCE	206
SCANNING ANGLE	206
DETECTORS	206
CALIBRATION	206
EXPOSURE FACTORS	207
OPTIONAL FACILITIES	207
Dynamic scanning	207
ECG trigger	207
Radiotherapy planning	208
Independent consoles	208
Dual energy scanning	209
ADVANTAGES OF CT SCANNING	209

BACKGROUND

Computerized tomography (CT) units produce cross-sectional images by the use of narrow beams of X-radiation, a series of electronic dose measurement devices and a computer. The first units were produced in Britain by EMI Medical Ltd. in 1973 and were designed by G. N. Hounsfield. These units were slow and crude by modern standards and could only be used for scanning heads. The system was able to differentiate more efficiently than conventional radiography between areas in the head with differing X-ray attenuation coefficients, these areas being displayed as shades of grey-scale on a television monitor.

Modern CT units use the same basic principles but are able to produce more detailed images of any part of the body in a fraction of the time required by the early machines.

The basic components of a CT scanner are shown in Figure 18.1. The X-ray generator must be capable of producing an exceptionally well controlled output, so that tube voltage and current are consistent throughout the exposure. Some units produce radiation in pulses but even those that produce a continuous exposure normally have some form of secondary control to ensure a uniform output. This may consist of a high resistance potential divider to monitor the output voltage and high voltage triode valves to control it. The gantry houses the X-ray tube and detectors which send dose measurement readings to the central processing unit (CPU).

The CPU is often a commercial main-frame computer of a type used for a range of applications. It is usually directly linked to a hard disc, for the storage of software and data, and to an operator console, for the viewing and manipulating of images. The computer memory is limited and is most unlikely to be able to store more than a few days worth of images. For this reason some form of long-term storage of scan data is essential. Frequently scans are archived on magnetic tape, though some users prefer 'floppy discs' particularly for head scans. A multiformat camera is useful for producing permanent images on photographic film or paper. A photograph of the Picker CT System is to be seen in Figure 18.2(a).

PLANNING A CT INSTALLATION

Figure 18.3 is a typical layout for a CT installation though it should be modified to suit the space available, the manufacturers requirements and the type of workload

200 EQUIPMENT FOR DIAGNOSTIC RADIOGRAPHY

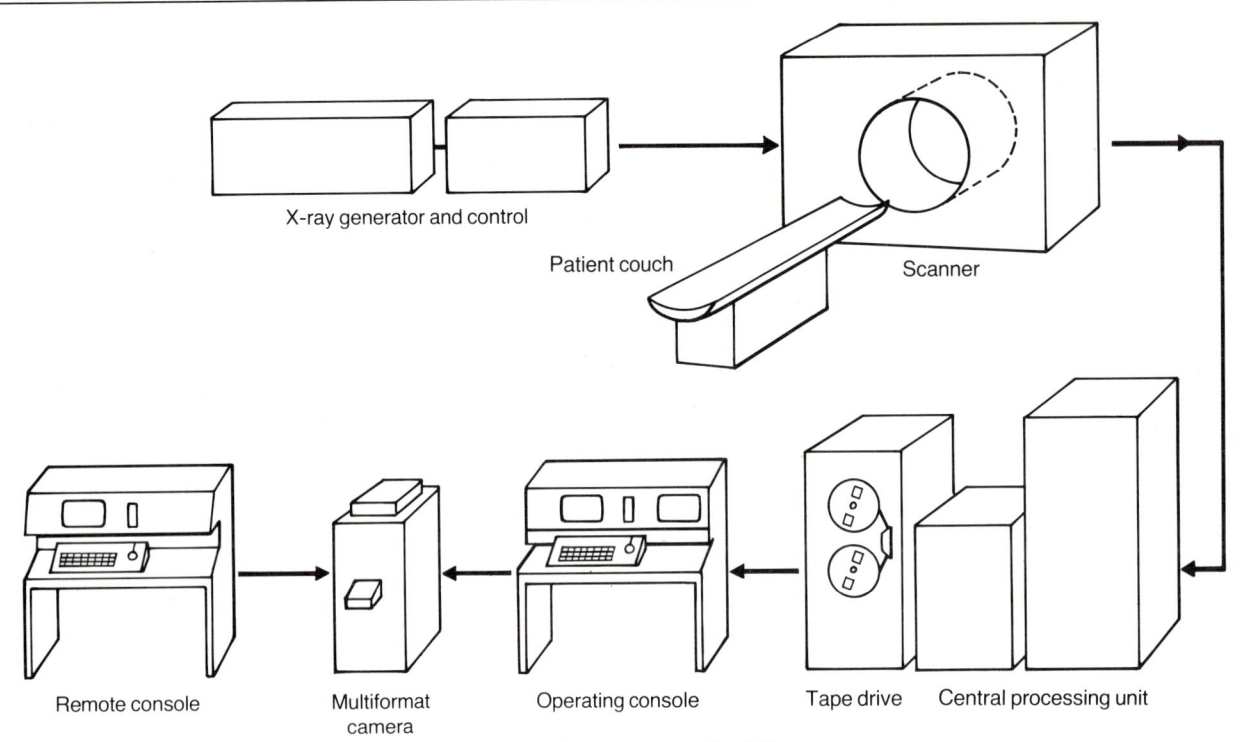

Figure 18.1 Basic components of a CT scanner

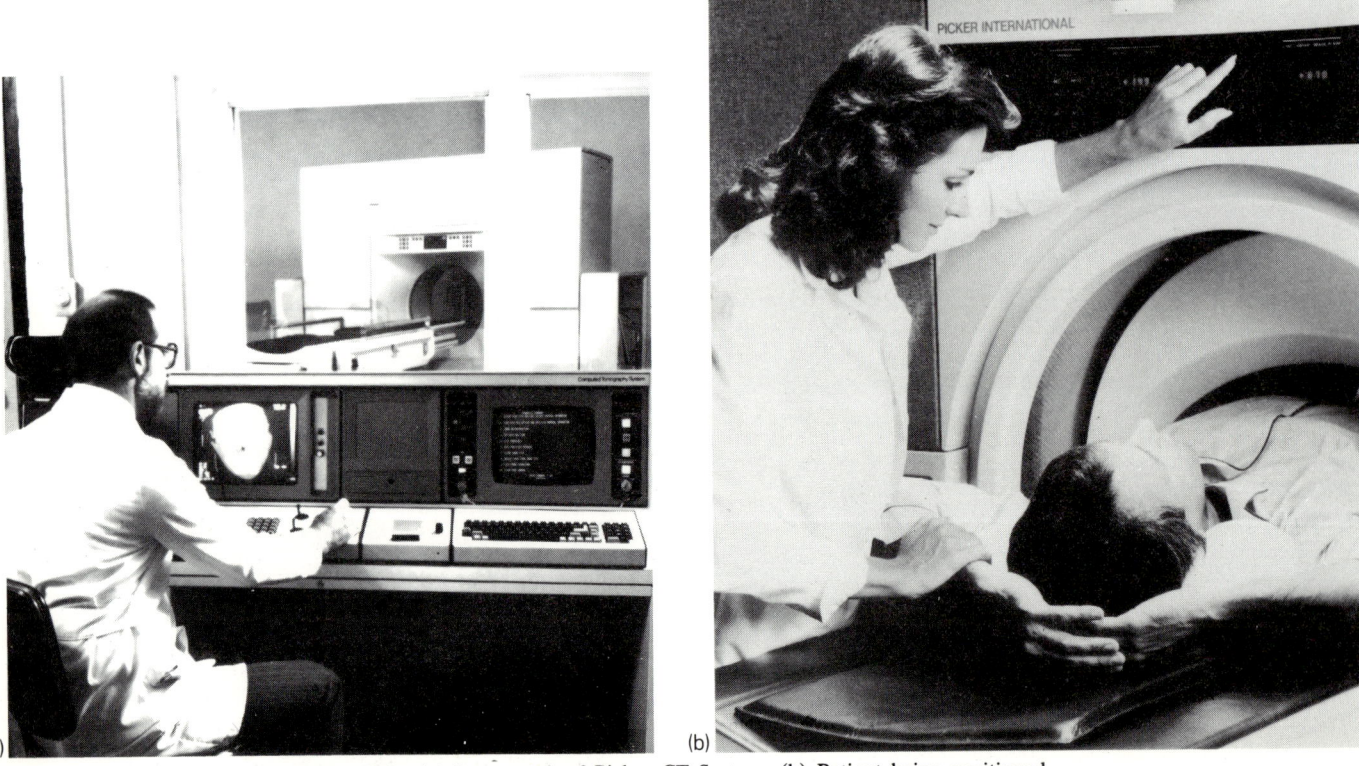

Figure 18.2 (a) Photograph of Picker CT System. (b) Patient being positioned

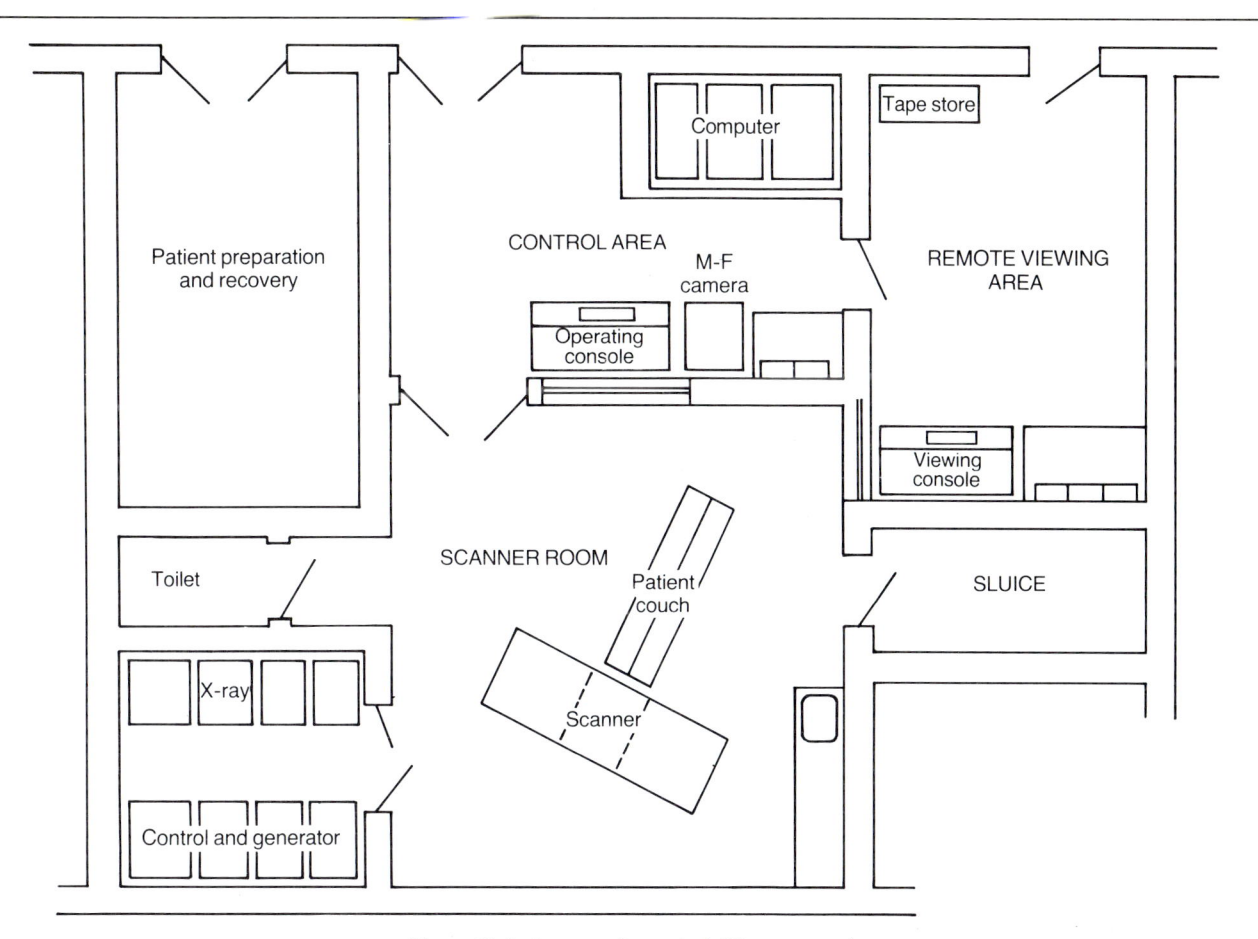

Figure 18.3 Layout of a typical CT scanner suite

envisaged, e.g. will some patients come to the CT room in their beds? If the CT suite is not adjacent to an X-ray department that already has those facilities, extra space will be required for patient waiting and preparation, film processing, storage of consumables and clerical support. Some thought must be given at an early stage to the location of the CT suite within the hospital complex. A typical scanner gantry is 2.2 m high, 3–4 m long, 1.5 m wide and weighs 2000 kg. Many hospital lifts, doorways and corridors are not designed for such heavy and bulky objects and this can create problems in delivering the scanner to its site. The gantry is arranged so that the operators can see through the aperture at an angle of approximately 15°. This enables them to see as much of the patient as possible. Some departments have found that a mirror positioned above the gantry enables the operators to see the further side.

It is usual for the manufacturer to require air conditioning in the computer area and the scanner room and a mains electricity supply that is free of 'spikes' (sudden temporary changes in voltage). As for any X-ray installation, the need for radiation protection must be considered.

TYPES OF SCANNER

The first scanners were of the 'translate/rotate' type (Figure 18.4). In these machines the X-ray tube and a single detector moved in parallel straight lines on either side of the object being scanned (translation). At the end of one movement the assembly would rotate through 1° and another parallel movement would follow. This process continued until sufficient dose measurements had been made. Since only one detector was used, the radiation was collimated to a narrow 'pencil beam' directed towards the detector. This first generation system was inherently slow and later second generation scanners had a number of detectors, but continued to 'translate/rotate'.

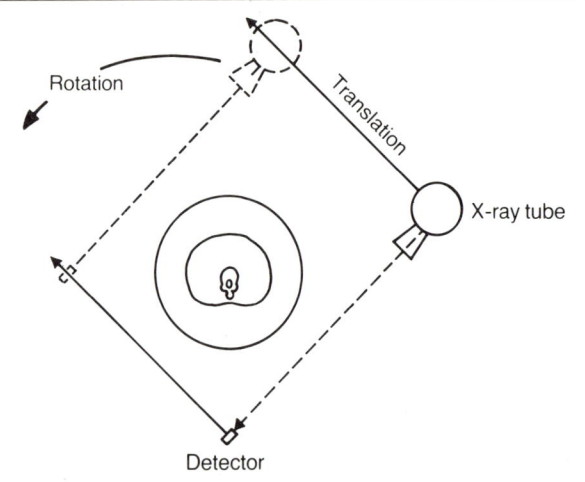

Figure 18.4 First generation translate/rotate scanner

Third generation scanners (Figure 18.5) are of the rotate/rotate type. In these machines the X-ray tube produces a 'fan beam of radiation' and is connected mechanically to a row of detectors. Both rotate around the plane to be scanned.

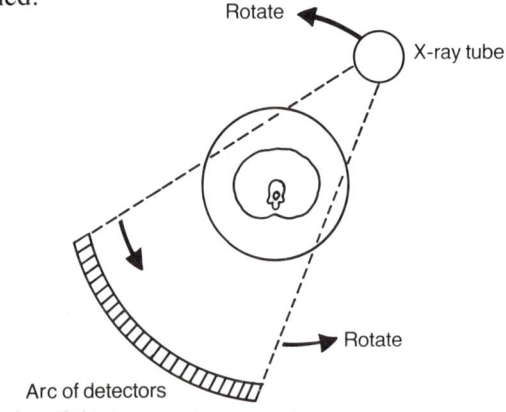

Figure 18.5 Third generation, rotate/rotate scanner

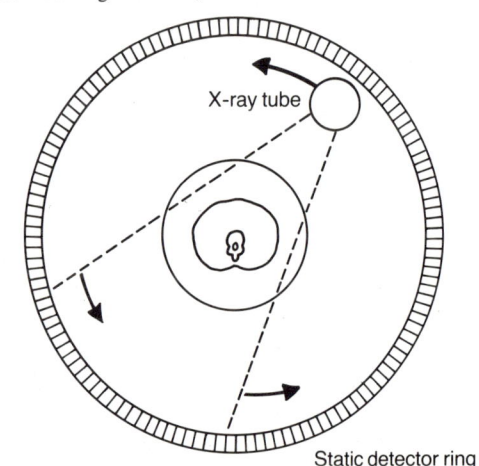

Figure 18.6 Fourth generation, rotate/static detector scanner

In fourth generation scanners (Figure 18.6) the detectors form a static ring around the gantry. The X-ray tube again produces a fan beam and rotates within this ring. Both types of unit continue to be produced, though at the time of writing the third generation machines appear to be more popular.

Comparison of third and fourth generation scanners

(1) With a fourth generation unit, the focus–object distance is shorter than the object–detector distance, since the tube rotates within the detector ring. This may contribute to a higher skin dose and necessitates the use of a smaller focal spot size to reduce geometric unsharpness.
(2) Detector failure and other faults produce 'ring artefacts' in third generation machines.
(3) Third generation detectors are always in the scanner beam and therefore cannot be individually calibrated during a scan. Since there are fewer detectors in a third generation unit, failure of one produces more noticeable results.
(4) It is easier to control scattered radiation in a third generation unit because the X-ray beam is always 'normal' to the detector face. With a fourth generation machine this will only be the case when the detector is in the centre of the beam. The 'air gap' inherent between patient and detectors in a fourth generation machine, though, will help to minimize this problem.
(5) Each CT X-ray detector is closely connected to its own amplifier to reduce 'electronic noise'. Thus in a third generation machine where the detectors rotate, the manufacturer must go to considerable lengths to ensure that these sophisticated electronics do not suffer from the continual movement and a large number of flexible electrical connections are required to link the detectors to the gantry and so to the computer.

X-RAY TUBE

With all CT scanners the X-ray beam is highly collimated and most of the radiation energy is wasted. Compared with conventional radiography, higher tube voltages and longer exposures are necessary. Thus a great deal of heat energy has to be dissipated from the anode. A typical exposure for an abdominal slice might be 130 kV and 300 mA s. In order to prevent artefacts on the images, the X-ray tube focus must follow a precise path. A small amount of anode 'wobble', that would be acceptable in a standard rotating anode tube, would render a CT tube useless. Modern CT scanners have very thick compound anodes with a heat storage capacity of the order of 1 million heat units. This is one of the factors that limit the rate of scanning, so that manufacturers are developing tubes with even greater anode thermal capacity. Focal spot size varies from one manufacturer to another; most now produce dual focus tubes with a fine focus of 0.6–1.0 mm and a broad focus up to 1.8 mm. Some units have high speed stators as an option. Their use should be limited because of the gyroscopic effect of a heavy anode rotating at high speed which is part of a tube which itself rotates around the patient. Continued use, especially for short scan times, where the tube moves quickly, would reduce tube life because of the wear on the anode bearings. Replacement tubes are a regular cost to any CT scanning department. They normally have a warranty life of 25 000–30 000 exposures and a working life measured in months rather than years.

FILTRATION

It is usual to use rather more added filtration for CT scanning than for conventional radiography. This helps to produce a more homogenous beam and reduces patient skin dose. The early scanners required the use of a water bath or 'bolus bags' of absorbent material, so that unattenuated beams did not fall on the detector(s). Modern scanners use detectors with a greater dynamic range, but it may still be desirable to use an added filter on the tube which is thicker at the ends than the middle. This will produce a beam-hardening effect at the edges of the beam whilst the absorption through the patient has a similar effect on the centre of the beam.

PATIENT DOSE FROM CT SCANNING

It is very difficult to be precise when answering the question, 'How much dose does the patient get from a CT scan?' Obviously this depends on the number of slices and the factors used. Skin dose is reduced by the use of high voltage and additional filtration. The beam is well collimated which helps to reduce scatter and the irradiation of parts of the body outside the scan plane.

VARIABLE GEOMETRY

At least one manufacturer produces third generation scanners where the tube-to-patient distance is variable. When a smaller diameter scan is required the tube can be brought closer to the patient. The resultant magnification of the image allows all the detectors to be used to record useful information. Most modern scanners are designed to tilt up to 20° either side of vertical. This is of particular benefit for scanning spines, where the slice through a disc space can be imaged. It also enables more difficult projections of the head to be achieved.

SCANOGRAM

With third and fourth generation scanners, it is possible to produce what amounts to a digital radiograph. An exposure is made with the tube stationary but the patient couch moving through the beam (Figure 18.7). This is normally done at the start of each investigation to provide a reference for the later axial sections. It can also be used to estimate the degree of tilt required for angled projections. The quality of these images is better with a third generation scanner since it is possible to use all of the detectors.

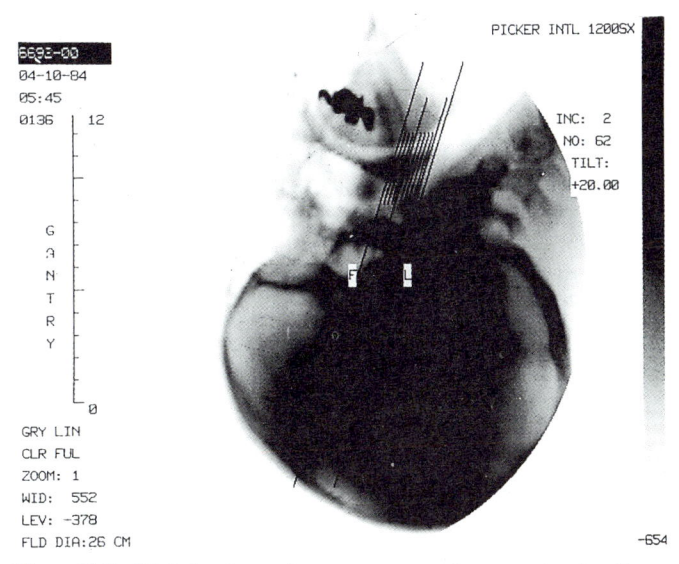

Figure 18.7 Digital radiograph, scanogram, or pilot scan, showing direct coronal brain slices

THE CT IMAGE

The CT image displayed on a television monitor are made up of a series of dots or *pixels*. Each pixel represents a *voxel*, that is the smallest volume of patient recorded as a separate CT number. The *image matrix* is the number of pixels (or voxels) in the images (e.g. 256×256, or 512×512). The CT number is a measure of the X-ray attenuation of the material in each voxel. The range is based on an arbitrarily chosen value of zero for water and −1000 for air.

IMAGE COMPUTATION

The first stage in producing CT images is a series of dose measurements. Many hundreds of thousands are required for each slice. For each dose measurement the computer has to know the positions of tube and detector and hence the voxels the measured beam has passed through. This total information is known as *raw data*, (i.e. unprocessed measurements). The computer then applies an *algorithm* to this data. This is a set of mathematical rules in an orderly sequence to change the raw data into *scan data* (i.e. CT numbers for each pixel). A choice of algorithms is normally available to produce optimum image quality in different parts of the body. The basic process used in many CT computers is *back-projection*. The dose readings are projected back in the computer's memory through those voxels involved in their measurement. Thus voxels with low X-ray attenuation will have high back-projected dose measurements. Unfortunately the process is not that simple and a *convolution* process is required to compensate for the fact that very high or very low dose readings will affect the neighbouring voxels. In addition some form of compensation must be made for voxels in the centre of the field which are involved in more dose measurements and therefore more back-projections. The body tissue will selectively absorb softer radiation with the result that emergent radiation will have shorter average wavelength. This *spectral hardening* must be compensated for in the algorithm.

RESOLUTION

An ideal CT image would accurately portray in its pixels the size, shape and X-ray attenuation of the structures scanned. It is also desirable to have the image in as short a time as possible. Inevitably, there has to be a compromise between the conflicting requirements of spatial resolution, contrast resolution and processing time. If the area being scanned has a high subject contrast, such as in the lung fields or in bony areas, an algorithm which gives good spatial resolution can be chosen. With a small scan field this can give resolution of the order of 11 line-pairs per centimetre. It may be desirable to demonstrate small variations in CT number, such as in the demonstration of liver metastases, where spatial resolution is less important than contrast resolution.

If the voxels of an image include tissues that have very different X-ray attenuation coefficients a mean value for each voxel will be recorded. This *partial volume effect* is quite noticeable in chest scans, where the voxel may include air (CT number, −1000) and soft tissue (CT number, 30–60). The resultant pixel will demonstrate any value between the two extremes).

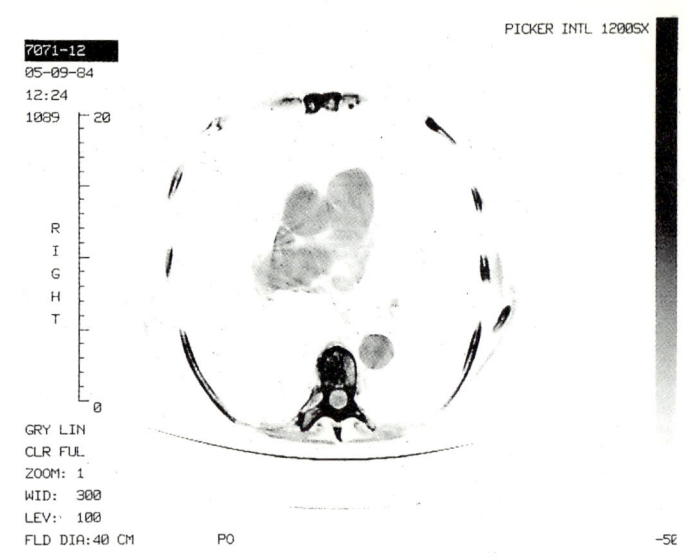

Figure 18.8 A section through lower thorax

WINDOW WIDTH AND LEVEL

An axial section through the thorax will display structures with a wide range of CT numbers, from air at −1000 to dense bone in the spine at up to 3000. By selecting the appropriate values of CT number, it is possible to demonstrate on one section a wide range of structures (Figure 18.8). This is achieved by varying the window width and level. If a window width of 300 is used at a window level of +100 the television monitor will display as shades of grey any pixels that have CT numbers between −100 and +200. Pixels below −100 will be black and pixels above

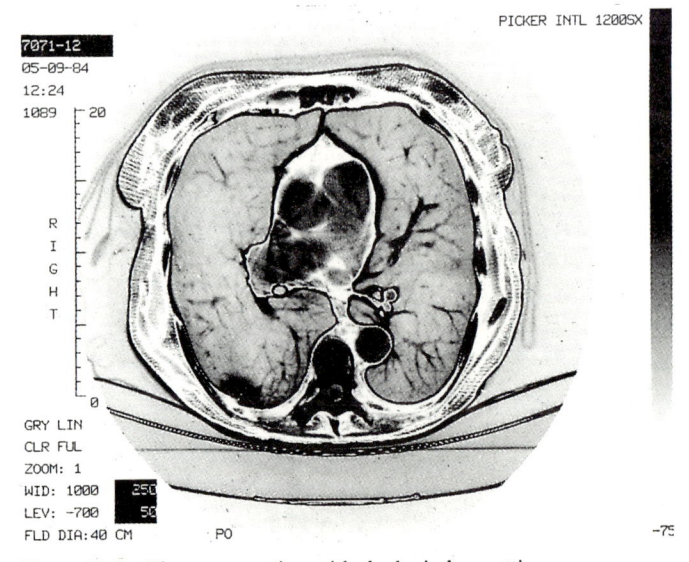

Figure 18.9 The same section with dual window settings

COMPUTERIZED TOMOGRAPHY 205

+200 will be white. Some units are able to employ two window settings simultaneously in order to display both lungs and soft tissue in the thorax (Figure 18.9).

IMAGE RECONSTRUCTIONS

Either by reference to the raw data or to processed data it is possible on many scanners to reconstruct and manipulate images in a number of ways. Busy scanning departments may feel that some of these functions are little more than gimmicks, but there are serious clinical applications for many. Figures 18.10–14 demonstrate some examples.

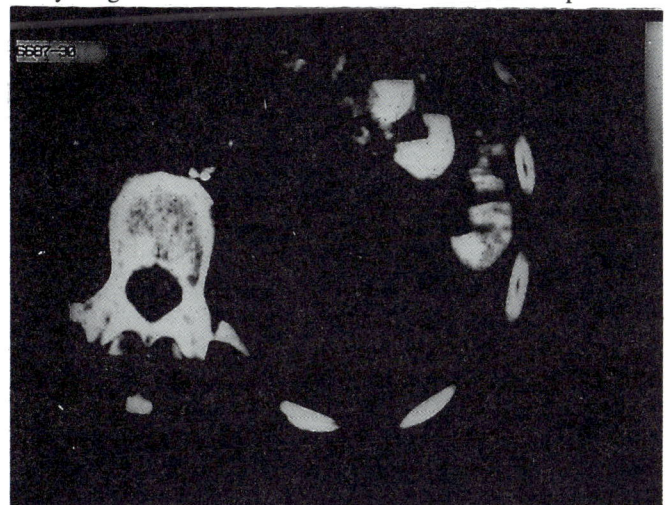

Figure 18.10 A ×2 zoom of an abdomen slice showing left kidney and renal arteries

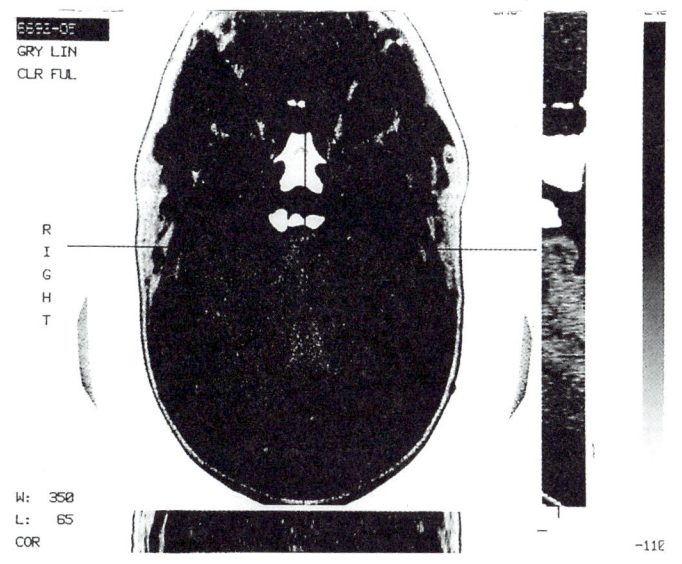

Figure 18.11 Reconstructions in two perpendicular planes of direct coronal slices through the pituitary area

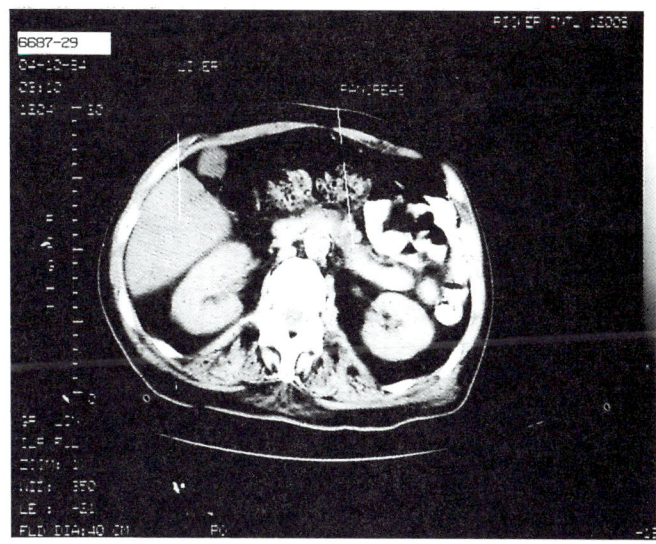

Figure 18.12 An annotated scan

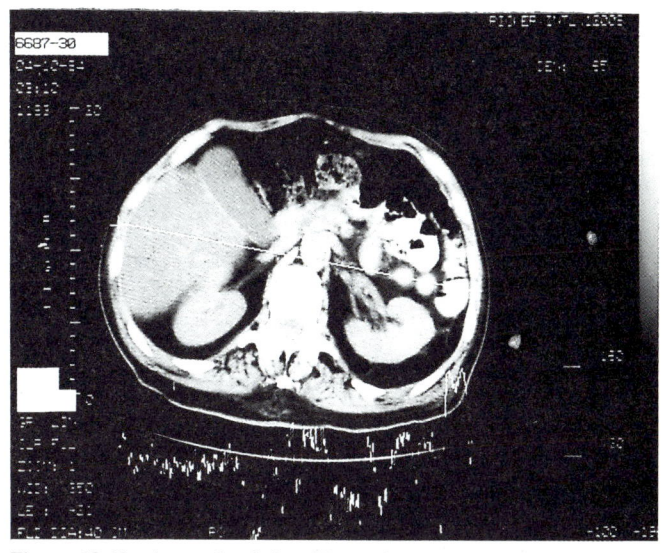

Figure 18.13 A graph of the CT numbers along a line through an abdominal slice

STORAGE OF CT SCAN DATA

As well as the memory of the computer itself, most CT scanners are connected to a computer disc memory for storing data on a relatively short-term basis. Systems vary widely but a typical unit will be able to store on the hard disc a few days' work. After this time the memory can be erased to make space available for new patient data. A wide range of cameras is available for recording images on photographic film or paper. This is very often the only

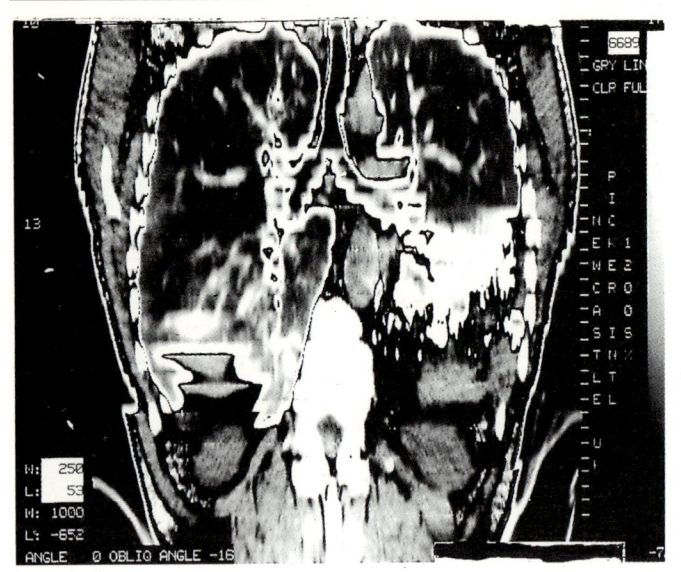

Figure 18.14 A coronal section produced by reconstruction from many axial sections through thorax and upper abdomen

way that clinicians who refer patients from other hospitals to the CT scanner can view the images. It also provides a permanent record, if required, for the CT scan department. In Newcastle we routinely produce two sets of film images on each patient. One set is retained in the department and the other is returned to the department which requested the scan. It is also possible to retain images on magnetic recording material. Flexible magnetic discs (floppies) were popular with the early EMI head scanners, because it was possible to record on one disc an entire series of head scan images. A 512×512 matrix body image has approximately ten times as many pixels as the 160×160 matrix head scan. There are likely to be many more slices in a scan of the abdomen so that floppy discs have become less popular for medium to long-term storage of data. Most departments now keep their archive scans on magnetic tape. The data is transferred from the computer disc memory to tape in a few minutes and can be recalled at a later date if required. The system at present used in Newcastle can store approximately 300 512×512 matrix images on one magnetic tape. At least one manufacturer offers the option of a laser-disc memory system to reduce the volume of the archive even further.

QUALITY ASSURANCE

The routine maintenance of a scanner will inevitably include some quality assurance checks, but it is usual to do simple checks each day. Most manufacturers supply a water phantom. This is a cylinder of water that can be scanned each day to ensure that the unit stays in calibration. We also regularly scan a contrast resolution phantom and a spatial resolution phantom.

SCANNING ANGLE

The tube of a third or fourth generation scanner produces a fan beam of radiation through an angle of up to 45°. On a third generation scanner this will irradiate all of the detectors, as both tube and detectors rotate around the patient. At least 200° of tube and detector rotation is required to provide sufficient information for a scan. It is usual to employ a greater scanning angle in order to improve the quality of the scan, unless patient movement is likely to be a problem. The detectors of a fourth generation scanner are stationary and therefore only a limited number are in the beam of radiation at any one time. The scanning angles are similar to third generation angles.

DETECTORS

The early scanners had detectors which consisted of sodium iodide crystals with a photomultiplier attached. Some modern machines use detectors containing xenon gas under pressure, others use crystal photodiodes containing materials such as cadmium tungstate. An ideal detector would be small, to enable a large number to be used, and would combine good sensitivity with a wide electronic dynamic range. (Electronic dynamic range is the ratio of the largest signal that does not saturate the system to the smallest detectable signal.) It is desirable to have an amplifier very close to the detector to reduce electronic noise and provide measurable signals for the computer.

CALIBRATION

It is essential that the X-ray detectors provide the computer with accurate and reproducible dose readings. Most scanners include a calibration scan in the warm-up sequence each morning before the unit is used for patients. This may take the form of a single slice scan through air to calibrate the detectors. If the slice width, filter or tube voltage is changed it may be necessary to recalibrate the detectors. On a fourth generation unit it is sometimes possible to calibrate the detectors whilst scanning by using the leading edge of the beam that is outside the scan diameter. On a third generation scanner this will always expose the same detectors, but may be used to compensate for very minor changes in tube voltage during the exposure.

COMPUTERIZED TOMOGRAPHY

EXPOSURE FACTORS

As with any use of ionizing radiation, the exposure to the patient must be reduced to the minimum. Unfortunately under or overexposure is not immediately apparent on the scan images since their effect is mainly on the amount of 'noise' in the image. Experienced radiographers will readily recognize a 'noisy' image produced by underexposure. The effects of overexposure are much less readily appreciated. Briefly, exposure factors when increased have the following effects:

(1) *kV.* It is important to use a high tube voltage combined with added tube filtration to reduce the artefacts produced by selective absorption of soft radiation in the patient. The range 100–140 kV is normal. Alteration of tube voltage may produce selective changes in CT numbers (see next section).

(2) *mA.* Increased tube current will reduce the amount of 'noise' in the resultant image.

(3) *Total exposure time per slice.* Increased exposure time will have a similar effect to increased current. Additionally, since each dose measurement will take place over a longer time, more accurate CT numbers may be possible.

(4) *Slice thickness.* If other factors remain the same, the dose reaching each detector will be proportional to the slice thickness. Increased 'noise' will be produced if the slice thickness is *reduced* unless other exposure factors are increased.

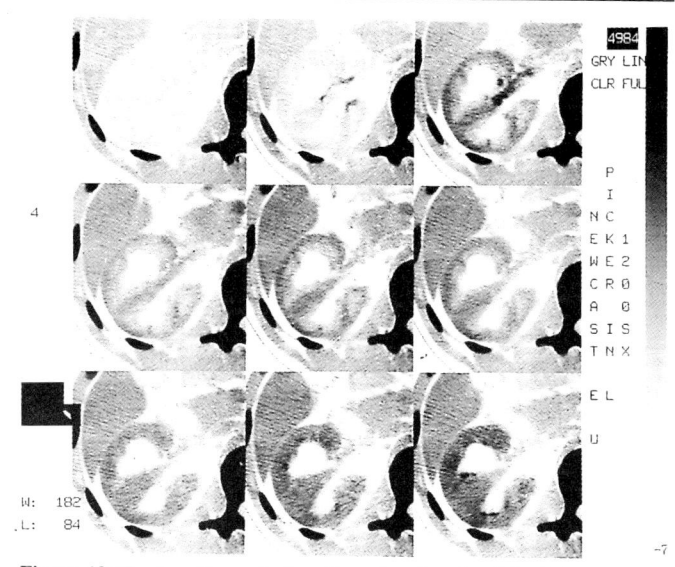

Figure 18.15 A collage of nine slices showing the right kidney before, during and after an injection of intravenous contrast medium

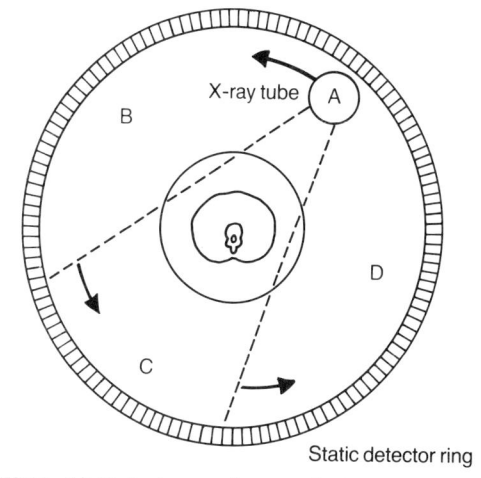

Figure 18.16 Multiple images from a single pass. It is possible to produce a number of images from one exposure. Each will demonstrate the same anatomical slice but will be slightly separated in time. In the diagram it is necessary for the tube to move through 180° to obtain enough data for one image. It would be possible to construct one image from the tube moving from A to B to C, a second image whilst the tube moved from B to C to D, and a third whilst the tube moved from C to D to A. Note that the first and third images are completely separated in time, but the second image uses part of the data from each of the other two

OPTIONAL FACILITIES

With CT scanners, as with most X-ray equipment, there are optional extra facilities that usually cost more money.

Dynamic scanning

It is possible with some modern scanners to repeatedly scan the same section in order to demonstrate the change in CT number produced by a bolus injection of intravenous contrast medium. This might demonstrate renal function (Figure 18.15), or the pathological circulation of a tumour. The scanner must be capable of rapid repeat exposures and it is desirable to have computer software that can divide each scan on a time basis into a number of images (Figure 18.16).

ECG trigger

If the start of each scan is triggered by a particular part of the electrocardiograph cycle it is possible to build up a series of images that demonstrate the cardiac cycle, by repeat scanning of the same section. Since the shortest scan times are of the order of 1 s there is inevitably a degree of movement artefact on scans of the lower thorax, which is overcome by this technique.

Radiotherapy planning

A number of radiotherapy centres have found the digital information contained in CT sections invaluable in treatment planning. This work is normally carried out on a separate console where the treatment isodose curves can be plotted (Figure 18.17).

Independent consoles

Many installations have a separate viewing console to enable previous patient images to be viewed without using the console on which images of the current patient are displayed. The console may be totally independent with its own computer or it may time-share with the main scanning computer. In the latter case it is possible to manipulate images on both consoles simultaneously but at slightly reduced speed.

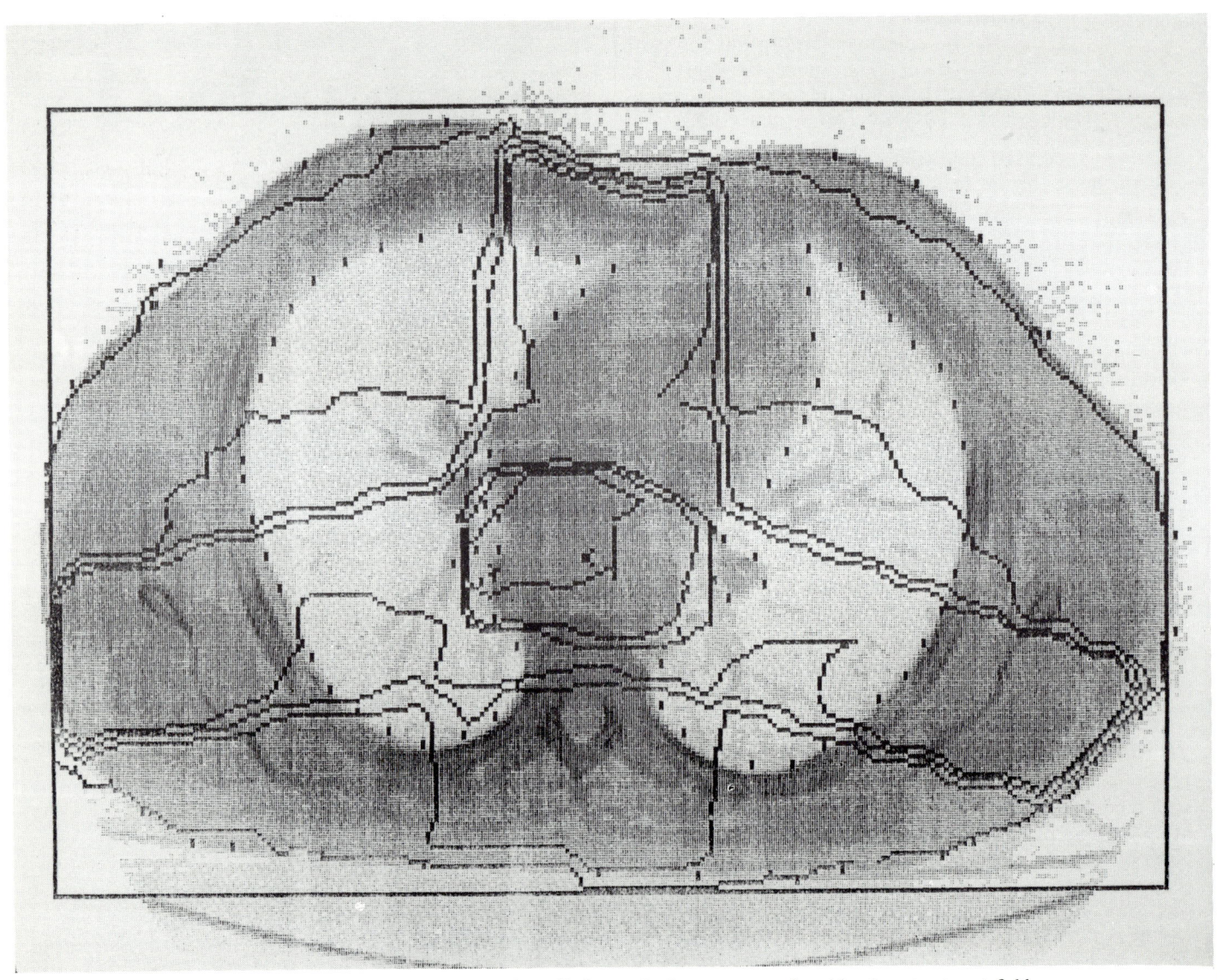

Figure 18.17 A chest CT slice showing the radiotherapy isodose curves produced by three treatment fields

Dual energy scanning

The basis of CT scanning is the ability to display tissues with differing X-ray attenuation coefficients. Since the attenuation coefficient of any material varies with the energy of the X-ray beam, the CT number is not an absolute measure of X-ray attenuation, but will vary with filtration, kV variation and, to some extent, with size of subject. A more consistent number could be produced by subtracting images produced at different kV settings. This would show the change in attenuation between the two beam energies for each voxel of the image. At the time of writing several manufacturers are experimenting with this idea, but as yet it is not commercially available. The most likely method to be used is to employ a pulsed X-ray beam, where alternate pulses are at the two different kV values. The computer could then be programmed to automatically subtract two images of the same slice produced with one pass of the X-ray tube.

ADVANTAGES OF CT SCANNING

CT scanning will always be an expensive technique and the patient throughput will be low, when compared with conventional radiography. Unlike ultrasound and MRI scanners which can also produce cross-sectional body images, there is a radiation hazard to be considered. The main advantage is that it can demonstrate relatively small differences in attenuation with a comparatively non-invasive technique. CT has considerably fewer artefacts than medical ultrasound and is able to image areas of tissue that cannot be imaged at all with ultrasound. MRI images, at the time of writing, require considerably longer data acquisition times and this is likely to remain a problem in those areas of the body with involuntary movement. The best CT images can display greater spatial resolution than the best MRI images.

The particular advantages for radiotherapy planning have been mentioned previously. CT as a non-invasive and readily reproducible technique has great advantages when it is desired to monitor disease during and after treatment. No doubt newer imaging techniques will continue to be developed, but for the foreseeable future CT will remain a valuable diagnostic tool.

19
Nuclear magnetic resonance imaging

D. MANNING

PRINCIPLES OF NUCLEAR MAGNETIC RESONANCE (NMR)	210
MRI SCANNERS	212
The magnet	212
Superconductive magnets	212
Resistive magnets	212
Installation	213
PRODUCING A MAGNETIC RESONANCE IMAGE	213
RADIOFREQUENCY (RF) COILS	213
APPLICATIONS	214
BIOLOGICAL HAZARDS AND PERMITTED EXPOSURE LEVELS	214
Static magnetic fields	216
Varying magnetic fields	216
Radiofrequency fields	216

Magnetic Resonance Imaging (MRI) is the most recent addition to the methods available for displaying organs and systems. The phenomenon of nuclear magnetic resonance (NMR) was first described in 1946 and found early application as a spectroscopic tool in investigating the properties of matter. But it was in the early 1970s that the technology and computation methods involved in CT scanners was fused with resonance techniques to make available a novel means of imaging biological systems. The recency of its arrival means that the place of MRI in the overall scheme of things in medical imaging has yet to be established – but it seems likely that the method will become a standard diagnostic aid and may even replace some of the established methods. Clear signs are emerging that indicate an enormous potential for anatomical, physiological and pathological studies using MRI. This chapter will outline the principles involved in the imaging process, possible future applications, developments and hazards.

PRINCIPLES OF NUCLEAR MAGNETIC RESONANCE (NMR)

Nuclei are composed of protons and neutrons. The proton number determines the element and its position in the periodic table while the neutron number can provide variation in mass between nuclei of atoms of the same element. This last point accounts for the existence of isotopes.

It is also true that both protons and neutrons spin on their axes, so if we consider that protons spin in one direction and neutrons in the other, then, in general, it will mean that nuclei of isotopes with even an even number of protons and neutrons (for example $^{16}_{8}O$) will not spin because the contra-rotation of their component particles will cancel out.

But isotopes with an odd number of nucleons will display net spin on their nuclei. These nuclei will behave like tiny bar magnets because they are, in fact, minute rotating charges. Materials made up of such isotopes will be unrecognizable from other materials under normal conditions because atoms tend to be orientated at random. They will show no evidence of magnetism. But, if an external magnetic field of sufficient strength is applied, some alignment of the magnetic moments will occur and it is under these conditions that certain isotopes can show NMR properties. Examples of the nuclei amenable to resonance are hydrogen (^{1}H), phosphorus ($^{31}_{16}P$), fluorine ($^{19}_{8}F$) and carbon ($^{13}_{6}C$).

Of these elements hydrogen is found in greatest quantity in living tissue because of the large amount of water present.

If a patient is placed in a static field, parallel with the Z axis in Figure 19.1 the hydrogen nuclei align themselves parallel with this field. They are in an equilibrium state with the external field but can be imagined to be *precessing* around the direction (Z) of the field. Figure 19.2 illustrates the situation and one can imagine similarities with the way a spinning top precesses around the vertical field of gravitation (Figure 19.3).

The nuclear precession will have a frequency of rotation related to (a) the magnetic field strength and (b) an inher-

NUCLEAR MAGNETIC RESONANCE IMAGING

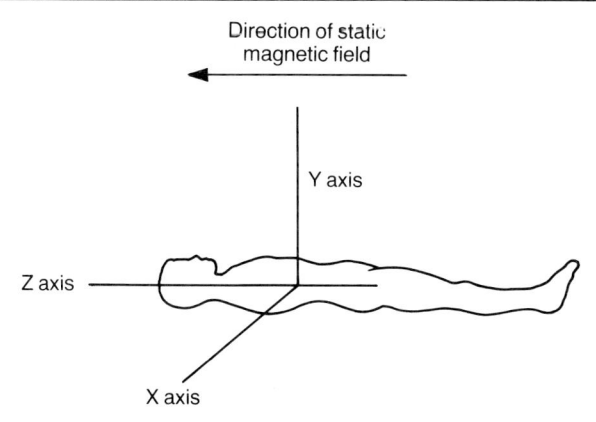

Figure 19.1 Patient in a static magnetic field parallel with the Z axis

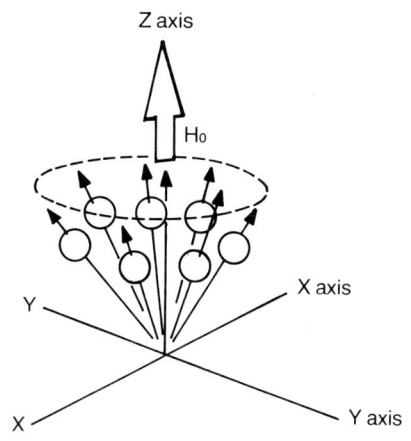

Figure 19.2 A group of nuclei precessing around main field axis (H₀) resulting in net magnetization (m)

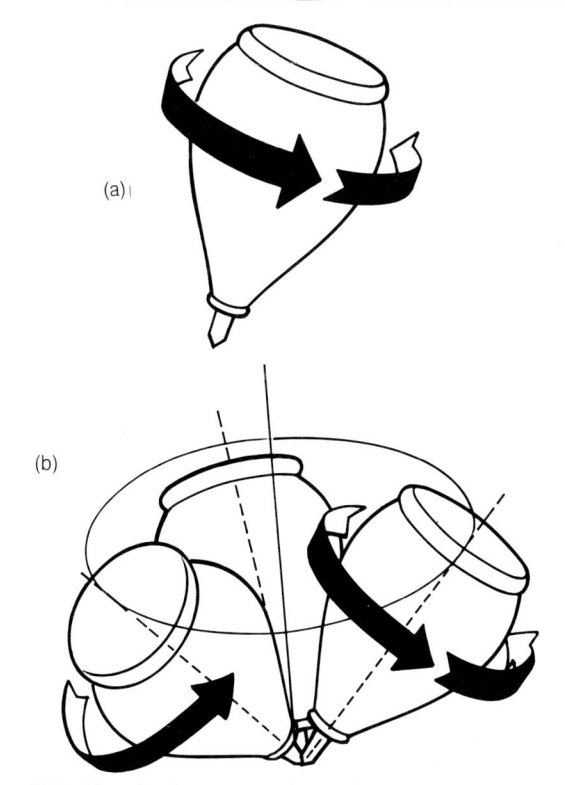

Figure 19.3 Two simultaneous motions take place when a top spins (a) spinning on its own axis (b) spinning and precessing around the vertical axis

ent feature of the nucleus called the gyromagnetic constant. The frequency is called the Larmor frequency and is found to lie in the radiofrequency (RF) part of the spectrum of electromagnetic radiation. Knowing the value of this frequency is important because it means that by applying a pulse of radiation of the equivalent (RF) energy, it will be possible to disturb the nuclei from their orderly precession. As soon as the disruptive pulse has ended nuclei return to their equilibrium state with the emission of radiofrequency radiation. But the return to magnetic alignment is not instantaneous and follows an exponential pattern. In fact, it is this measurable *relaxation time* that allows observation of the events to take place.

For magnetic resonance there are two simultaneously occurring relaxation times that are of interest for diagnostic imaging. The first is sometimes called the spin–lattice relaxation time (T_1) and describes the time taken for nuclei to shed the energy they gained from the RF pulse, into their immediate environment (lattice). The second is called (T_2), the spin–spin relaxation time and comes about because of a phenomenon called coherence. When the RF pulse is applied it not only adds energy to the precessing nuclei but induces a sort of ordered 'ringing' of the excited nuclei in a way analogous to the way tuning forks vibrate. At the end of the pulse application the nuclei begin to lose this coherent 'ringing' because of individual interactions between themselves. Some slow down while others speed up, and the result is that the nuclei gradually slip out of phase with each other. They eventually slip into a random orientation and then back into alignment with the static external magnetic field.

During the coherent phase, the nuclei emit a detectable signal of RF, but the duration of this signal (T_2) is generally about one-tenth of the T_1 relaxation time in tissues. So there are two quite separable and distinct relaxation time pulses that can be detected and measured after RF excitation, and the practice of MRI exploits this. What is more, a distinct difference is seen between various body tissues when relaxation times are compared and the ratios of T_1/T_2 are variable too. This forms a basis for 'contrast differences' between tissues in the MRI sense in a similar fashion to contrast difference between the attenuation properties of tissue in conventional radiography and computed tomography.

MRI SCANNERS

From the brief discussion on the principles of nuclear magnetic resonance it should be clear that several items of equipment are vital for the process (Figure 19.4). A magnet is essential for producing the initial conditions of nuclear alignment. A generator of radiofrequency (RF) pulses is needed to perturb the precessing nuclei, and an RF receiver is also necessary to detect the resulting 'return pulse' signals from the patient.

In addition to this basic hardware, it is important to have a means of identifying the position of the source of an RF signal when it is emitted from the body. Without this facility a MRI scanner would have no method of separating in space the signals emerging from a volume of tissue. It is performed by computerized encoding of signals in respect of their point of origin in a magnetic field gradient.

The magnet

The imaging process requires a magnetic field that is uniform and static and of sufficient size to accommodate an adult human being. Magnetic fields can be produced either by electromagnets or by permanent magnets, but in practice it is only the first type that have found general application in MRI scanners. The field strengths necessary are in the order of 0.1–0.3 tesla and the required uniformity is 1 part in 10^6. This is generally too high a requirement for permanent magnets. Electromagnets are therefore the choice, but there are two competing types available.

Superconductive magnets

These are electromagnets where the coils carrying the current are made of metals or alloys which have zero resistivity at very low temperatures. Such conductive coils will circulate a current for ever, without a driving voltage for as long as the temperature remains low. The metal alloys used are niobium/titanium and the temperature is kept at $-269\,°C$ by immersion in liquid helium. The whole device is called a cryostat and is itself immersed in a vacuum-shielded liquid nitrogen bath at $-200\,°C$. Despite all this the liquid helium requires regular replenishment because of boil off and is the cause of the very high running costs for this type of equipment.

Resistive magnets

These magnets have conventional, thick copper windings carrying a heavy current. They are usually arranged in four pancake-shaped coils called a Helmholtz arrangement and

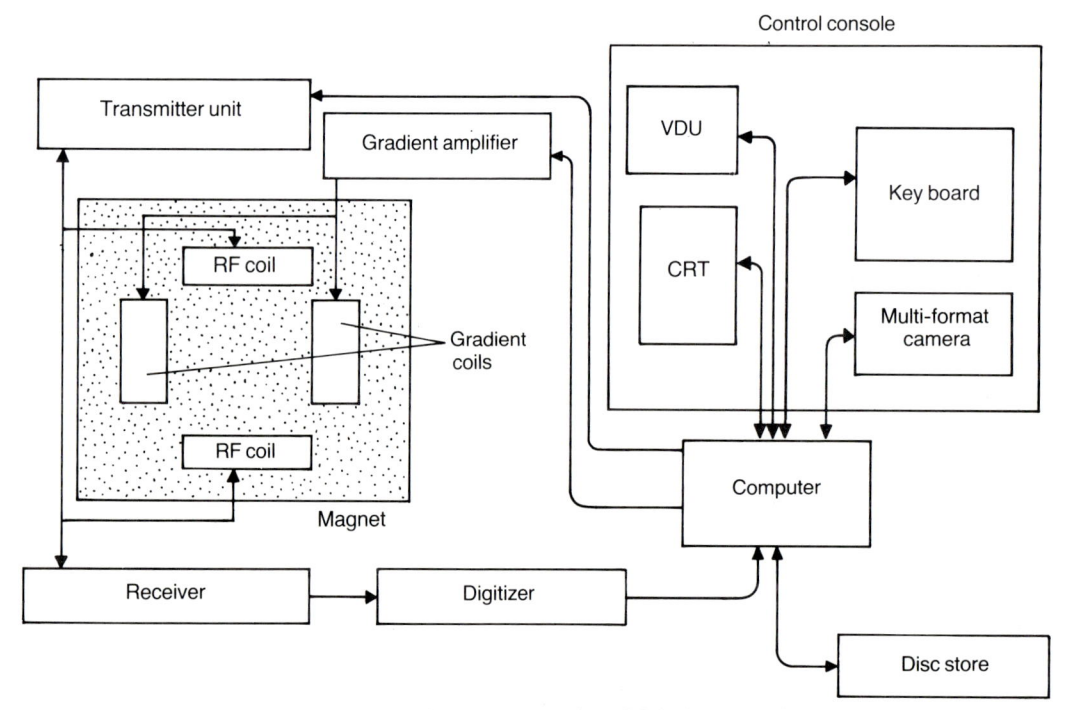

Figure 19.4 Block diagram to show the main components of a MRI device. Note the various methods of display and storage: VDU (video display unit), CRT (cathode ray tube), multi-format camera and disc store

maintain good field stability only if the current is left on continuously. There is a great deal of heat generated by this type of equipment and the coils must be permanently cooled by water linked to a heat-exchanger and pump. It is a very expensive process unless the waste heat can be put to good use by some recycling method. Power consumption is naturally very high and is typically about 30 kW continuous so the cost of running a resistive magnet is not appreciably different from the superconductive type.

Installation

Large magnets with stable field and high levels of field uniformity require special environments. It is important that the immediate area surrounding the magnet should remain at a constant level of magnetic permeability. In practice this means that no large masses of ferrous metal should be mobile in the vicinity. An example of the problem might be the close proximity of the MR installation to a car-park or roadway. Moving vehicles, representing a volume of higher magnetic permeability than the surrounding air, would seriously affect the field uniformity of the magnet and disrupt the progress of an examination. Careful thought is given to the position of an MRI unit because of this.

PRODUCING A MAGNETIC RESONANCE IMAGE

It was mentioned briefly that a means of identifying the origin of a radiofrequency signal within the body is essential for successful imaging. The task of identification is given to a computer which is programmed to abstract the data necessary for image formation. But the way in which that data is encoded so that it is recognized by the computer program requires some explanation.

Nuclear magnetic resonance frequencies are known as Larmor frequencies (see above) and are proportional to the applied, static magnetic field (H_0). Now if the value of H_0 is constant throughout the volume of the object being imaged and during the collection of RF pulses, then the frequency of the NMR signals will remain constant too. Their value will be the same no matter where in the object and static field they originated. In this case there will be no means of identifying one signal as being different from another.

However, if the value of H_0 is varied during the data collection stage then there will be recognizable differences in the value of the MRI signals. The differences will be proportional to the changed value of H_0. If a *gradient* magnetic field is used, the position on the gradient will provide a MRI signal value that is characteristic of that position in the field. It provides a means of spatially encoding the origin of a resonance signal which can be recognized by the computer program.

Once this identification has been made then the image can be reconstructed on a display unit in a very similar way to the method used by other computerized tomography imaging units.

The gradient fields are usually three in number and are generated by coils which have their own power supplies. These supplies can be switched under computer control to reconstruct images in all dimensions within the body (Figure 19.5). The stability of these gradient fields is a major factor in the determination of image quality in MRI.

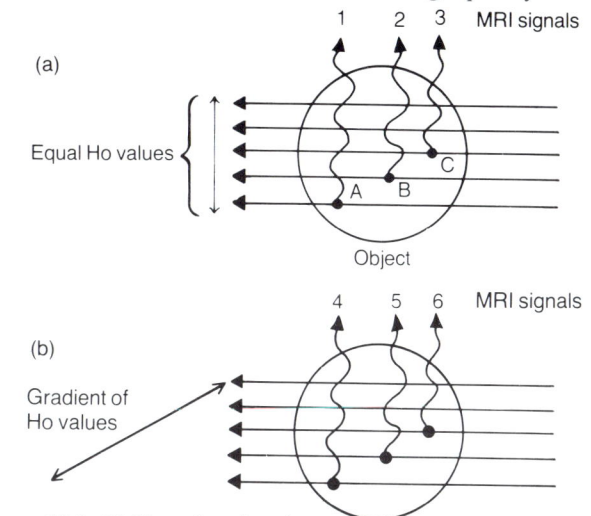

Figure 19.5 Field gradient imaging.
(a) In a *uniform* field Ho, MRI signals 1, 2 and 3 are of equal value of frequency despite their different points of origin, A, B and C
(b) If a magnetic field *gradient* is applied during data collection the MRI signals 4, 5 and 6 will be of different frequency values because of their different positions of origin in the non uniform field

RADIOFREQUENCY (RF) COILS

These coils produce the excitation of the static magnetic field and also pick up the emitted signal on decay. They are usually saddle-shaped and direct their field perpendicularly to the direction of the main field of magnetization.

They receive pulsed excitation for radiofrequency (RF) generation from a transmitter unit which delivers its energy in bursts. The coils also collect the return signal from the patient, and it is by selection of different combinations of pulse transmissions and collection times that contrast is produced between different tissues (Figure 19.6). These combinations are called *sequences*. The return signal from the patient induces a small microvolt pulse in the RF coils which is then amplified and digitized ready for computer acquisition. It is vital that through this detection path for the return signal there is no deterioration in the signal-to-noise ratio by interference from outside sources.

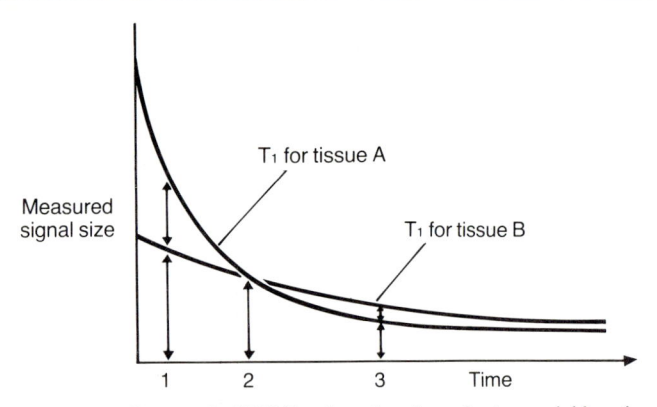

Figure 19.6 *Contrast in MRI.* T_1 relaxation times for two neighbouring tissues A and B are shown and illustrate origins of contrast in resonance images. This will depend on the time of acquisition. Contrast between A and B will be highest at time 1, lowest at time 2, and reversed at time 3. This gives MRI a flexibility unique in computed tomography by the ability to change pulse sequences and collection times

APPLICATIONS

Because the field of magnetic resonance imaging is so new it is a rapidly changing one. Any written word on the subject runs the risk of being outdated before it goes to print, so one can only make statements on the 'state of the art' in the certain knowledge that it will be different tomorrow!

Already it is possible to produce images of any part of the body in any section direction imaginable. The images produced can have the most spectacular anatomical detail if certain relaxation times are used for signal acquisition and there is a natural temptation to make comparisons with CT images. It is perhaps an unfair comparison and certainly one that is not free of prejudice. Protagonists of X-ray CT would no doubt point out that the examination times for comparable areas are much greater for MRI than for their own methods.

But, as a summary of the current applications of MRI the following statements can be made:

(1) Outstanding anatomical detail can be produced with certain signal acquisition sequences. Images showing such spectacular structural information require examination times of about 30 minutes at present, and some workers have suggested that these images may not be using MRI to its best advantage.

(2) Different signal acquisition sequences can produce images that look less anatomically informative, but display pathological tissue more clearly because of major differences in its relaxation time.

(3) Contrast in MRI images can be made to depend on physiological as well as structural differences. For example, the flow of blood in vessels can be detected and quantified.

(4) Discrimination between areas of different chemical composition or concentration is possible (e.g. concentrations of metabolites such as ATP). This technique has been described as 'human spectroscopy' and may have important applications in fields such as the assessment of patients with ischaemic heart disease. The chemical difference between normal and poorly perfused tissues is provided by spectral display instead of images.

(5) Tissue characterization with its powerful implications for tumour diagnosis and histology is currently being investigated in some centres. It is based on the idea that all tissues display relaxation times that are unique to themselves. Pathological changes in these tissues will change the relaxation times thus providing an index of disease. It will be necessary to accumulate a great store of 'normal' tissue information before this technique becomes established, but points towards a major application for MRI.

Looking to the future and the prospects for MRI is difficult, but it seems likely that unless capital costs *and* running costs are reduced, then these instruments will not be available to everyone. Certainly nuclear magnetic resonance techniques will be the medicine of the technological nations and not the third world in the immediate future! This is disappointing when one considers the potential for early, non-invasive diagnosis that the techniques could offer as screening methods for high risk fractions of populations.

BIOLOGICAL HAZARDS AND PERMITTED EXPOSURE LEVELS

It is quite natural that any investigative procedure should be scrutinized for possible damaging bioeffects. This is especially so in procedures where, traditionally, radiations that are potentially lethal have been used. Radiography is steeped in this background and there is therefore a clear requirement for workers and patients to be protected and informed if any hazards exist.

In 1981 the report of a Working Party on the subject set up by the UK National Radiological Protection Board (NRPB 1981) was published. It stated that there were three *possible* (but unconfirmed in large clinical trials) biological hazards. These were radiofrequency heating, the formation of static magnetic fields and electromagnetic

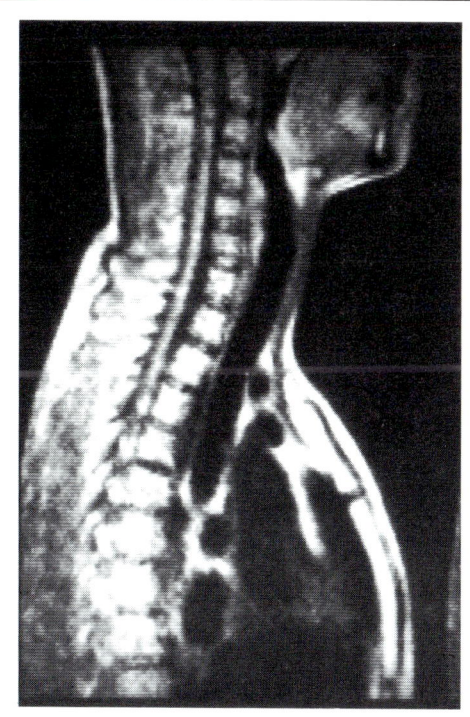

Figure 19.7 MRI of normal spinal cord

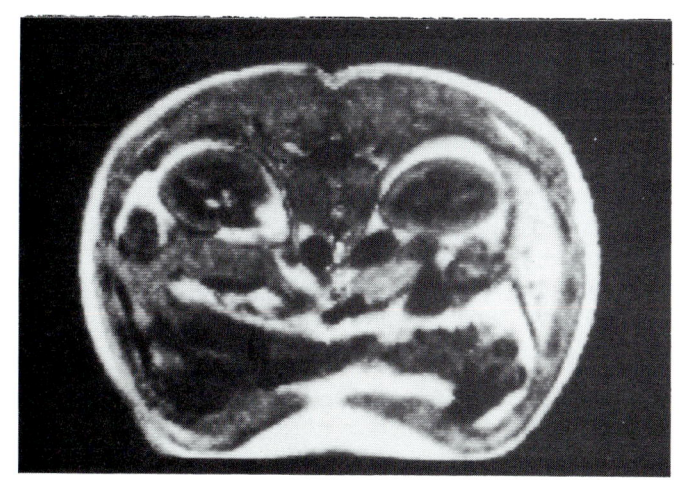

Figure 19.8 Normal kidneys showing tissue differences of cortex and medulla

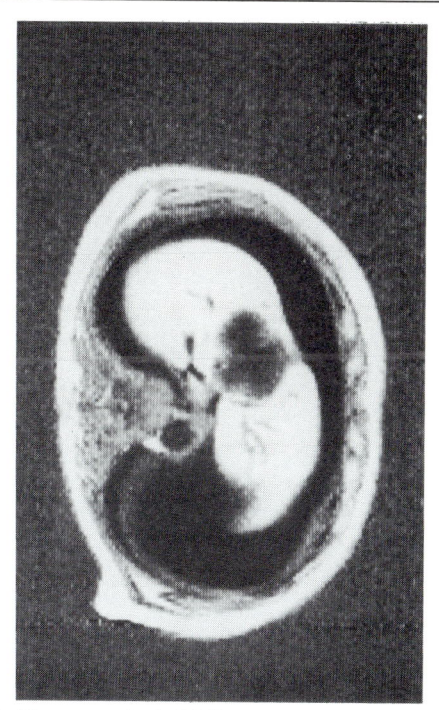

Figure 19.9 Transverse body MRI section showing a large liver metastasis from carcinoma of the breast

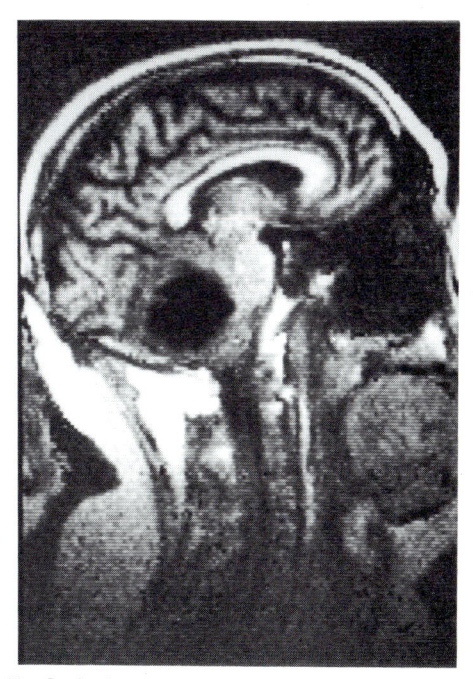

Figure 19.10 Sagittal section using T_2 relaxation time imaging. Notice the posterior fossa tumour

induction in tissues. Studies have shown no adverse biological effects from static magnetic fields below 5 T and it is worth noting that all current instruments operate at about or below 0.5 T. One effect of magnetic field alteration inducing an electric current has been recorded as the heating of dental fillings or hip prostheses, but this has been to a level below discomfort.

Possible magnetic effects of NMR have been studied

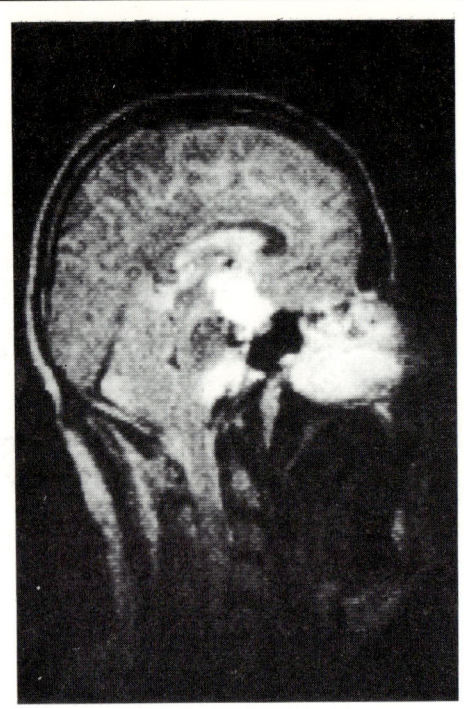

Figure 19.11 Sagittal brain section showing a bright area of recurrent tumour

with the use of bacteria and lymphocytes in cell culture and these observations have shown no DNA damage. The investigations are being continued on human tissue and genetic material to assess any possible long-term effects.

In 1983 a revised guidance on acceptable limits of exposure during MRI was published by the NRPB. In essence, this relaxed some of the previously laid down guidelines indicating an increased confidence in the innocence of NMR and advised the following:

(1) Volunteer subjects with heart disease or epilepsy are no longer excluded.
(2) No medical practitioner with resuscitation experience is required to be present.
(3) Higher frequency fields are allowed.

Exposure conditions were laid down as follows.

Static magnetic fields

Static field strength to the patient should not exceed 2.5 T.

Staff exposure should be less than 0.02 T whole body (long periods) or 0.2 T (for less than 15 min).

These short exposures are not accumulative if reasonable periods of time interspace them.

Varying magnetic fields

For periods of magnetic flux density change of 10 m sec or more exposure is restricted to less than 20 T/s.

Radiofrequency fields

These should be limited so that a temperature rise in any part of the skin surface should not exceed 1 °C.

In conclusion to these findings it seems unlikely that any of the biological hazards experienced in ionizing radiation exposure is to be expected from MRI.
It is wise to take a cautious view of the subject, of course, and such bodies as the NRPB and the World Health Organization make reliable and vigilant institutions in this. But the indications are that this new type of imaging provides a noninvasive and non-hazardous means of investigating disease processes. The future for magnetic resonance imaging looks very exciting.

20
Digital Radiographic Systems

OVERVIEW	217
HISTORY – BACKGROUND	217
SUBTRACTION PRINCIPLES	218
SYSTEM COMPONENTS	219
TV camera	219
The analogue-to-digital converter	219
Image acquisition	220
Static mode	220
Dynamic mode	220
The image processor	221
Image storage	221
Current storage	221
Archival storage	221
Image processing	221
Image analysis	222
Image viewing	222
RADIOLOGICAL APPLICATIONS	222
Digital intravenous angiography	223
Digital arteriography	224
RADIOGRAPHIC REQUIREMENTS AND CONSIDERATIONS	224
Exposure factors	224
Field size selection	224
Input dose	224
kVp choice – optimal beam quality	224
Summary	224
CONCLUSION	224
FUTURE DEVELOPMENTS	225
ACKNOWLEDGEMENTS	226

OVERVIEW

Digital radiography is a very general term which encompasses systems in which X-ray photon transmission is detected, and the resultant range of signals is converted from the hitherto analogue or continous spectrum into a digital or numerical one. Once numerical values have been ascribed, the image-forming pattern can be manipulated mathematically and in a variety of ways by a computer, in both on line, real time, or as a postprocessing interrogative exercise. Because very discrete changes in adjacent photon transmission are now made perceptible by this technology, digital radiography can be considered to be synonymous with low contrast detectability. Consider, for example, an analogue scale of 1000 shades from black to peak white. If two adjacent shades were to be viewed in isolation, it is very doubtful whether the eye could perceive any difference. However, if the two adjacent shades were given numerical values, these would be different.

HISTORY – BACKGROUND

Digitisation of radiographs represents one of the earliest adventures in this field. Although the results were encouraging the limitations were quickly realized. Digital imaging activities are, of course, already well advanced in the fields of nuclear medicine and ultrasound, but most particularly in computerized tomography, and the scout view which involves the use of a slit beam to produce a scanned projected image.

It could be said that the most rapidly developing form of digital radiography at the present time is in the vascular field, involving digital subtraction angiography, by means of digital fluorography, and temporal subtraction. Many titles are used – digital vascular imaging (DVI) and digital subtraction angiography (DSA) to name but two.

An example of the specialized equipment needed for D.S.A. is shown in Figures 20.1 and 20.2.

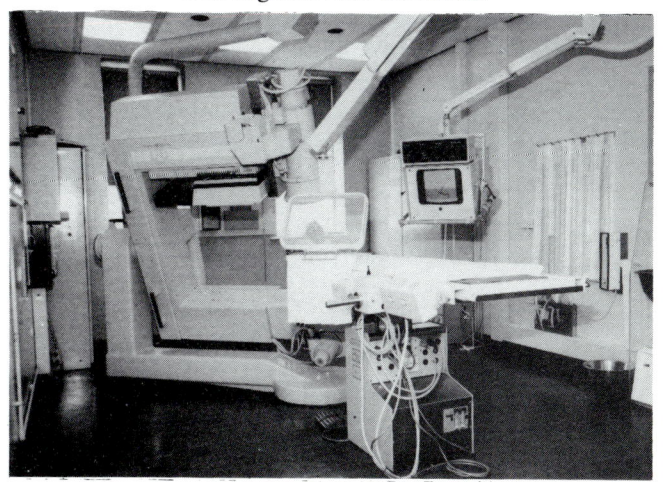

Figure 20.1 Base unit IGE LUA system

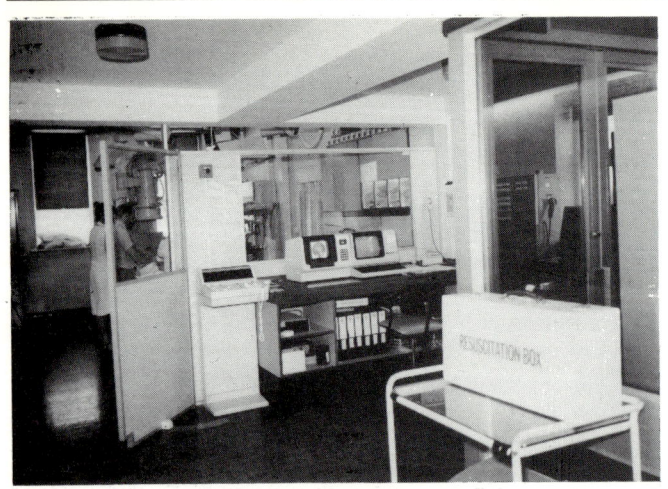

Figure 20.2 Control area. Fluoricon 3000 digital system housed in air conditioned cabinet in right foreground

SUBTRACTION PRINCIPLES

For many years photographic subtraction has been an integral part of vascular radiography as a means of isolating the blood vessels from their bony background by a simple cancellation process.

A series of radiographs is taken whilst an intravascular contrast injection is made. The first film in the series precedes the advent of the contrast injection, and a copy of this radiograph is made in equal but opposite tones – black-to-white reversal. When this new image is laid upon any one of the subsequent series, the elements which are common to both radiographs are cancelled, leaving only that which is different – the contrast medium – clearly visible (Figure 20.3). The print which is made from this superimposition may be made using a high contrast photographic emulsion thus amplifying the final difference image.

Although this simple and comparatively inexpensive technique is very effective when carried out with care and accuracy, it is extremely time consuming, especially if addressed to the series as a whole. Furthermore, the cancellation is very rarely complete. No matter how accurately the exposures are matched in both making the mask or the final print, in no way can the single emulsion of the mask film match the duplicised one of the series in its maximum density. Double order subtraction can go some way towards remedying this discrepancy, but the final image may well suffer degradation derived from the multiplicity of processes involved.

Digital subtraction is an electronic process and is performed by a computer. In addition, having obtained a numerical difference value, this can be enhanced by multiplication twice, three times, four times or whatever is necessary to make the difference more readily perceptible when the image is viewed again in analogue form (Figure 20.4).

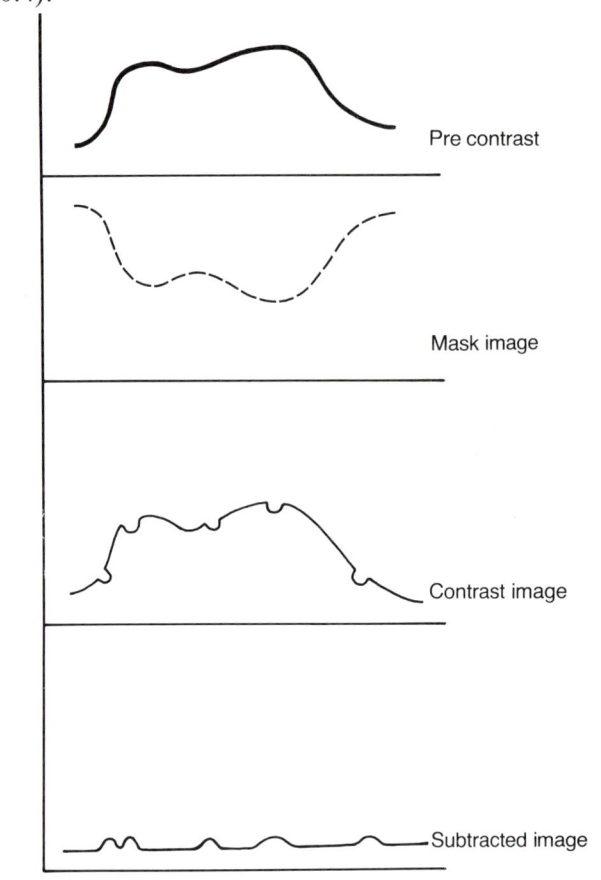

Figure 20.3 Photographic subtraction principles

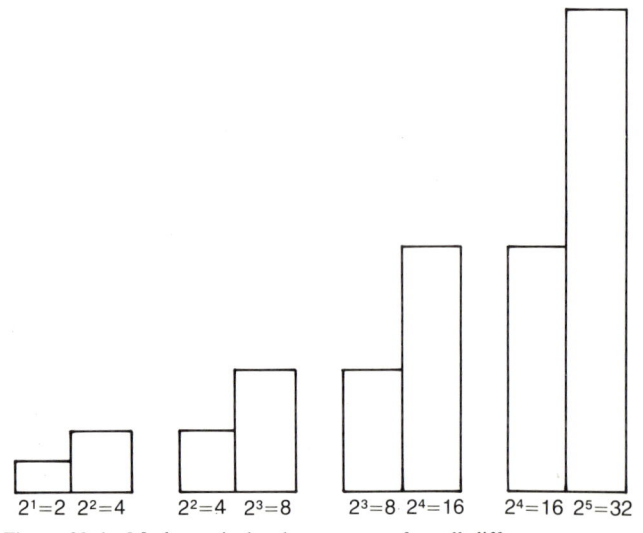

$2^1=2$ $2^2=4$ $2^2=4$ $2^3=8$ $2^3=8$ $2^4=16$ $2^4=16$ $2^5=32$

Figure 20.4 Mathematical enhancement of small differences

DIGITAL RADIOGRAPHIC SYSTEMS

SYSTEM COMPONENTS

Figure 20.5 shows a simplified block diagram featuring the major components of a digital fluorographic system. Although manufacturers vary in the disposition and capacity of their hardware, the main elements which are common to all systems are represented.

The digital system can be said to start at the television camera.

TV camera

Image forming X-radiation efficiency is greatest when the signal-to-noise ratio (SNR) of the television camera is low, i.e. when electronic noise from the camera makes a minimal contribution to the image. See Figure 20.6.

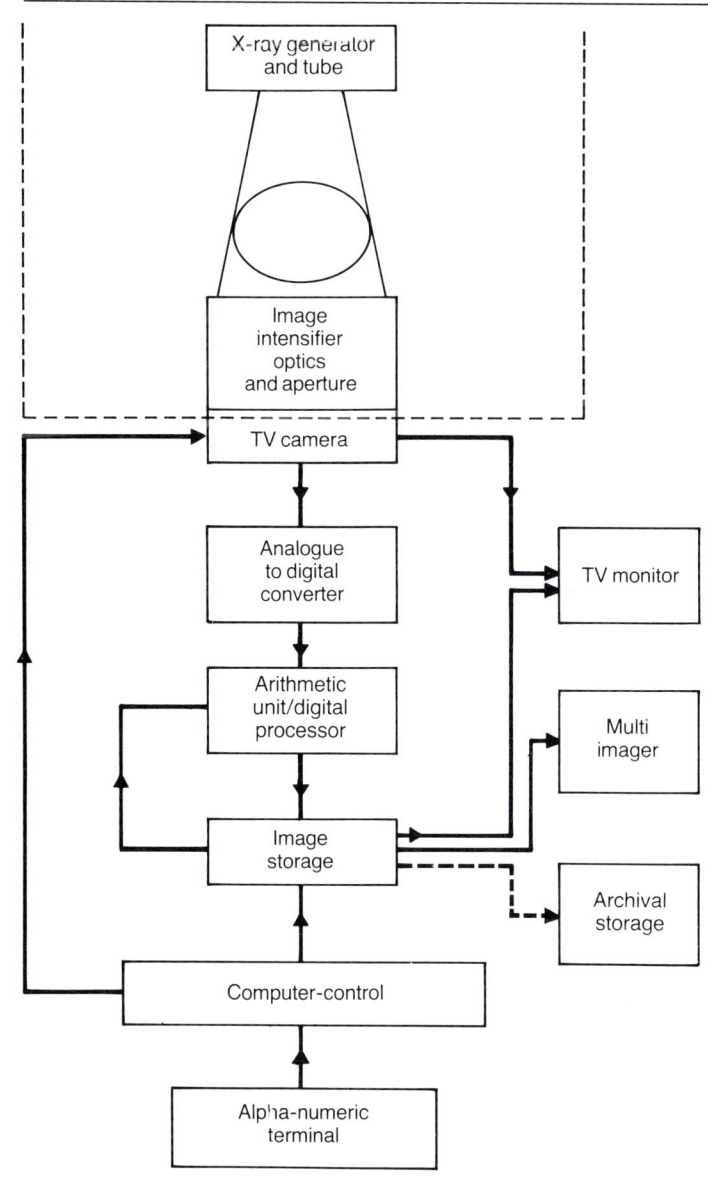

Figure 20.5 Simplifed block diagram of the major components of a digital fluorographic system

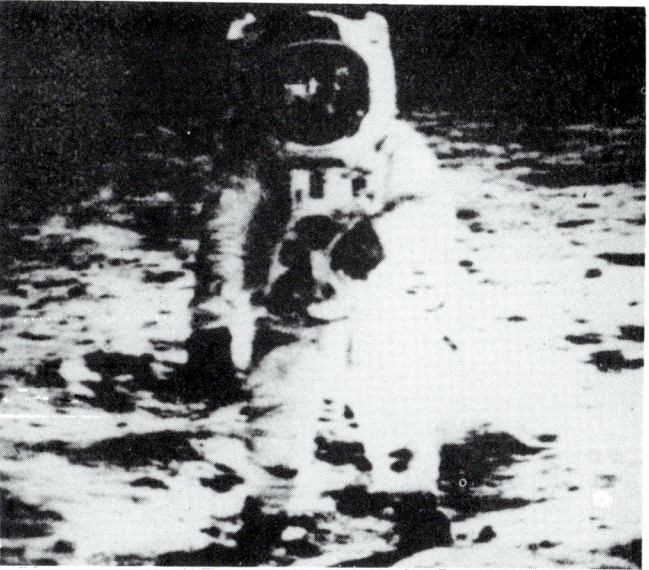

Figure 20.6 This photograph of a spaceman is an example of low SNR low signal-high noise

The television camera of a DSA system is a high quality plumbicon with a signal-to-noise ratio now universally quoted as 1000:1. It is optically linked to the image intensifier by a standard lens system with variable aperture.

The analogue-to-digital converter

This converts electronic signals from the television camera into numerical values (Figure 20.5). The number of numerical levels available is referred to in terms of binary digits (bits). Ten bits means a total of 1024 levels. This figure is derived from 2^{10}. Similarly, eight bits refers to 256 levels. The greater the number of numerical levels, the more accurate will be the capability of the system in distinguishing subtle image differences.

Whilst digital subtraction is founded upon the same principles as those of photographic subtraction, it provides a very much more sensitive system, with real-time difference images. These images can be mathematically enhanced, stored in both the short term on magnetic disc, or in the long term on magnetic tape, or possibly laser disc. They can be reprocessed, remasked, reregistered, integrated and interrogated in all manner of ways by suitable computer programs (software).

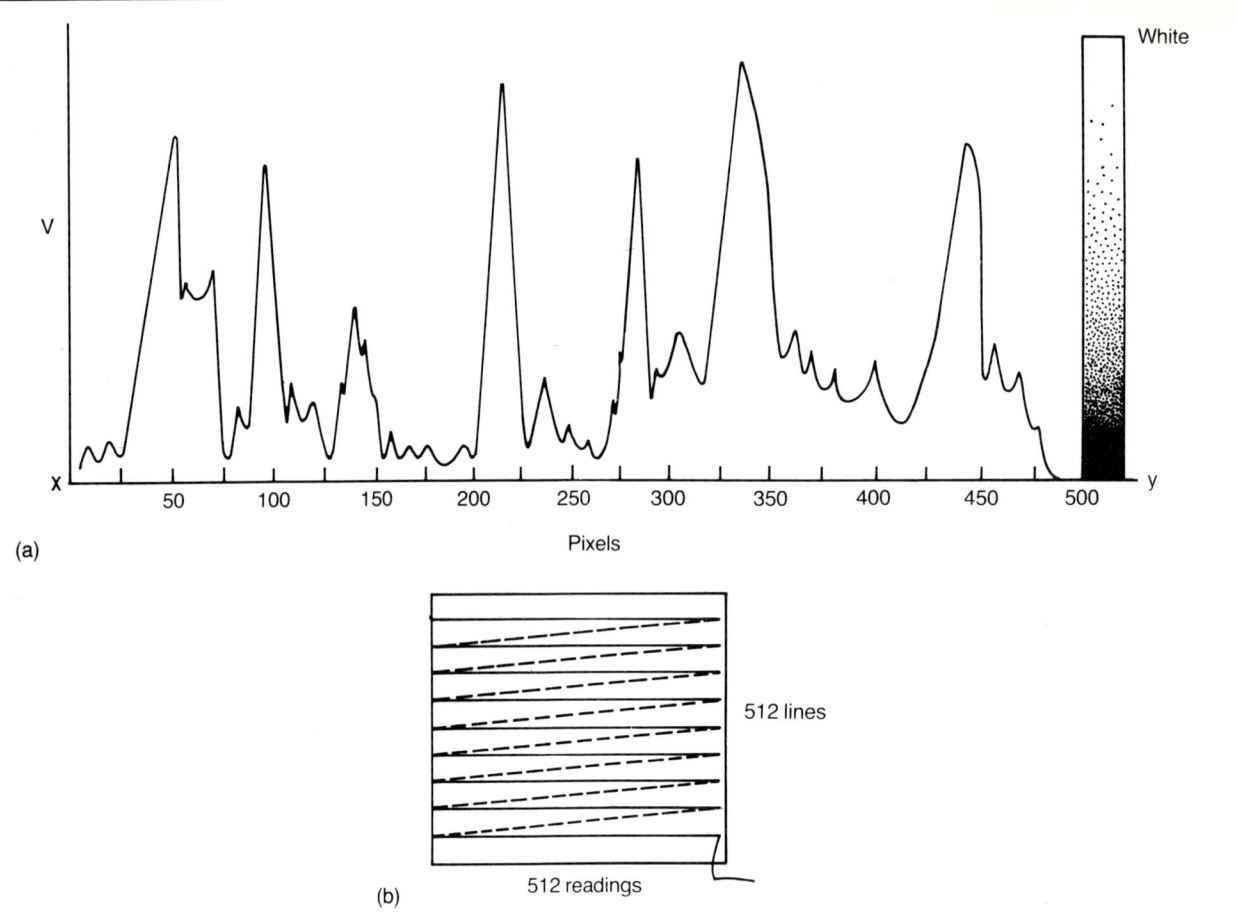

Figure 20.7(a) Image acquisition. x···y represent one horizontal T.V. line **(b)** Image matrix

Image acquisition (see Figure 20.7)

Images are acquired in two modes – static and dynamic. Although there are other variations, an understanding of these two modes will provide a sound base for the alternatives.

Static mode

Static mode uses a single pulse of radiation of required duration in milliseconds. The operator selects the input radiation dose, the kVp, mA and a suitable TV camera aperture.

The latter is commensurate with the image brightness, and the dynamic range of image intensities. A reading is obtained by a trial exposure. Where the range is found to be exceptionally high, appropriately positioned filters will effect local X-ray beam hardening, so that the relevant anatomy can be visualized within the dynamic range of the system.

The television camera face is read progressively by a scanning electron beam and it is from these readings that the image matrix is built up. The matrix represented in Figure 20.7(b) has 512 elements per line and 512 lines. It is therefore a 512×512 pixel matrix. Each pixel is a picture point in the resultant image. The higher the concentration of picture points, the greater will be the image resolution. This sampling rate is the ultimate dictator of the spatial resolution capability of the digital system and this statement cannot be overemphasized. In practice, the use of the static acquisition mode is comparable with using a spot film camera in conventional photofluorography, or an automatic film changer.

Dynamic mode

Dynamic mode is fundamentally a fluoroscopic method of acquisition. A continuous X-ray exposure is subjected to similar treatment as above, but with an interlaced readout – odd numbered TV lines are read from top to bottom, followed by even numbered lines. With a mains frequency of 50 Hz, 50 'course' fields can be blended by the interlacing to provide 25 whole frames per second. Dynamic mode can be compared with cinefluorography and its application is mainly in cardiovascular studies, but it may be used where fast blood flow and rhythmic organ movement appertain. Multiple images can be integrated to form a composite 'blurred' mask and subtraction achieved by the presence within that group of a matching mask for each of the ensuing series of images.

The image processor

The image processor comprises the arithmetic unit and includes the capacity to convert the incoming digital values into logarithmic ones. The large numerical range is thus compressed without affecting its difference accuracy. Logarithmic conversion has a further important effect in that it renders the difference values independent of density changes across the image (Figure 20.8).

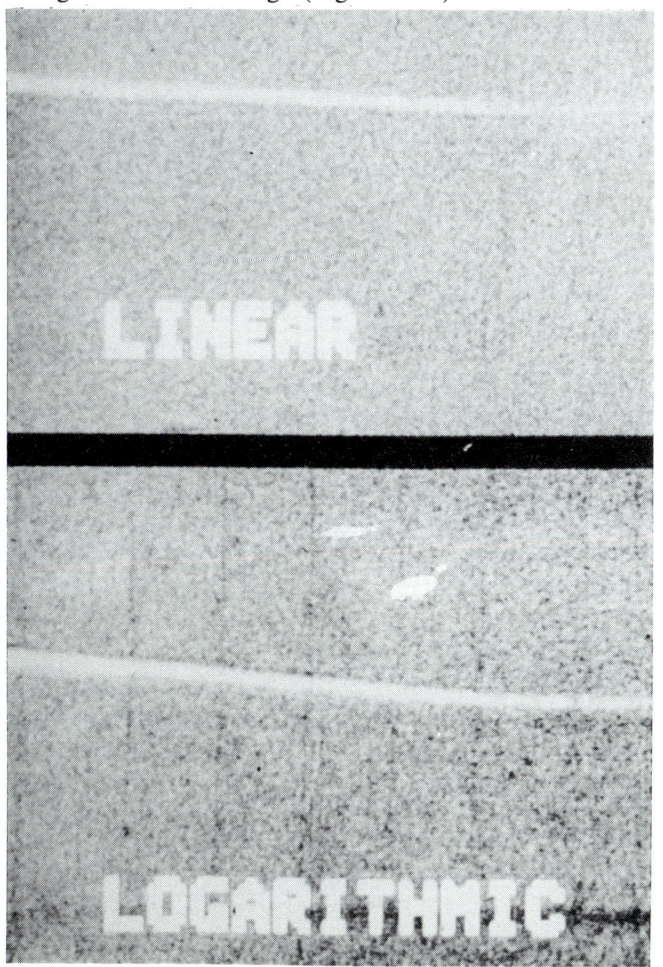

Figure 20.8 Examples of linear and logarithmic acquisition

It is in this part of the system that enhancement, subtraction, integration, averaging and all mathematical functions are executed. Some of these functions may be incorporated into the real-time image, and some may be part of the postprocessing modality.

The mask image is stored in the computer memory and it is subtracted from each subsequent image. By cancellation, if there has been no change, the result is nothing. All subsequent equalities are cancelled out and only differences are seen on the final image.

In order to accelerate data handling, the digital processor may well have more than one memory. Furthermore, if the system incorporates image integration on acquisition, it must have a binary digit depth greater than that of the analogue-to-digital converter.

Image storage

Current storage

Arithmetically processed images can be stored on an analogue video disc, from which they may be viewed on the TV monitor. Alternatively, the data may be stored in digital form on a high capacity magnetic disc – a Winchester disc. The further development of magnetic disc capacity and computer processing rates has made raw data storage on magnetic disc a financially viable proposition. Originally, acquisition rates and real-time viewing of images had to be sacrificed in the interests of the sophisticated reprocessing functions which raw data storage and the digital disc make possible.

Archival storage

Long-term storage of complete image sequences is generally handled by transfer of data to magnetic tape, although the laser disc could well emerge for such purposes with great economy of archival space.

In nearly all clinical situations, there is a demand for hard copy of the most informative images derived from the examination. To this end a multi-imager, incorporating a slave video monitor, is part of all digital subtraction angiographic units.

Image processing

Having acquired a series of images it is then possible to reprocess the data in a number of interesting and useful ways. These facilities may include such refinements as enlargement or 'blow up' together with smoothing to remove image 'noise', edge enhancement and pixel shift. Currently, pixel shift or reregistration of images is only available using the X and Y axes – rotational reregistration is without doubt on the way. However, the most frequently used postprocessing facility is remasking. This allows the operator to select a later image as a mask, should slight movement of the patient have occurred immediately prior to the arrival of the contrast injection. It is also possible to integrate or average images and see small time interval differences. All these funtions are available in the postprocessing mode.

Image analysis

Good computer programs have made it possible to calculate vessel size and calibre, blood flow, vessel wall motion and ejection fraction. The latter are usually related to cardioangiography. All these functions may be executed and represented either in numerical or graphical form.

Image viewing

Image display is optimized by manipulation of the grey scale (Figure 20.9). Consider all image densities being represented by the shades between black and white. A good smooth overall image will result, but very small discrete density differences will not be perceptible. Alternatively, let the entire black to white scale be addressed to a mere portion of the density range. Now small density differences are much more noticeable. These controls are referred to as window controls and they generally take the form of either a two-speed button operation or a variable slide type of control, by which window width and height are varied. The window width refers to the proportion of the density range to be encompassed by the grey scale. In practical terms, it will be found that window width will govern the degree of contrast seen in the processed image. Moving the contracted window up and down the density range will produce the effect of changing image brightness (Figure 20.10). The operator will quickly become aware of the limits to which he can exploit the window control, since as he decreases the width and increases the processed image contrast, he begins to see the individual pixels, giving rise to a more 'noisy' picture.

RADIOLOGICAL APPLICATIONS

It would be true to say that the most exciting and important application of DSA is the capacity to visualize iodinated blood in the arterial system, from an intravenous injection. This was attempted at the very dawn of the angiographic era, but failed hopelessly because insufficient sensitivity existed in radiological imaging equipment at that period.

Intravenous angiography is a comparatively less invasive technique, but issues the greatest challenge to both operator and equipment in DSA. It demands a very sensitive system, with high spatial resolution and minimal electronic noise. It also requires a fully co-operative patient who is capable of absolute stillness throughout the contrast injection and the image series acquisition.

The effect of patient movement is reflected in misregistration of the mask upon the subsequent images. Although some slight degree of movement can be overcome by a rescue operation in remasking and reregistration, there is no way in which progressive and rotational patient motion can be overcome. Image 'chaos' is the only result here.

In intravenous angiography it must be mentioned that all vessels are seen simultaneously. Although this can be a diagnostic advantage in some instances, e.g. whole tumour blood supply and drainage, it can also make individual vessels difficult to examine throughout their course by reason of superimposition. In consequence, a series of cunningly devised projections involving oblique views are necessary. If comparison is to be made between right and left sides, then those oblique projections must be exactly comparable and readily reproducible. Clinical follow-up frequently demands accurate reproduction of original projections, in both positioning and geometrical enlargement.

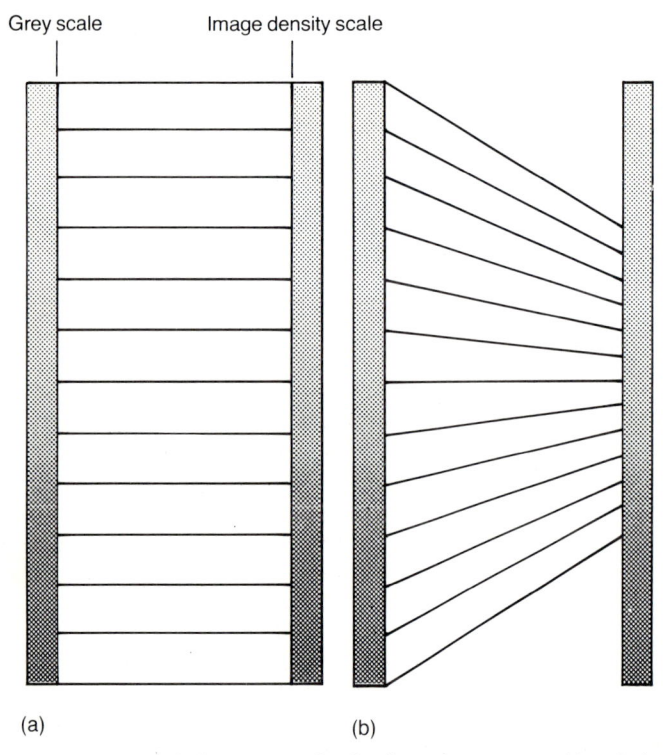

Figure 20.9(a) Window open entire density scale represented by whole of grey scale. (b) Window partially closed portion of density scale represented by whole of grey scale. This portion can be moved up or down

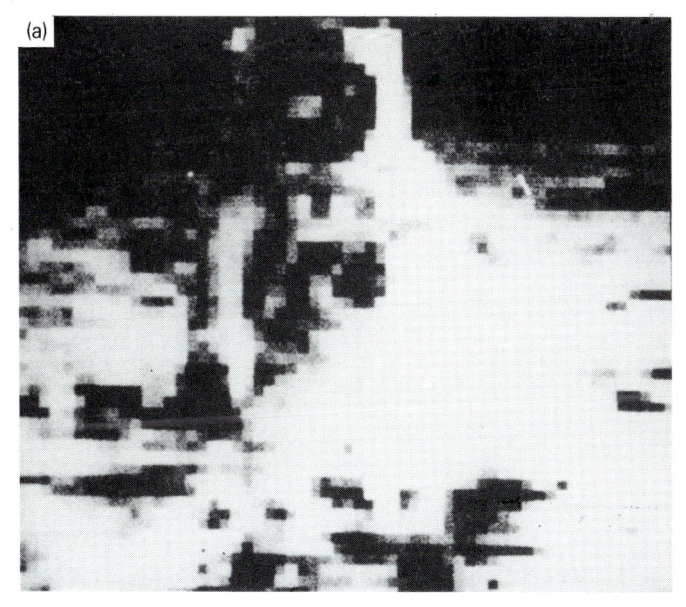

DIGITAL RADIOGRAPHIC SYSTEMS

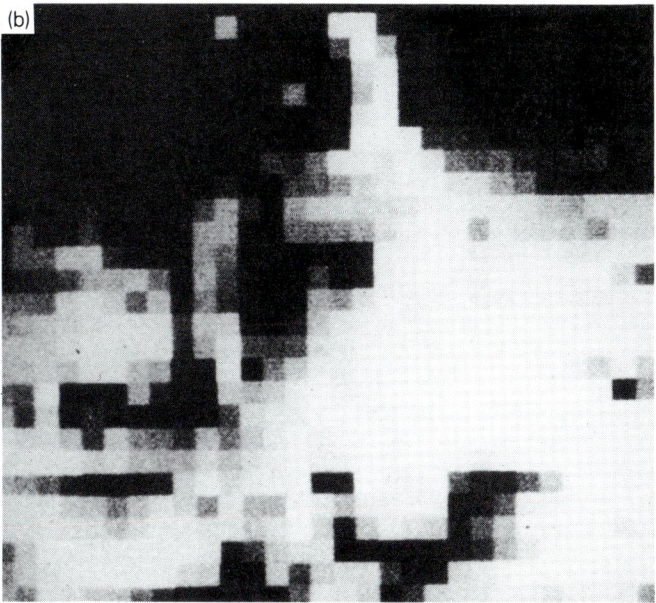

Figure 20.10 (a) Window open, (b) window partially closed

There is, therefore, a considerable advantage in using an isocentric radiographic technique. Here the patient lies in a comfortable supine position upon the X-ray couch. All radiographic projections are obtained by rotation of the X-ray system, in an orbit about the patient the angles and geometric enlargement are recorded. Angiographic equipment of this type has been available for some years now and radiographers are familiar with its operation.

There are two types of DSA digital intravenous angiography and digital arteriography.

Digital intravenous angiography

This involves the injection of a bolus of contrast medium into a suitable vein. This may be delivered using a single cannula (the larger the better) into an arm vein, or by a straight or pigtail catheter into the superior or inferior vena cava.

The injection is carried out preferably by an automatic injector, which can be electrically linked with the digital angiography system. This ensures a consistent and accurate bolus delivery, in which the injector can be made to initiate the imaging sequence. Once the vein has been cannulated the equipment is positioned and the patient is immobilized and given his instructions. Emphasis is placed upon the necessity of remaining absolutely motionless. The cannula/catheter is coupled with the injector.

An appropriate protocol is composed by the operators using the alpha-numeric key board. The protocol is in essence a set of instructions to be carried out by the system (Figure 20.11).

```
PROTOCOL CRANIAL I.V.__   2
PATIENT ID .............  SN +20
DIFFERENCE GAIN ........  12
EXPOSURES/IMAGE ........  1 EXP
INJECT BEFORE MASK? ...   Y (Y
   INJ-MASK DELAY ......  5.0 S
MASK-RUN DELAY .........  0.4 S
GROUP1 RATE ............  1.0 I
GROUP1 TOTAL ...........    2 I
GROUP1-GROUP2 DELAY ...   0.4 S
GROUP2 RATE ............  2.0 I
GROUP2 TOTAL ...........   14 I
GROUP2-GROUP3 DELAY ...   0.4 S
GROUP3 RATE ............  1.0 I
GROUP3 TOTAL ...........   12 I
APERTURE: ACTUAL/RECOMM  30 /3
MAXIMUM IMAGE RATE ....   4.1 I
PEAK VIDEO .............   85%
RUN NUMBER .............  1400
SPACE AVAIL/START IMAGE 249/
```

Figure 20.11 Sample protocol

The radiographic exposure factors – kVp, mA, input dose to the image intensifier, and focal spot size – are selected. A trial exposure is made so that the TV camera aperture can be tuned to the video signal, and the exposure in milliseconds checked against the tube loading charts. Local beam hardening by means of spot filters or bolus bags may be necessary where extremely low densities are overcontributing to the video signal.

The patient is given his respiratory instructions and the injection is made. The image series is visible in real time via the TV monitor, and the sequence can be terminated the instant the necessary information has been displayed. This is an important feature in DSA since by it the patient is saved unfruitful X-radiation dose, and the expensive equipment is saved from unnecessary wear and tear.

Digital arteriography

If DSA equipment, by reason of its high sensitivity, is capable of visualizing the extremely low concentrations of iodine which success in intravenous arteriography implies, only a moment's consideration will be required to realize the obvious advantages when intra-arterial injection is made. Small volumes of diluted contrast medium can be injected through a small calibre catheter. The examination can be viewed in real time, and the images stored upon a magnetic disc. No longer is it necessary to await film processing in order to view the images, or even to use, a great quantity of hard copy film. A multi-imager will provide as many as 12 images upon one piece of 43 cm × 35 cm film.

Catheterization of any artery still implies a degree of invasiveness, but with fast and efficient DSA technique, general anaesthesia is very rarely necessary. Also, since there is now a move to use finer and finer intra-arterial catheters, some radiological centres are considering the possibility of conducting digital arteriography on a day case basis. The merits of instant arteriography cannot be overstated in interventional radiology, and DSA could well play a very important role in the more venturesome areas of this fast developing field.

RADIOGRAPHIC REQUIREMENTS AND CONSIDERATIONS

Having mentioned the current applications of DSA systems, a look at some of the radiographic parameters may assist in providing some enlightened yardstick whereby basic equipment specifications can be assessed.

Exposure factors

There is no doubt that this imaging system exerts considerable constraints upon the X-ray generator, but most particularly upon the X-ray tube. Each of the following parameters represents a demand for an increase in X-ray photons and in practice, the operator finds himself in the inevitable 'trade-off' position.

Field size selection

At the outset of this account it was stated that spatial resolution in the image is ultimately a function of the sampling frequency – pixel density per unit of image area. Whilst maintaining a matrix of 512×512 pixels, spatial resolution will improve as the image intensifier field size is decreased. However, for every decrease in field size, the demand for photons may double. Furthermore, as the anatomical area covered by each image series is smaller, it is possible that more sequences will be required.

Input dose

The figure of 1000:1 SNR of the T.V. camera refers to an input dose of some 1 mR to the image intensifier. Clearly, the nearer the input dose is to this figure the greater will be the conspicuity of the system. By conspicuity is meant the ability of the system to visualize small vessels with lower concentrations of iodine. Indeed, the almost universal claim of current DSA systems is the capability of visualizing a 1% iodine concentration in a vessel of diameter 1 mm, at an input dose of 1 mR. The highest conspicuity, then, can be achieved by employing a high input dose. These selections challenge the heat loading capacity of the X-ray tube, especially if a high frame rate is needed. Compromises are nearly always necessary.

kVp choice – optimal beam quality

Practically, a very good case can be made for exploiting the increase in photon mass attenuation coefficient which is known to occur at and immediately above the electron 'K' shell energy of the iodine – 33 keV. In terms of beam quality, this would suggest a choice of 75 kVp or thereabouts. Adhering to this figure tends to demand high mA values when short exposure times are required, for instance in order to 'freeze' pulsating vessels or for high frame rates to be obtainable.

Summary

A brief look at these basic radiographic parameters can only serve to endorse the fact that constant referral to tube loading charts is essential, and the inclusion of a tube heat integrator within the system is advantageous. Although, of itself, the heat integrator is no protection against tube overload, a 'cut-out' switch and warning hooter are usually incorporated for this purpose. The heat integrator at least allows the operator to know the percentage of total heat load which is available for use.

CONCLUSION

Success in digital subtraction angiography hinges upon the following important issues.

(1) The equipment must be capable of the task.

It must comprise:

(a) A high quality image intensifier system;

(b) A TV camera with high signal-to-noise ratio (high signal:low noise);

(c) A high powered efficient and stable generator;

(d) An X-ray tube of suitable calibre, with high loading capacity on a small focal spot, and high speed rotating anode and efficient fast cooling;

(e) Computer processing capacity in keeping with high frame rates, fine image matrix and real-time viewing;

(f) Computer hard and software which will not only handle today's investigative projects, but be suitable for developments in fulfilling tomorrow's needs.

(2) The operators of this equipment must have a thorough understanding of the concepts of basic radiographic imaging, together with a special knowledge of the individual DSA system. There is no substitute for meticulous radiographic technique, scatter control, and patient immobilization. Radiologist and radiographer must work as a team, the one to be aware of the strengths and weaknesses of the intravenous angiographic technique in particular and the other to execute his requirements in producing the best possible images. Lastly, but most importantly, the team must gain the confidence of the patient.

FUTURE DEVELOPMENTS

No discussion entitled 'Digital Radiography' would be complete without a glimpse towards the future. Technology in the field of computers is clearly leaping forward daily, as more and more information can be stored in less and less space and microchips expand in capacity.

Currently, the main developments are in temporal subtraction and DSA. Digital fluorography has been at the heart of this discussion, but the scanned projected image using solid state detectors as in the 'scout view' in computerized tomography is undergoing development. However, at the present time the image resolution obtainable by this method on a 512×512 matrix is of the order of 1 line pair/mm.

The other fast developing form of digital radiography is dual energy subtraction. Here subtraction is used to separate different body tissues. The basis for the technique is the exploitation of the physical variation in differential absorption of different tissues to different photon energies. If two images are made, one at a suitable low kVp, e.g. 80, and the other at perhaps 140, subtraction of these digitized images followed by mathematical manipulation is capable of permitting selective cancellation of various tissues. For instance, bone can be subtracted from soft tissue and vice versa. Then by grey scale interrogation each of these tissues can be analysed and such information as calcium content can be 'teasled' out.

Dual energy subtraction is being developed for use in angiography. Two images are made in rapid succession – high and low kV, one pair prior to the arrival of the contrast injection, and the others in pairs with contrast. If soft tissue is eliminated on all these images, followed by further subtraction, only the contrast medium remains. This is called hybrid subtraction, and its main advantage is that it can eliminate artifacts caused by soft tissue motion, such as bowel gas and the so-called 'swallow' artifact much in evidence in neck vessel studies in temporal subtraction.

Hybrid subtraction is in the course of development and its advantages are currently offset by limitations such as a reduction in signal-to-noise ratio and a definite increase in patient radiation dose. Technical problems are multiple but no doubt will be conquered. These involve the accurate control of pulse width and mA. The short exposure times, required to minimize motion artifacts and deliver sufficient photon intensity at low and high kV values, demand very stable mA values of 1000+. Consequently, the tube must tolerate very high loading and have high heat storage capacity. These are but some of the problems.

Digital imaging has already begun to show itself in departments of diagnostic imaging – a noteworthy change of name. Computerized tomography, ultrasound, nuclear medicine, magnetic resonance and DSA – digital radiography could very well constitute a Department of Diagnostic Digital Imaging.

On the next page are examples of DSA taken at Manchester Royal Infirmary (Figure 20.12).

ACKNOWLEDGEMENTS

To International General Electric Medical Systems, most particularly to Mr Ray Joyner for his valuable help and advice with the manuscript and the diagrams. To Mr Philip Wilson of the Royal Victoria Infirmary, Newcastle upon Tyne, Mrs Susan Rouse, The General Infirmary at Leeds, and Miss Rosemary Dennett, of the Middlesex Hospital, London, radiographic colleagues involved in DSA from whom I acquired helpful information with regard to other DSA systems. Finally to the Department of Medical Illustration, Manchester Royal Infirmary for the photographs.

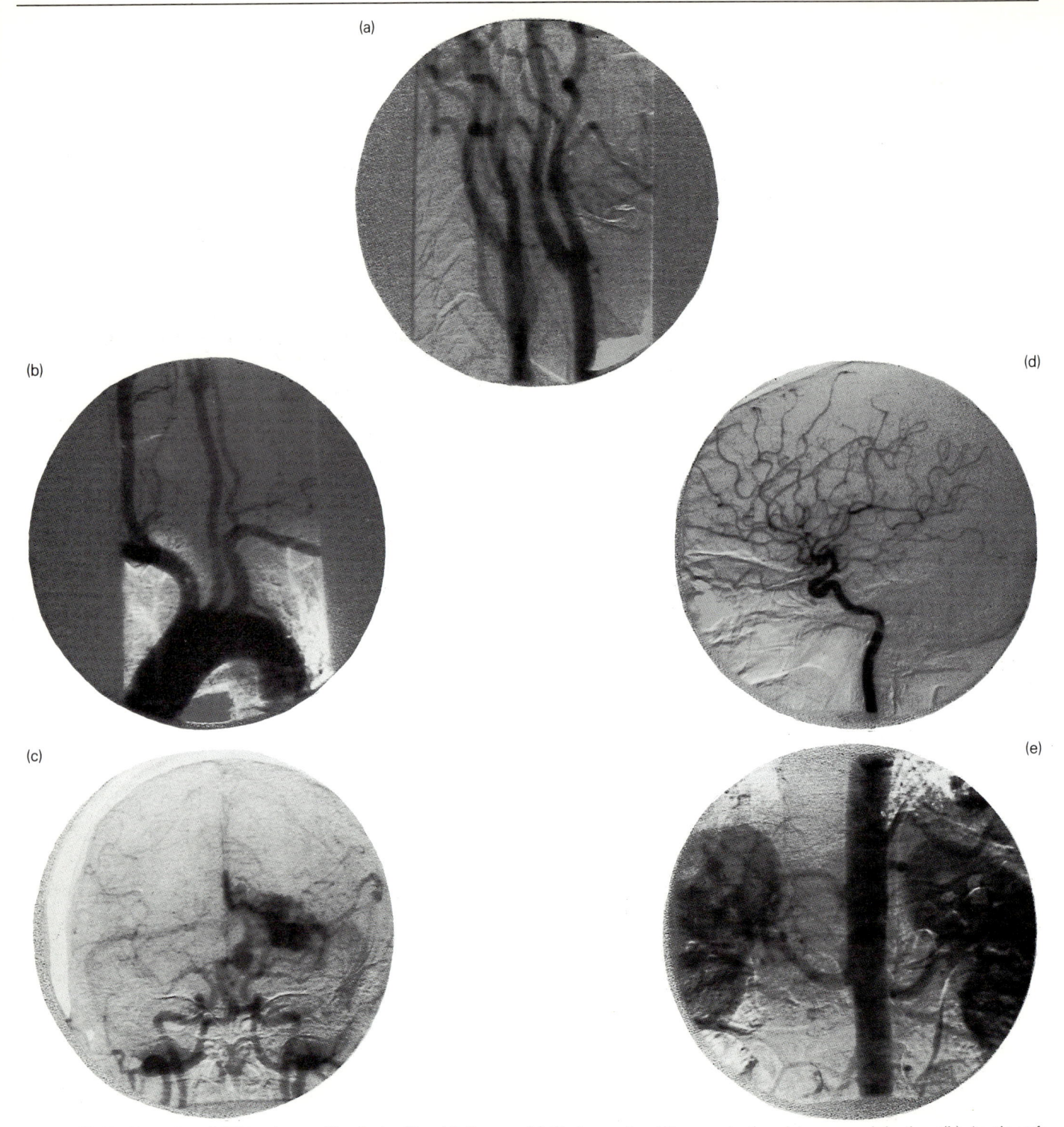

Figure 20.12 Examples of DSA taken at Manchester Royal Infirmary: (a) Neck vessels, oblique projection, intravenous injection; (b) Aortic arch and vessel origins, intravenous injection; (c) Intracranial vessels showing angioma and aneurysm; (d) Intracranial vessels in capillary phase, left internal carotid arterial injection (e) Renal artery study, intravenous injection, prospective live renal donor

Appendix 1
Calculation of power

(1) In a purely resistive direct current (constant potential) circuit, the power in watts is calculated by the simple multiplication of v and i.

power in watts = volts × amperes

(2) In a similar circuit using alternating current (a.c.) however, the root mean square (rms) factor must be used. The *rms factor* for a sinusoidal waveform is 0.707 of the peak value and the peak value of v and i must therefore be multiplied by 0.707.

power in watts = $V_p \times 0.707 \times i_p \times 0.707$

(3) If the a.c. circuit in addition to resistance has capacitive and/or inductive components v and i may be out of phase with respect to one another and the power dissipated in the circuit will be determined by the extent to which they are out of phase. The *power factor* (cos φ) is the factor by which v and i must be multiplied to calculate the power expended in such a circuit.

power in watts = $V_{rms} \times i_{rms} \times \cos \phi$

It should be noted that for a purely resistive circuit v and i are in phase; $\phi = 0$ (cos $\phi = 1$) and power expended is therefore $V_{rms} \times i_{rms} \times 1$.

(4) It should also be noted that the rms value 0.707 of peak is *not* the same as the average value which is 0.637 of peak. As an mA meter registers an average value it is necessary to multiply the current by the *form factor* which is the rms value divided by the average value and for a sinusoidal wave = 1.11.

Appendix 2
Measurement of angles

Phase angle, rotation of the anode etc. may be measured in degrees or radians, the relationship between the two units is as follows:

360 degrees = 2π radians = 6.28 radians

A phase angle of 45° might therefore also be expressed as 0.785 rad.

In the same way an anode rotating at 50 revs. per second might be said to rotate 360° or 6.28 rads × 50 per second. Therefore 50 revs/s can also be expressed as 315 rads/s.

Appendix 3
Symbols in common use on imaging equipment

Symbols in common use on fluoroscopy units, tables, etc. and in descriptive literature

Symbol	Meaning	Symbol	Meaning	Symbol	Meaning
	Direct radiography		Table top rotating about its longitudinal axis *cradle*		Longitudinal movement of layer radiographic unit
	Indirect radiography *formerly used for all radiography*		Layer radiography movement *tomography and planigraphy*		Setting layer level *tomography and planigraphy*
	Fluoroscopy		Bucky table		Adjust layer in direction of arrow
	Ultrafine focus		Bucky wall stand		Raise table top
	Fine focus		Layer radiographic unit *tomography or planigraphy*		Lower table top
	Broad focus		Limited field illumination *full-field indicator for beam defined by diaphragms*		Tilting table with overtable tube
	Thin patient (yellow)		Slot diaphragm or collimator open		Tilting table with undertable tube
	Average patient (blue)		Slot diaphragm or collimator closed		Photofluorographic unit
	Fat patient (red)		Iris diaphragm open		TV *television in general or X-ray television*
	Moving scattered radiation grid		Iris diaphragm closed		TV monitor
	Stationary scattered radiation grid		Light-beam indicator *direction of radiation is indicated by lines or dashes of light*		Brightness *picture controls*
	Without scattered radiation grid		Decompression		Contrast *picture controls*
	Table tilting about a horizontal axis *Tilting table movement*		Compression		Image intensifier
	Tilting table move to vertical		With compression cone *for operation with compression cone*		Image intensifier *normal-sized image in use*
	Tilting table move to horizontal		Without compression cone *for operation without compression cone*		Image intensifier *enlarged image in use*
	Tilting table move into adverse tilt (head down position)		Oblique setting of a layer radiographic unit		Move table top or footrest longitudinally

APPENDIX 3

Symbol	Meaning	Symbol	Meaning	Symbol	Meaning
↑	Move footrest towards head (upwards)	↔↕	Movement in four directions, vertical and horizontal		Lock disengaged – free
↓	Move footrest downwards		Movement in four directions, horizontal		Mid position *movement to locate the central position*
←	Movement in direction of arrow *to a limit position*		Free movement of table top in four directions *floating table top*		Brake ON
→	Movement in direction of arrow *away from a limit position*		Stepped table top movement towards the head		Brake OFF
←	Movement in direction of arrow		Stepped table top movement towards the feet		Clamp, secure, press
↔	Movement in two directions		Rotational movement in two directions, pendulum		Release *make free*
↕	Movement in two directions, vertically		Rotational movement in two directions about an axis		Transport of mobile X-ray units
↗	Movement in two directions to and from the operator		Lock engaged		

Spotfilm devices; format selection

Symbol	Meaning	Symbol	Meaning	Symbol	Meaning
	Spotfilm device		Cassette vertical 2 exposures (one above the other)		Cassette vertical 4 exposures
	Cassette vertical 1 exposure (survey)		Cassette horizontal 2 exposures (side by side)		Cassette horizontal 4 exposures
	Cassette horizontal 1 exposure (survey)		Cassette vertical 3 exposures (side by side)		Cassette vertical 6 exposures
	Cassette vertical 2 exposures (side by side)		Cassette horizontal 3 exposures (side by side)		Cassette horizontal 6 exposures

Miscellaneous

Symbol	Meaning	Symbol	Meaning	Symbol	Meaning
	X-ray tube		Acoustic signal (bell)		Red lamp *for darkroom lighting not for infra-red*
	X-ray tube emitting radiation		Intercom – speak		Signal lamp *optical signal*
	Tube assembly *on an accessory to show the side to be placed towards the tube*		Intercom – listen		Calibration mark *scales*
	Timer		Lamp *white light or room lighting*		Warning (general) Danger *check the operating instructions*

Symbol	Meaning	Symbol	Meaning	Symbol	Meaning
	Loudspeaker		Green lamp		Indirect lighting *for scales, controls etc.*
	Intercom		Blue lamp *not for UV*		

Examination units

Symbol	Meaning	Symbol	Meaning	Symbol	Meaning
	Urology table		Mammography		Biplane X-ray unit, simultaneous exposure
	Skull unit		Cutfilm changer Cassette changer *single plane*		Biplane X-ray unit, without simultaneous exposure
	C-arm unit		Cutfilm changer Cassette changer *biplane*		

Automatic exposure

Symbol	Meaning	Symbol	Meaning	Symbol	Meaning
	Ionization chamber		Blackening *film density*		Three-field chamber of automatic exposure device *the dominant can be filled in or Roman numerals inserted as required*

Appendix 4
SI units used in radiography

Table to show the relationship between traditional and the new SI units

Quantity	Traditional unit (symbol)	SI unit (symbol)	SI units in which measured	Conversion factor
Exposure	roentgen (R)	roentgen (R)	coulombs/kg ($C\,kg^{-1}$)	$1\,C\,kg^{-1} = 3876\,R$
Absorbed dose	rad	gray (Gy)	joules/kg ($J\,kg^{-1}$)	$1\,Gy = 100\,rad$
Dose equivalent	rem	sievert (Sv)	joules/kg ($J\,kg^{-1}$)	$1\,Sv = 100\,rem$
Activity	curie (Ci)	becquerel	Disintegrations per second (s^{-1})	$1\,Bq = 2.7 \times 10^{-11}\,Ci$

* An exposure of 1 R is equivalent to an air kerma of 8.7 mGy (0.87 rad)

Index

A-mode 182, 183
Abdominal angiography 144
Absorbed dose 196
Acceptance testing 168
Accident radiography equipment 125–7
Added filtration 62
Air gap technique 87
All metal grid 90
Alternating current (a.c.) power supply 1–4
Analogue-to-digital converter 219
AND gate 158
Angiographic rating chart 80–1
Angiography equipment 144–5
Angle measurement 226
Anode 59
  "cracked" 63
Anode angle 59, 63
Anode compound 63, 65
Anode cooling chart 49, 78–9
Anode delay circuit 49
Anode diameter 63
Anode rotation 58, 63
Anode rotation speed 62, 76–7
Anode surface crazing 60
Anode temperature monitoring 64
Anode thermal load indication 52
AOT cut film changer 141–3
  mode of operation 142
  motor drive 142
  punch card control 142
  simultaneous biplane operation 143
AOT roll film changer 143
Ardran and Crooks penetrameter 175
ASCII code 160
Assessment parameters 168–79
Automatic beam collimation 96
Autotransformer 11, 12, 29, 31
Avalanche diode 40
Axial resolution 184

B-mode 183
Babix immobilizer 150
Back-projection 204
Bar phantom 174
Batteries 1
Beam alignment 115
Beryllium window 66
Beta-particles detection 191
Bimetal strip 7–8
Binary arithmetic 157–8
Binary code 157
Binary coded decimals (BCD) 157

Binary number 157
Binary system 156–7
Biological half-life 191
Bipod tube support 129
Bistable multivibrator 160
Blood flow detection 187
Blood vessels 144
Bone marrow, radiation damage 163
Brightness control 114
Bucky assemblies 98–100
Bucky radiography 135
Bucky table 97
Bucky tomographic system (Philips BTS4) 133

Cable resistance compensation 5, 18, 119
Cables
  high tension 9–10
  inspection 117
  low tension 9
  testing 171
Capacitor discharge with time 120
Capacitor discharge unit 119–21
  control panel 120
  simplified circuit 120
  small mAs values 121
Capacitor smoothed voltage 23
Carcinomas, radiation-induced 162
Cassette carrier 126
Cassette changer 141
Cassette holder 135
Cassetteless radiography 150–3
Catapult grid movement 93
Catheterization 223
Cathode ray tube, TV monitor 111
Central processing unit (CPU) 156, 160, 199
Central ray 58
Cephalostat 124
Cerebral angiography 129, 144
Chest radiography 152
Cine cameras 113
Cine fluorography 113–14
Cine pulsing 113
Cine radiographic rating chart 81–2
Cine recording 112
Circuit breakers 7–9
  bimetal strip 7–8
  electromagnetic 8
  operation of 8–9
  thermal 7
Clocks 160
Closed circuit television 101

Code of Practice for the Protection of Persons against Ionizing Radiation 163, 171, 198
Collimation test 115, 148
Collimator test tool 169
Collimators 94, 151, 194
Compton scatter 85
Computerized tomography (CT) 199–209
  advantages of 209
  background 199
  basic components 199
  calibration 206
  detectors 206
  dual energy scanning 209
  dynamic scanning 207
  ECG trigger 208
  exposure factors 207
  filtration 203
  image computation 204
  image matrix 203
  image reconstructions 205
  independent consoles 209
  installation planning 199–201
  optional facilities 207–9
  patient dose 203
  quality assurance 206
  radiotherapy planning 208
  resolution 204
  scanning angle 206
  scanogram 203
  storage of scan data 206
  types of scanner 201–2
  variable geometry 203
  window width and level 204
  X-ray tube 202–3
Computers 156
  analogue 161
  digital 156
Conduction 70
Conduction band theory 38
Cones 94
Constant potential circuit 23
Constant potential equivalent 175
Constant potential unit 22
Contrast medium injectors 145
Contrast resolution 204
Control panel or console 55
Convection 70
Conversion factor 117
Convolution process 204
Copper filter 175
Copper reference number (CRN) 176
Cordless mobiles 121

Craniostat 124
Cross-hatch grid 87, 90
Crossed light beam centering device 97
Cut film camera 112
Cut film changer 141

Densitometric analysis 176
Density control 47, 114
Dental radiography equipment 123–5
Dental tomograph unit 124
Diac 42
Diamentor 105, 167
Diaphragms 94
Digital arteriography 223
Digital fluorography 115, 219
Digital intravenous angiography 222, 223
Digital radiography 217–24
   history and background 217
   overview 217
   subtraction principles 218–19
   system components 219–22
   use of term 217
Digital readout 161
Digital subtraction angiography (DSA) 217–19, 222
   applications 222–4
   archival storage 221
   current storage 221
   exposure factors 224
   field size selection 224
   image acquisition
      dynamic mode 220–1
      static mode 220
   image analysis 222
      image processing 221–2
   image processor 221
   image storage 221
   image viewing 222
   input dose 224
   kVp choice 224
   radiographic requirements and considerations 224
   radiological applications 222–4
   television camera 219, 220
Digital switching circuits 158
Digital vascular imaging (DVI) 217
Doppler effect 187
Double interlacing 110
Dulac system 127

Earth continuity 171
Earthing 9, 10
ECG trigger 208
Effective half-life 191
Effective kilovoltage 175
Electric shock protection 9, 10
Electrical conductors 9, 38
Electrical energy 76

distribution 4
Electrical insulation 9, 16, 171
Electrical insulators 38
Electrical safety 171
Electricity supply and distribution 1–10
   cable resistance compensation 5, 18, 119
   to hospital 5
Electroacoustic transducer 184
Electromagnetic induction 2
Electromagnetic waves 180–2
Electromagnets 212
Electromotive force (e.m.f.) 1–2
Electron current 37
Electron emission 36
Electron migration 39
Electron motion 35
Electronic calipers 186
Electronic devices 35–43
Electronic lens 185
Electronic stabilizer 27
Electronic switching, primary circuit 36–7
Energy expenditure 71
Energy resolution 195
Enlargement factor 173
Enlargement techniques 135
Exclusive OR gate 160
Exposure area 141
Exposure dose variation with change in field size 115
Exposure factors 18
Exposure switching 33–4
Exposure time 63, 93, 177–8
Exposure timers 44–8
   clockwork 44–5
   electronic 45–6
   fluoroscopic 105
   guard timer 47–8
   mAs control (timer) 47
Extra focal radiation 58
Eye, radiation damage 163

Falling load generator 52–3
Fetal heartbeat 182
Fetus, radiation damage 163
Fibre optic coupling 109
Field effect transistor (FET) 42–3
Field size, reduction in 115
Field uniformity 195
Filament heating current 72
Filament heating curves 72
Filament step-down transformer 32–3
Film badges 165–7
Film holder 166–7
Film magazine 141, 153
Film transport systems 150
Flip flops 160
Floating top tables 98

Fluoroscopic density control 114
Fluoroscopic equipment 101–5
   code of practice 105
   protection 105
   quality assurance tests 115–17
   radiation dose 101–2
   range of forward and adverse tilt 102
   remote controlled 103
   screening assembly 102
   serial changer 103
   switching from radiography to fluoroscopy 104
   switching to radiography 104
Fluoroscopic timer 105
Fluoroscopy 77
   principle of 101
Focal area 76, 77
   actual and apparent 58
Focal film distance (FFD) 131, 169, 170
Focal spot dimension 173
Focal spot size 66, 76, 171–3, 174, 175
Focused grid 87, 89–90
Frame 110
Free wheeling spinning top 177
Full wave rectified (2 pulse) circuit 22
Fuse wire 6, 7
Fuses and holders 6–7

Gamma camera 193–7
Gamma camera collimator 194
Gamma camera computer 197
Gamma camera images 198
Gamma-ray detection devices 191, 193
Gas counters 191
Gas-filled triode valve 37
Geiger-Müller counters 192
Generators
   direct current (d.c.) 1
   falling load 52–3
   high frequency 54
   medium frequency 54
   shared 53–4
   three-phase 3, 25
Genetic effects of X-radiation 162
Gonads, radiation damage 162, 163
Grid alignment 170
Grid cassette 90
Grid-controlled X-ray tube 64–5
Grid efficiency assessment 91
Grid factor 86
Grid lattice 87
Grid loss 90
Grid movement 92
Grid ratio 86, 91
Grid selectivity 91
Guided fine-needle biopsy 148

Handlebar control unit 83

INDEX

Heart valve movement 182
Heat 69–70
Heat capacity 69
Heat energy 69, 77
Heat exchange unit 63
Heat sensor 64
Heat transfer 70, 78
   through X-ray tube 77–82
Heat transfer rate 71
Helmholtz arrangement 212
High tension circuits 18–25, 53
   advantages of three-phase over single-phase 25
   single-phase constant-potential 22–4
   three-phase (six-pulse) 24–5
   12-pulse (12 rectifier) 25
High tension current 10
High tension transformer 12, 14–16, 31
Horizontal resolution 110

Image formation 85–7
Image intensifier tube 101, 105–7, 135
   for fluoroscopy 114
   for radiography 114
   magnification (dual field) 107
   mobile 116, 122
   triple field 35 cm 108–9
   viewing output image 108
   with cut film and TV camera 112
Image memory (or retention) systems 112, 123
In vitro tests 190
Information display 161
Inherent filtration 62
Initial delay circuit 48–9
Insulation. *See* Electrical insulation
Interchangeable grids 93
Interlocked circuits 48
International Commission on Radiological Protection (ICRP) 163
Inverse square law 165
Inverse voltage reducer circuit 21–2
Ionization chamber 166, 178, 179, 191

Kidneys 197
Kinescopy 112
kV compensator 28–31
kV control 14, 24

Larmor frequencies 213
Lateral resolution 184–5
Lead leaves 95
Lead zinconate titanate (PZT) 184
Lenz's Law 62
Light beam diaphragm 94–6
   alignment 169–70
   with automatic exposure control 96

Light emitting diode (LED) 40
Light pen caliper 187
Line focus principle 57–8
Line voltage 4
Linear array scanners 185
Linear array transducers 183
Lithium fluoride 166
Loadix system 52, 64
Logic gates 158–60
Longitudinal waves 180
Lysholm system 127

M-mode 182
mA control 31
Magnetic field 2, 14, 62
Magnetic flux 14
Magnetic resonance imaging (MRI) 210, 212–14
Mains supply. *See* Electricity supply
Mains switch 5
Mains voltage compensation, automatic 13–14
Mains voltage compensator 12–14
Mammography 145–50, 163
   equipment quality assurance tests 148
   X-ray tube insert for 66
Maximum kVp 71
Maximum mA 71
Maximum power 72
Mechanical assessment 169–70
Metal filter 91
Meters
   Position in X-ray circuit 26–7
   prereading kV 26, 29
   prereading kVp 29, 30
   reading 26–7
   tests 117
Microprocessors 156
Mobile equipment 118
Molybdenum anode 147
Molybdenum filter 66
MOSFET (metal oxide semiconductor) FET 43
Motor-driven spinning top 177
Moving grids 92–3, 97
Multilayer cassette 135
Multipin-hole images 173

NAND gate 159
Negative feedback 161
Non-stochastic effects of radiation 163
NOR gate 160
NOT gate 159
Nuclear magnetic resonance 210–16
   biological hazards 214–16
   magnetic effects 215–16
   permitted exposure levels 214–16
   principles of 210

Nuclear medicine 189–98
   applications of 196–7
   radiation problems and hazards in 197
   scope of 189–90
   therapeutic 189

Oil-filled tube casing 64
Operational amplifier 161
Optical viewfinder 96
OR gate 159, 160
Organ imaging techniques 190
Organ programmed units 140–1
Organ uptake measurements 189
Orthopantomograph (OPG) unit 123
Oscillating transducer 183
Oscillating vibrating grid movement 92–3
Overload protection circuits. *See* X-ray tube

Paediatric radiography equipment 149
Parallel circuit 6
Parallel grid 87–8
Partial volume effect 204
Patient identification 113, 152
Patient trolley 129
Peripheral angiography 144
Peripheral interface adaptor (PIA) 161
Peripheral interface input/output chip (PIO) 161
Permanent magnets 212
Phase angle 4
   measurement of 226
Phase voltage 4
Philips BTS4 tomographic and general unit 133
Philips Cephalix unit 124–5
Philips Polytome U 133–5
Photoelectric absorption 85
Photographic subtraction 218–19
Photomultiplier 192, 194–5
Photons 71
Picker 'Care' system 126
Picker CT System 199
Piezo-electric effect 184
Pin-hole camera 172–5
Pixels 203, 205
Plate diaphragm 94
Plumbicon camera tube 110
Polytome U3 135–6
Portable X-ray units 118
Positioning electronics 194–5
Positron emission tomography (PET) 196, 197
Power calculation 226
Power supply, portable and mobile equipment 119
Primary barriers 164–5
Primary contactor circuit 48

proximal diaphragm 66
Puck film changers 143–4
Pulse-echo technique 180, 184, 185, 187
Punch card control of AOT 142

Quality assurance 168–79
   computerized tomography 206
   fluoroscopic equipment 115–17
   mammography equipment 66

Radiation, heat transfer by 70
Radiation detection 191
Radiation dose 101–2, 162–3, 196
   assessment of 167
   measurement of 105, 165, 167
Radiation hazards 162, 197–8
Radiation-induced carcinomas 162
Radiation intensity 74
Radiation leakage 170
Radiation monitoring of staff 166
Radiation monitoring film 167
Radiation output tests 115
Radiation protection, primary and
   secondary barriers 163–5
Radiation quality 175
Radiation safety 170–1
Radiation survey 170
Radiation survey meter 165
Radioactivity spills 198
Radiofrequency (RF) coils 213
Radioisotope imaging 195
Radiological Protection Advisor (RPA)
   165, 198
Radionuclides 190–1
   imaging 196
Radiopharmaceuticals 190–1
Radiotherapy isodose curves 208
RAM (random access memory) 160
Random phantom 148
Raw data 204
Reaction time 47
Real-time 183
Real-time scanners 183–4
   electrical method 183
   mechanical method 183
Receiving box 141
Reciprocating grid movement 92
Rectification 19, 21, 22, 71–82
Renal function 207
Renogram function curves 197
Resistive magnets 212
Resolution in ultrasound 184–5
Resolution of CT image 204
Resolution methods 174–5
Resolution phantoms 174
Resolution tests 116, 148
Respiramet X 151
Roll film cameras 112

ROM (read only memory) 160
Rotalix metal tube and casing 65
Rotalix metal tube insert 66
Rotating anode tube 56–63, 77, 78, 121
Rotating transducer 183
Rotor assembly 60–1

Safety precautions 9–10
Saturation current 27
Scales, accuracy of 169
Scan data 204
Scanning gamma camera 196
Scattered radiation 85–7, 164
Scintillation detectors 192–3
Secondary barriers 164–5
Secondary radiation grid 86
Self-rectified circuit 19, 21, 32, 74, 75
Semiconductors 38–40
Sequences 213
Serial changer 103
Series circuit 6
Series connection 26
Shift register 160
Siemens catapult bucky 93
Siemens Infantoskop 149
Siemens Mammomat 145
Siemens Mammomat B 147
Siemens Mobilett mobile unit 121–2
Siemens Siregraph-C unit 145
Siemens Thoracomat 149, 150
Siemens Thoramat 153
Signal-to-noise ratio (SNR) 219
Silicon-controlled rectifier (SCR) 41–2
Single-phase voltage 3
Single photon emission tomography
   (SPECT) 196, 197
Skull unit 127–9
   attachments 128
   generator 128
   grid rotation 128
   spring loaded manually operated
     cassette changers 128
Slot technique 93
Soft radiation 66
Solid state devices 35, 37
Solid state rectifier 37
   forward biased 39
   reverse biased 39–40
Somatic effects of X-radiation 162
Sound waves 180
Space charge compensator 27
Spatial resolution 194–5, 204
Specific heat capacity 69
Spectral hardening 204
Split intensity distribution 173, 175
Stability assessment 169
Stalloy 15
Star phantom 174

Static stabilizer 27
Stationary anode tube 77, 78
Stationary grids 87–91
Stator operation
   50 cycle 77
   150 or 180 cycle 77
Stator supply circuit 62
Stator windings 61–2
Stepped moving top table 144
Stochastic effects of radiation 163
Superconductive magnets 212
Sussex cassette 175
Switches
   circuit breaker 8
   exposure 33–4
   high tension changeover 53
   interlock 48
   mains 5
   mechanical (electromagnetic)
     contactor 33–4
   'on' and 'off' 8

Technetium-99m 190–1
Telescopic tube support 83
Television camera 109, 135, 219, 220
Television monitor 111
Temperature 69–70
Temperature scales 69
Temporal resolution 195
Thermionic diode valve 35–6
Thermionic emission 35, 36
Thermistor sensing device 151
Thermoluminescent powders 166
Three-phase rectified circuit 75
Three-phase supply 3
Thyratron valve 36–7
Thyristors 36, 41–2
Time gain compensation (TGC) 185
Timer test tool 178
Timers. *See* Exposure timers
Tomographic attachment 130–3
Tomographic camera 196
Tomographic units 133–6
Tomography 130–9
   automatic exposure control 136–7
   exposure control 135
   fan test 138–9
   frequency of testing 139
   inclined plane 133
   linear movements 130
   quality assurance tests 137–9
   reciprocal movements 130
   sequential 131
   simultaneous multisection 131–3
   test tool for layer height 138
Total filtration 62
TP-mode 182
Transformer

INDEX

filament step-down 32–3
high tension 14–16, 31, 53
Transformer rating 16–18
Transformer regulation 16
Transistors 41
Transverse waves 180
Triac 42
Trimmer resistance 32
Triple interlacing 110
Tube housing cooling chart 79–80
Tube rating chart 71, 72
Tungsten, electron energy 36

Ultrasound 180–8
  amplitude 181
  displaying returning echoes 182–4
  frequency 182
  imaging sequence 185–6
  postprocessing 185
  postprocessing measurements 186–7
  power output 188
  preprocessing 185
  production 184
  resolution 184–5
  safety 187
  transducers 184–5
  velocity 181
  wavelength 182
Undercouch tube 96

Vacuum triodes 37
Variable aperture diaphragm 95
Variable height table 98
Versatilt bucky 98
Vertical bucky 98
Vertical resolution 110
Video signal 110

Video tape recording 111–12
Video test pattern generator 117
Vidicon camera tube 108–10
Visual image 109
Voltage drop, compensation for 17

Wave travel 181
Wisconsin beam alignment tool 169
Wisconsin focal spot test tool 174
Wisconsin X-ray test cassette 175

Xeroradiography 147–8
X-radiation, effect on human body 162–3
X-ray beam parameters 171–5
X-ray circuits 11–34
  position of meters 26–7
  primary 11–14
  secondary 11, 23
  see also High tension circuits
X-ray detectors 206
X-ray equipment
  care of 154
  choice of, installation of 154–5
  servicing 154
X-ray generator
  2-pulse 74, 75
  6-pulse 66, 75, 144, 147
  12-pulse 66
  constant-potential 73
  tomography 135
X-ray output 178
X-ray tables 97–100
X-ray tube characteristics 75
X-ray tube filament 56–7
X-ray tube filament boost 49
X-ray tube filament heating circuit 27–8
X-ray tube filament interlock 49

X-ray tube insert 19, 56, 61, 63, 64, 66, 67
X-ray tube loading 72, 82
X-ray tube overload protection circuits 49–52
  against multiple exposures 51–2
  against single exposure 50
  percentage tube load indication 51
X-ray tube shield 62
X-ray tube supports 82–4
  'C' arm 84
  ceiling-suspended 82–4
  floor stands 82
  floor to ceiling stands 82
  motorized movements 84
  telescopic 83
X-ray tubes 19, 56–8, 147, 171
  casing 19, 63
  code of practice 66
  computerized tomography 202–3
  grid controlled 25, 64–5
  heat produced at target 21
  heat transfer through 77–82
  heavy duty 63–4
  high tension changeover circuit 53
  inherent and added filtration 62
  microfocus 66–7
  rating of 71–2
  rotating anode 56–63, 77, 78, 121
  stationary anode 19, 56
  super Rotalix ceramic-120 67
  super Rotalix metal 65–6
  tomography 135
  voltage applied to 16, 29

Zener diode 40
Zonography 133, 134